THERAPEUTIC STRATEGIES IN HEART FAILURE

THERAPEUTIC STRATEGIES IN HEART FAILURE

Edited by

Clyde W. Yancy
James B. Young

CLINICAL PUBLISHING

OXFORD

Clinical Publishing
an imprint of Atlas Medical Publishing Ltd

Oxford Centre for Innovation
Mill Street, Oxford OX2 0JX, UK
Tel: +44 1865 811116
Fax: +44 1865 251550
Email: info@clinicalpublishing.co.uk
Web: www.clinicalpublishing.co.uk

Distributed in USA and Canada by:

Clinical Publishing
30 Amberwood Parkway
Ashland OH 44805 USA
Tel: 800-247-6553 (toll free within U.S. and Canada)
Fax: 419-281-6883
Email: order@bookmasters.com

Distributed in UK and Rest of World by:

Marston Book Services Ltd
PO Box 269
Abingdon
Oxon OX14 4YN UK
Tel: +44 1235 465500
Fax: +44 1235 465555
Email: trade.orders@marston.co.uk

© Atlas Medical Publishing Ltd 2008

First published 2008

A catalogue record for this book is available from the British Library.

ISBN-13 978 1 904392 40 8
ISBN-10 1 904392 40 7

The publisher makes no representation, express or implied, that the dosages in this book are
correct. Readers must therefore always check the product information and clinical procedures
with the most up-to-date published product information and data sheets provided by the
manufacturers and the most recent codes of conduct and safety regulations. The authors and
the publisher do not accept any liability for any errors in the text or for the misuse or
misapplication of material in this work.

Project manager: Gavin Smith, GPS Publishing Solutions, Hitchin, Hertfordshire, UK
Typeset by Mizpah Publishing Services Private Limited, Chennai, India
Printed and bound in Great Britain by Biddles Ltd, King's Lynn

Contents

Editors and Contributors   vii

Preface   xi

Section I: The prevention of heart failure   1

1   The treatment of hypertension as a strategy to prevent heart failure   3
    S. D. Nesbitt

2   Insulin resistance: implications for the failing heart   23
    B. Drabicki, S. Carr, R. P. Shannon

Section II: Established pharmacologic therapies for chronic heart failure   37

3   Digoxin therapy: does it still have a role in the management of heart failure?   39
    J. Kalman

4   Neurohormonal activation in heart failure: ACE inhibitors   47
    D. W. Markham

5   Neurohormonal activation in heart failure: angiotensin receptor
    antagonists   57
    A. E. Atchley, G. Michael Felker

6   Neurohormonal activation in heart failure: β-blockers   69
    S. A. Kamath, C. W. Yancy

7   Neurohormonal activation in heart failure: aldosterone antagonists   81
    E. Hsich, R. C. Starling

Section III: Emerging pharmacologic therapies for heart failure   91

8   Nitric oxide biology and oxidative stress in heart failure: heart failure in
    African-Americans   93
    C. W. Yancy

9   B-type natriuretic peptides in heart failure   105
    J. Patel, J. Thomas Heywood

Section IV: Future pharmacologic therapies for heart failure   123

10 Arginine vasopressin antagonism in heart failure   125
    J. Finley, O. Hedrich, M. A. Konstam, J. E. Udelson

11   Extracellular remodeling in heart failure – potential use of MMP inhibitors   141
     D. S. Feldman, F. G. Spinale

12   Erythropoietin analogs in the treatment of anemia in heart failure   151
     Y-D. Tang, S. D. Katz

Section V: Special topics in heart failure   163

13   Applying data from registries to improve outcomes in heart failure   165
     G. C. Fonarow

14   Device therapy in heart failure   177
     P. B. Adamson

15   Ventricular replacement therapy for heart failure   191
     R. Bogaev

16   Palliative and hospice care in heart failure   213
     P. J. Hauptman, P. Mikolajczak

Postscript   223

List of Abbreviations   225

Index   231

Editors

CLYDE W. YANCY, MD, FACC, FAHA, FACP, Medical Director and Chief, Cardiothoracic Transplantation, Baylor Heart and Vascular Institute, Baylor University Medical Center, Dallas, Texas, USA

JAMES B. YOUNG, MD, FACC, FAHA, FACP, Vice Chairman, Cardiovascular Medicine, The Cleveland Clinic, Cleveland, Ohio, USA

Contributors

PHILIP B. ADAMSON, MD, FACC, Medical Director, Adjunct Associate Professor, The Heart Failure Institute at Oklahoma Heart Hospital, Oklahoma Foundation for Cardiovascular Research, Department of Physiology, University of Oklahoma Health Sciences Center, Oklahoma City, Oklahoma, USA

ALLEN E. ATCHLEY, MD, Cardiology Fellow, Division of Cardiovascular Medicine, Duke University Medical Center, Durham, North Carolina, USA

ROBERTA C. BOGAEV, MD, FACC, FACP, Medical Director, Advanced Heart Failure and Cardiac Transplantation, Texas Heart Institute at St Luke's Episcopal Hospital, Assistant Professor of Medicine, Section of Cardiology, Department of Medicine, Baylor College of Medicine, Houston, Texas, USA

STEVEN J. CARR, MD, Department of Medicine, Allegheny General Hospital, Drexel University College of Medicine, Pittsburgh, Pennsylvania, USA

BRANDY DRABICKI, MD, Department of Medicine, Allegheny General Hospital, Drexel University College of Medicine, Pittsburgh, Pennsylvania, USA

DAVID S. FELDMAN, MD, PhD, FACC, Associate Professor of Medicine, Director of Heart Failure and Cardiac Transplant, Division of Cardiology, Departments of Medicine, Physiology and Cell Biology, The Ohio State University, Columbus, Ohio, USA

G. MICHAEL FELKER, MD, MHS, FACC, Assistant Professor of Medicine, Division of Cardiovascular Medicine, Duke University Medical Center, Durham, North Carolina, USA

JOHN J. FINLEY IV, MD, Chief Medical Resident, Department of Medicine, Tufts-New England Medical Center, Boston, Massachusetts, USA

GREGG C. FONAROW, MD, FACC, Eliot Corday Professor of Cardiovascular Medicine and Science, Director, Ahmanson-UCLA Cardiomyopathy Center, UCLA Division of Cardiology, David Geffen School of Medicine at UCLA, Los Angeles, California, USA

PAUL J. HAUPTMAN, MD, Professor of Internal Medicine, Saint Louis University School of Medicine, Division of Cardiology, Saint Louis University Hospital, St. Louis, Missouri, USA

OLAF HEDRICH, MD, Cardiology Fellow, Department of Cardiology, Tufts-New England Medical Center, Boston, Massachusetts, USA

J. THOMAS HEYWOOD, MD, FACC, Director, Heart Failure Recovery and Research Center, Scripps Clinic, Department of Cardiology, La Jolla, California, USA

EILEEN HSICH, MD, Heart Failure and Transplant Cardiologist, Department of Cardiology, Section of Heart Failure and Cardiac Transplant Medicine, Cleveland Clinic, Cleveland, Ohio, USA

JILL KALMAN, MD, Associate Professor of Medicine, New York University Medical Center, Director, Cardiomyopathy Program, Chief, Cardiac Service, Tisch Hospital, New York, USA

SANDEEP A. KAMATH, MD, Cardiology Fellow, University of Texas Southwestern Medical Center, Dallas, Texas, USA

STUART D. KATZ, MD, Associate Professor of Medicine, Yale University School of Medicine, New Haven, Connecticut, USA

MARVIN A. KONSTAM, MD, Chief, Division of Cardiology, Professor of Medicine, Division of Cardiology, Tufts-New England Medical Center, Tufts University School of Medicine, Boston, Massachusetts, USA

DAVID W. MARKHAM, MD, Assistant Professor of Medicine, Department of Internal Medicine, Division of Cardiology, Heart Failure/Transplant Program, University of Texas Southwestern Medical Center, Dallas, Texas, USA

PETER C. MIKOLAJCZAK, MD, Cardiology Fellow, Department of Medicine, Saint Louis University Hospital, Saint Louis, Missouri, USA

SHAWNA D. NESBITT, MD, MS, Associate Professor of Internal Medicine, University of Texas Southwestern, Dallas, Texas, USA

JIGAR D. PATEL, MD, Fellow, Heart Failure Program, Scripps Clinic, Department of Cardiology, La Jolla, California, USA

RICHARD P. SHANNON, MD, Interim Chairman, Department of Medicine, University of Pennsylvania School of Medicine, Hospital of the University of Pennsylvania, Philadelphia, Pennsylvania, USA

FRANCIS G. SPINALE, MD, PhD, Professor of Surgery and Physiology, Department of Surgery, Medical University of South Carolina, Charleston, South Carolina, USA

RANDALL C. STARLING, MD, MPH, Medicak Director, Kaufman Center for Heart Failure, Section Head, Heart Failure and Cardiac Transplantation, Department of Cardiology, Section of Heart Failure and Cardiac Transplant Medicine, Cleveland Clinic, Cleveland, Ohio, USA

YI-DA TANG, MD, PhD, Associate Research Scientist, Department of Internal Medicine, Section of Cardiovascular Medicine, Yale University School of Medicine, New Haven, Connecticut, USA

JAMES E. UDELSON, MD, Associate Chief, Division of Cardiology, Tufts-New England Medical Center, Tufts University School of Medicine, Boston, Massachusetts, USA

CLYDE W. YANCY, MD, FACC, FAHA, FACP, Medical Director and Chief, Cardiothoracic Transplantation, Baylor Heart and Vascular Institute, Baylor University Medical Center, Dallas, Texas, USA

Preface

"Knowing is not enough; we must apply; willing is not enough; we must do"

Johann Wolfgang von Goethe

Why another book on heart failure? The important discoveries in heart failure (HF) over the last 10–20 years have greatly enhanced our opportunities to improve outcomes for this disease but have also significantly expanded the knowledge base. The everyday busy clinician is now presented with an almost impossible task of reviewing, digesting and synthesizing this knowledge and in turn, applying it correctly in the care of patients with heart failure. This is a daunting task and captures the exact reason for *Therapeutic Strategies in Heart Failure*.

This book is not an in-depth review of the pathophysiology of heart failure. That has been done well by many of our peers. It is also not a re-capitulation of prevailing guidelines that have been expertly prepared by the guideline-writing committees of major organizations. Multiple iterations and reformulations of those guideline statements are readily available and it would have been redundant to revisit the guideline statements.

Rather, this book is written by clinician scholars for clinicians and is topical, contemporary and relevant. By design, we intended to bring forward a book that was strategic, not encyclopedic. The areas addressed represent many of the 'nuts and bolts' in the everyday management of heart failure and encompasses several of the major questions of the day. It was our aim that, after reading each chapter, the clinician would have a clear, updated and renewed perspective on an important HF issue and a template for *applying* that information in the care of patients with HF.

We begin with a scholarly section on hypertension and diabetes as two of the most pervasive causes of heart failure and a discussion of how we can incorporate a preventive approach in the management of heart failure. Section II is straightforward and eminently practical as it addresses the established pharmacological therapies for heart failure and presents the rationale, supporting data and a summary algorithm of clinical recommendations for each chapter. Sections III and IV cover therapies that are relevant in the field of heart failure that are either recent additions in the clinical domain for which some uncertainty exists or may be likely to enter the clinical arena in the near future. Where an indication for therapy already exists, a summary algorithm is once again presented. Thus, the information in Sections II–IV empowers the bedside clinician with an easily accessible database presented from a clinical perspective with clear recommendations on how best to proceed with established, new and emerging therapies. Finally, there are a number of special topics that we felt were important to include in such a book: the use of registries as a new data source in heart failure; device therapy in heart failure; ventricular replacement strategies; and a very important chapter on palliative and hospice care.

A word about our contributors – in putting together this book, we sought out a group of authors who are clinically active, deeply involved in clinical investigation and who for each of the assigned topics represent one of the current or emerging thought leaders in the field. Our contributors are active in the field of heart failure now and we believe that they will continue to be so over the intermediate and long term. It has been our pleasure to work with each contributor and it is our hope that you will agree that each is representative of the discipline of heart failure and has already made important contributions to the areas addressed by their chapters.

We hope that you enjoy this book, recognize the unique place we tried to occupy and that, most importantly, the information shared with you in this book is of benefit to you and your patients.

Clyde W. Yancy, MD
James B. Young, MD
October 2007

Section I

The prevention of heart failure

1

The treatment of hypertension as a strategy to prevent heart failure

S. D. Nesbitt

INTRODUCTION

Heart failure is the most frequent diagnosis for cardiovascular hospitalizations in the US. Although treatment strategies for heart failure have evolved in the past decade which has led to an improvement in survival, the best strategy for heart failure is prevention. To that extent, it is important to examine the most frequent contributor to the development of heart failure, specifically hypertension. The most recent classification of heart failure recognizes hypertension as stage 1, i.e., at-risk for the development of heart failure in the progression from asymptomatic to symptomatic left ventricular (LV) dysfunction [1]. In this chapter, the treatment of elevated blood pressure (BP) will be addressed as a preventive measure for heart failure.

EPIDEMIOLOGY

Hypertension is diagnosed when the systolic and diastolic BP is ≥140 mmHg, and/or 90 mmHg respectively, on at least two occasions; or if systolic pressure is >160 mmHg and/or diastolic pressure ≥100 mmHg on one occasion [2]. In the US, 65 000 000 adults suffer from hypertension, disproportionately affecting African-Americans [3]. In addition, the incidence increases with age, such that in those >55, the risk of developing hypertension is 90% [4].

Although the focus has been on BPs above 140/90 mmHg, the risk associated with cardiovascular (CV) events is apparent well before the diagnosis of hypertension. From a BP of 115/75 mmHg, the risk of CV mortality doubles with every 20/10 mmHg increment in systolic and diastolic BP respectively [5]. In recognition of this fact, the classification of BP now includes 'Prehypertension' which is defined as untreated BPs in the range of 120–139/80–85 mmHg [2] (Table 1.1). The prevalence of prehypertension in the US is 45 000 000 [6]. Normal BP refers to BPs <120/80 mmHg. Hypertension precedes heart failure in over 90% of individuals, and it is associated with a 2–3 times higher risk for developing heart failure [7]. Elevated BP contributes to the two leading etiologies for heart failure: ischemic coronary disease and hypertensive heart failure [8]. The population attributable risk of hypertension in heart failure is 39% for men and 59% for women. Furthermore, the risk of heart failure increases with the severity of BP elevation [9]. Since African-Americans develop hypertension earlier and have poorer rates of BP control, it is not surprising that the rate of heart failure presumably due to hypertension is also over-represented in this population [1].

Shawna D. Nesbitt, MD, MS, Associate Professor of Internal Medicine, University of Texas Southwestern, Dallas, Texas, USA

Table 1.1 Classification and management of BP for adults (age ≥18 years)[2]

BP classification	Systolic BP (mmHg)		Diastolic BP (mmHg)
Prehypertension	<120	and	<80
Normal	120–139	or	80–89
Stage 1 hypertension	140–159	or	90–99
Stage 2 hypertension	≥160	or	≥100

Several large clinical trials demonstrate that controlling BP to optimal levels decreases the risk of new onset heart failure by approximately 50% [10]. Despite multiple therapeutic options for hypertension and a concerted focus on optimizing medical care over the past three decades, the success rate in achieving BP treatment goals remains less than acceptable, particularly in the elderly, diabetics and African-Americans [3] (Table 1.2). Accordingly, greater focus should be given to developing better strategies to control BP. In several clinical trials, BP control requires multiple medications, yet even in these settings achieving goal BP reductions remains well below 100% [11]. While it is clear that combination therapy is necessary for most stage 2 hypertensives, many of these patients already have target organ damage. Perhaps the best opportunity for reducing the target organ damage from escalating BP is to focus on prevention. The recently published TRial Of Preventing HYpertension (TROPHY) demonstrated that treatment in prehypertension is safe and well-tolerated with a low-dose angiotensin receptor inhibitor [12].

MECHANISM OF HYPERTENSION LEADING TO HEART FAILURE

The earliest evidence of vascular damage associated with hypertension begins with endothelial dysfunction and inflammation [13]. Early BP elevation initiates a risk of heart failure by beginning with multiple stimuli including activation of the sympathetic nervous system, activation of the renin–angiotensin–aldosterone system (RAAS), excessive mineralocorticoid activity, and several other neuroendocrine maladaptations. These stimuli may raise BP initially, however these factors alone may not necessarily sustain the BP elevation. The pathway of the progression from normotension to hypertension, as described by Alexander, is characterized importantly by changes in the morphology of resistance blood vessels [14–17]. Increases in BP lead to adaptive changes in the microvasculature. These changes manifest as an increase in the mass of the medial layer of vascular smooth muscle or through remodeling of the vascular smooth muscle medial layer. This alteration in the vasculature further propagates hypertension through increased vascular resistance. Angiotensin stimulates both hypertrophy and hyperplasia of the smooth muscle of resistance arteries through cellular signaling, inflammation, endothelial dysfunction and vasoconstriction [18]. Thus, interrupting these changes in the morphology may attenuate the progression of hypertension. The TROPHY study investigated the interruption of these mechanisms on the vasculature of prehypertensives with a low-dose angiotensin receptor inhibitor. After 2 years of treatment, compared to placebo, prehypertensive participants who were treated with candesartan developed hypertension less frequently over the subsequent 2 years of observation on placebo. These findings provide new insight into the mechanisms of early hypertension, however additional studies are needed to clarify the role of pharmacologic treatment in prehypertension. As well, it is not known, but might be presumed, that earlier reductions in the development of hypertension might lead to a reduction in the incidence of heart failure but this will require further clinical investigation.

Table 1.2 Major clinical trials

Drug class	Drug name	Dose range (mg/day)	Outcome studied — CVD	Stroke	CHF	LVH	Pre-hypertension	Renal	Trial
ACE-Is	Benazepril Captopril	20–40 QD; BID 37.5–450 TID	■	■				■	UKPDS, CAPPP, Captopril in DM type 1, STOP2, SAVE [47, 48, 69, 78, 82]
	Enalapril	20–40 QD; BID	■	■	■			■	SCAT, ABCD, STOP2, HOT, ANBP2, TOHMS, SYST-Eur, SOLVD [39, 49, 52, 54, 69, 83, 95]
	Fosinopril Lisinopril Moexipril Perindopril	40–80 QD 40–80 QD 7.5–30 QD 4–16 QD	■	■	■ ■			■	FACET [64] ALLHAT, STOP2 [5, 69] PROGRESS, EUROPA, PREAMI [59, 65, 67]
	Quinapril Ramipril Trandolapril	10–40 QD; BID 10–20 QD 1–4 QD	■		■ ■			■	QUIET [68] HOPE, AASK [63, 75] PEACE [73]
ARB	Candesartan	16–32 QD	■	■	■		■	■	CHARM, SCOPE, TROPHY [13, 71, 87]
	Eprosartan Irbesartan Losartan	400–600 QD; BID 150–300 QD 50–100 QD; BID	■	■	■	■		■ ■	IDNT [78] LIFE, RENAAL, ELITE [76, 77, 86]
	Olmesartan Telmisartan Valsartan	20–40 QD 40–80 QD 160–320 QD; BID	■ ■	■	■	■		■	ONTARGET (in progress) [95] VALUE, VALIANT, MARVAL, ValHEFT [74, 80, 88, 89]
Diuretics	Thiazides Chlorthiazide	125–1000 BID	■					■	

Table 1.2 (continued)

Drug class	Drug name	Dose range (mg/day)	CVD	Stroke	CHF	LVH	Pre-hyper-tension	Renal	Trial
	Chlorthalidone	12.5–50 QD	■	■					TOMHS, ALLHAT, VHAS, SHEP, HDFP, HAPPHY, ANBP2 [5, 46, 54, 72, 84, 90, 95]
	Hydro-chlorothiazide	6.25–50 QD	■	■		■			SYST-Eur*, STOP, ANBP2, VA Coop, MAPHY, EWPHE, SYST-China* [29, 49, 51, 54, 92]
	Indapamide	1.25–5 QD							
	Methylclothiazide	2.5–10 QD							
	Metolazone	0.5–1 QD							
	Polythiazide	1–4 QD							
	Trimethiazide	1–4 QD	■	■					NICS-EH [57]
Loop diuretics	Bumetanide	0.5–2 QD							
	Ethacrynic acid	50–600 BID							
	Furosemide	40–160 BID							
	Torsemide	5–10 QD							
K+ sparing	Amiloride	10–20 QD	■						INSIGHT [55]
	Eplerenone	25–50 QD; BID							Eplerenone Study [32]
	Spironolactone	100–300 BID			■				HDFP, RALES*** [31, 90]
	Triamterene								HDFP [90]
Calcium channel blockers	Dihydropyridines*								
	Amlodipine	5–10 QD	■	■	■			■	VALUE, AASK, ALLHAT, PRAISE, PREVENT [5, 63, 79, 80, 94]
	Felodipine	10 QD	■	■	■				HOT, STOP2, VHEFT [39, 50, 69]
	Isradipine; XL	10–20 QD; BID	■	■					STOP2 [69]
	Nicardipine	90–120 BID	■	■					NICS-EH [57]
	Nifedipine XL	60–120 QD	■	■					INSIGHT, ACTION [53, 55]

	Drug	Dose				References
Peripheral sympatho-lytics	Diltiazem CR	30–60 QD; BID	■	■	■	NICOLE, ABCD [52, 62]
	Verapamil	240–540 QD	■	■		NORDIL [58]
	Nisoldipine ER	240–480 QD; BID	■	■		CONVINCE (incomplete), VHAS [60, 70]
α-blockers	Doxazosin	8–16 QD	■	■		ALLHAT, TOMHS [5, 85]
	Prazosin	8–20 TID				
	Terazosin	5–20 QD				
Cardioselective β-blockers	Acebutolol	QD; BID	■			TOMHS [88]
	Atenolol	QD	■	■	■	LIFE, MRC, STOP, STOP2, SHEP, MAPHY, HAPPHY [45, 46, 69, 76, 92, 95]
	Betaxolol	QD				
	Bisoprolol	QD				
	Esmolol (IV only)	QD				
	Metoprolol (XL)	QD/BID	■	■	■	AASK, STOP, STOP2, MAPHY [63, 69, 91, 92]
Non-selective β-blockers	Carteolol	QD				
	Nadolol	QD				
	Penbutolol	QD				
	Pindolol	QD/BID/TID				
	Propranolol	BID	■	■		STOP [91] BHAT, MRC, MAPHY [45, 92, 95]
α-, β-blockers	Timolol	QD/BID				
	Carvedilol	QD/BID	■	■	■	Carvedilol in HF Study** [61]
	Labetolol	BID/TID				
Central sympatho-lytics	Clonidine (po, patch)	0.6–1.8 TID; weekly				
	α-methyldopa	500–2000/BID	■			EWPHE [93]
	Guanabenz	32–64/BID				
	Guanfacine	2–6/QD				

Table 1.2 (continued)

| Drug class | Drug name | Dose range (mg/day) | Outcome studied | | | | | | | Trial |
			CVD	Stroke	CHF	LVH	Pre-hyper-tension	Renal	
Direct acting vasodilators	Hydralazine	50–300/BID	■						VA-Coop, HDFP [29, 90]
	Minoxidil	10–80 QD/BID							

*Both SYST-Eur and SYST-CHINA investigated the dihydropyridine nitrendipine, which is not available in the US.

**Carvedilol Study enrolled primarily heart failure patients.

***RALES Study enrolled primarily heart failure patients.

BID = twice a day; QD = every day; TID = three times a day

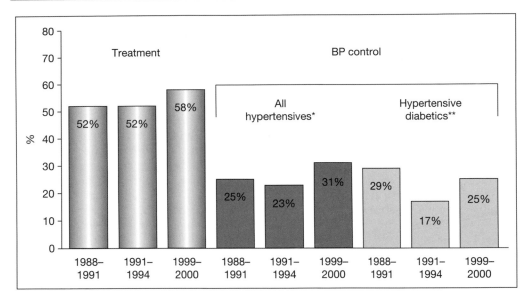

Figure 1.1 US treatment and control of hypertension. *BP <140/90 mmHg; **BP <130/85 mmHg. With permission [3].

As hypertension progresses, elevated afterload pressures as well as neurohumoral stimuli contribute to the development of left ventricular hypertrophy (LVH). In the American College of Cardiology/American Heart Association (ACC/AHA) classification, stage 2 includes both LVH and myocardial injury as precursors to symptomatic heart failure through myocardial remodeling [1]. In the cascade of events from the initial vascular changes to fulminant heart failure, BP treatment is a key component in preventing progression, halting ventricular remodeling and improving the functional status of heart failure patients.

Assessment of blood pressure

Effective treatment for hypertension requires proper measurement. BP should be measured with a patient in a seated position, back supported, and feet on the floor after 5 min of quiet rest. It is best to perform at least two measurements and use the average of these measures. Most clinical trial data are based on clinic measurements however, more recently, 24-h ambulatory monitoring and home BP measurements demonstrate a stronger correlation to clinical outcomes [19–21]. These measurements are often helpful in treatment decisions particularly in white coat hypertension, symptomatic episodes, and labile BP. White coat hypertension is defined as BPs of >140/90 mmHg in the clinic, while BPs are normal outside of the clinic. The reported prevalence of white coat hypertension is 10–15%; however the white coat effect in which clinic BP is higher than home BP is likely more common [22, 23]. Recommended standards for normal ambulatory BP values currently include: daytime BP <135/85 mmHg, nighttime BP <120/70 mmHg, and 24-h BP <130/80 mmHg [24]. Self-taken home BP measurements are helpful in managing hypertension by inviting patients to participate in their healthcare, as well as providing additional measures for a more complete assessment of BP control. Patients should be instructed to perform these measurements in a similar manner to office-derived BP measurements and their devices should be calibrated with an office device. In prehypertension, especially individuals with BPs of 130–139 mmHg systolic and/or 85–89 mmHg diastolic, home BPs are helpful in early detection of progression to frank hypertension (Figure 1.1).

TREATMENT OPTIONS

RAS blockade

The renin–angiotensin system (RAS) plays a crucial role in hypertension and heart failure, therefore blockade of this system is important to reduce BP, and minimize target organ damage. These agents consist of angiotensin-converting enzyme inhibitors (ACE-I) and angiotensin receptor blockers (ARB). ACE-Is block the effect of angiotensin by reducing the conversion of angiotensin I to angiotensin II which is the active form of angiotensinogen. While the primary BP effects are mediated through reduction of angiotensin, additional effects are mediated through the upregulation of bradykinin. The primary effect of ARBs is to antagonize the effects of angiotensin II through blockade at the angiotensin II type 1 (AT1) receptor level, however additional benefits may be rendered through binding at the angiotensin II type 2 (AT2) receptor [25]. Currently, trials are underway to investigate renin inhibitors as a treatment for hypertension. Preliminary data suggest that renin inhibitors may be especially effective at lowering systemic BP. How that will translate into additional clinical benefits, if at all, remains under investigation.

■ Clinical trials have clearly demonstrated the benefit of these agents targeting the RAAS in reducing BP, improving cardiovascular morbidity and mortality, and correcting renal disease in hypertension (Table 1.3). These agents should be strongly considered in any treatment algorithm for hypertension – especially stage 2 hypertension or when a second agent and/or a combination regimen is required to effectively treat stage 1 hypertension. There are no treatment recommendations for 'prehypertension' per se. However, the TROPHY data previously referenced do suggest the potential benefit of an angiotensin receptor antagonist for this circumstance.
■ Overall, these agents are well-tolerated and have the highest reported adherence rates for any single antihypertensive drug. The most common side-effect with ACE-Is is cough and there is also a small risk of angioedema. These effects are not necessarily dose-dependent but are minimal with ARBs [26].

DIURETICS

Diuretics are one of the oldest drug classes for the treatment of hypertension. The mechanism of action is primarily volume control, however there are implications that these drugs may also have chronic vasodilatory effects. Currently in the US, the average intake of sodium is higher than the recommended amount [27]. High sodium intake may cause increased fluid retention and thus higher BP. In studies of salt sensitivity, African-Americans and elderly patients have a higher prevalence of this condition and are thus more likely to have a more robust response to these drugs. However, these drugs effectively lower BP in most patients, irrespective of race, gender or age. Caution must be exercised when utilizing them as they may elicit hypokalemia, exacerbate glycemic control, adversely affect lipid profile, and cause dehydration and hyponatremia particularly in the elderly [28, 29]. These effects are dose-dependent.

The most commonly used classes of diuretics are thiazides, loop diuretics and potassium-sparing diuretics. Thiazides act by inhibiting tubular sodium and chloride reabsorption resulting in loss of salt and water. They become progressively less effective with worsening renal function, and have limited efficacy at estimated glomerular filtration rate (eGFR) <30 ml/min. An advantage of these drugs is that they are effective with once daily dosing for the treatment of hypertension.

■ The loop diuretics block sodium reabsorption in the ascending loop of Henle [30]. These agents are effective in causing rapid diuresis when given once daily, however for effective

Table 1.3 Combination drugs

Drug Combination	Drug ratios	CVD	Stroke	Renal	Trials
Combination antihypertensives					
*ACE/CCB**					
Amlodipine/ benazepril	2.5/10, 5/10, 5/20, 5/40, 10/20, 10/40	■	■		ACCOMPLISH (in progress)
Enalapril/ felodipine	5/2.5, 5/5				*ASCOT [35, 81]
Trandolapril/ verapamil	2/180, 1/240, 2/240, 4/240			■	BENEDICT, INVEST [56, 66]
ACE/diuretic					
Benazepril/ hydrochlorothiazide	5/6.25, 10/12.5, 20/12.5, 20/25				
Captopril/ hydrochlorothiazide	25/15, 25/25, 50/15, 50/25				
Enalapril/ hydrochlorothiazide	5/12.5, 10/25				
Lisinopril/ hydrochlorothiazide	10/12.5, 20/12.5, 20/25				
Moexipril/ hydrochlorothiazide	7.5/12.5, 15/12.5, 15/25				
Quinapril/ hydrochlorothiazide	10/12.5, 20/12.5, 20/25				
ARB/diuretic					
Cadesartan cilexetil/ hydrochlorothiazide	16/12.5, 32/12.5				
Eprosartan mesylate/ hydrochlorothiazide	600/12.5, 600/25				
Irbesartan/ hydrochlorothiazide	150/12.5, 300/12.5, 300/25				
Losartan potassium/ hydrochlorothiazide	50/12.5, 100/12.5, 100/25				
Telmisartan/ hydrochlorothiazide	40/12.5, 80/12.5, 80/25				

Table 1.3 (continued)

Drug combination	Drug ratios	CVD	Stroke	Renal	Trials
Valsartan/hydrochlorothiazide	80/12.5, 160/12.5, 160/25, 320/12.5, 320/25				
β-blocker/diuretic					
Atenolol/chlorthalidone	50/100/25				
Bisoprolol fumarate/hydrochlorothiazide	2.5/6.25, 5/6.25, 10/6.25				
Propranolol LA/hydrochlorothiazide	40/25, 80/25				
Metoprolol tartrate/hydrochlorothiazide	50/25, 100/25, 100/50				
Nadolol/bendroflumethiazide	40/5, 80/5				
Centrally acting drug/diuretic					
Methyldopa/hydrochlorothiazide	250/15, 250/25, 500/50				
Reserpine/hydroflumethiazide	0.125/25, 0.125/50				
Reserpine/hydrochlorothiazide	0.125/25, 0.125/50				
Diuretic/diuretic					
Amiloride Hcl/hydrochlorothiazide	5/50	■	■		STOP, STOP2, MRC, INSIGHT [45, 55, 69, 91]
Spironolactone/hydrochlorothiazide	25/25, 50/50				
Triamterene/hydrochlorothiazide	37.5/25, 50/25, 75/50	■	■		EWPHE [93]

*ASCOT studied amlodipine/perindopril vs atenolol/bendroflumethiazide on cardiovascular events and stroke, showing significant reduction in events with amlodipine/perindopril. These specific combinations are not commercially available as a single pill.

BP treatment, shorter acting agents such as furosemide need twice daily dosing (see Table 1.2). Loop diuretics are usually required in heart failure and renal failure for volume control and should be the preferred diuretic for patients with heart failure or renal failure who remain hypertensive.

■ Potassium-sparing diuretics are useful in patients who are at risk for hypokalemia as the effects of the agents are mediated through the distal tubule where they reduce potassium excretion and increase sodium excretion. One common practice to improve diuresis and reduce the concern of hypokalemia is to use these agents in combination with a thiazide or loop diuretic.

Calcium channel blockers

Calcium channel blockers (CCBs) are one of the most commonly used drug classes to treat BP and have the advantage of high response rates across various patient populations [31]. The major subtypes are dihydropyridine (e.g. nifedipine and amlodipine), and non-dihydropyridines (e.g. diltiazem and verapamil). Both types block the influx of calcium into the smooth muscle cell walls of the vasculature leading to vasodilation. However, there are differences between these subtypes. The non-dihydropyridines bind to the calcium channels located on myocardial cells as well as vascular cells, which leads to slowing of the heart rate and negative myocardial contractility.

■ Dihydropyridines have the strongest affinity for the vasculature and have little effect on the contractility and conduction of the heart. The potent vasodilation rendered by these agents leads to the most common side-effect of lower extremity edema which is dose-dependent. This edema is not due to fluid overload but rather to excess precapillary vasodilation relative to postcapillary vessels. Thus, diuretics may have little effect on this edema. For similar reasons, dihydropyridines as monotherapy in diabetics and renal disease may cause transient proteinuria which can be averted with combination therapy with ACE-Is [32]. Dihydropyridines may also cause nocturia in men and gingival hyperplasia. The non-dihydropyridines also cause bradycardia. In heart failure patients, caution should be used when prescribing any calcium channel blocker due to potentially important cardiodepressor effects.

Sympathetic nervous system blockers

The sympathetic nervous system plays an important role in the regulation of BP. Activation of the sympathetic nervous system (SNS) leads to multiple hemodynamic changes and these effects may be exaggerated in hypertensives. The primacy of the sympathetic nervous system in hypertension is still a source of debate, yet the effects on hemodynamics are an important target of therapy in reducing BP. Both central and peripheral stimulation of the sympathetic nervous system lead to elevated heart rate and BP, thus blockade is a plausible approach. Specific types of hypertension may be more responsive to these agents, in particular states of excess catecholamines such as pheochromacytoma and paraganglionic tumors, baroreceptor dysfunction, and autonomic dysfunction.

β-blockers

β-blockers are among the older therapies for hypertension. The mechanism of action is blockade of the peripheral β receptors. The antihypertensive effects are primarily related to the β_1 receptor blockade which leads to a reduction in cardiac output and reduction in renin, release. Cardioselective β-blockers have a stronger affinity for β_1 than β_2 receptors. Ideally, minimizing the β_2 receptor effects reduces adverse effects such as bronchoconstriction in the lungs and peripheral vasoconstriction. However, at higher doses these effects may still occur.

Some of the reported negative effects of β-blockers are worsening of insulin sensitivity, increase in triglycerides and decrease in (high-density lipoprotein) HDL-cholesterol. However these effects appear to be less in newer agents such as carvedilol and nebivolol. Clearly, β-blockers, in particular bisoprolol, metoprolol succinate extended release and carvedilol, offer specific benefits in the setting of heart failure and patients with both hypertension and left ventricular dysfunction should have one of these agents incorporated in the treatment regimen [1].

Although these agents have been widely used in hypertensives, recent meta-analyses call into question whether β-blockers are the best agents as first line of therapy in particular groups such as the elderly. However, a newer agent, nebivolol, has been demonstrated to have favorable effects in an elderly population with heart failure. Nebivolol is currently under investigation in the US but it has been used in other countries for several years.

α-blockers

Peripheral α-blockers offer an alternative mechanism as add-on therapy in the treatment of uncontrolled hypertensives. Through blockade of the vascular target of norepinephrine and epinephrine, these drugs reduce peripheral vasoconstriction. α-blockers, e.g. phenoxybenzamine and phentolamine, are clearly the drugs of choice in patients with very high circulating catecholamines, particularly in preparation for surgery. However, the Anti-hypertensive and Lipid-Lowering Treatment to Prevent Heart Attack Trial (ALLHAT) [33] study demonstrated worsening of heart failure symptoms in patients assigned an α-blocker as primary therapy. This finding may be confounded by the design of the study restricting the addition of diuretics to other agents. Nevertheless, it is reasonable to reserve these drugs as add-on therapy after RAS blockade, diuretics, calcium channel blockers and β-blockers. The most common side-effects are orthostatic hypotension, dry mouth and fatigue. Longer-acting versions of these drugs are typically given at bedtime which reduces certain side-effect complaints, e.g. dizziness. These drugs are commonly used in low doses to relieve prostatic hypertrophy symptoms in men, however, at these doses, minimal BP effect occurs. Beneficial effects of α-blockers include small increases in HDL-cholesterol, slight reduction in triglycerides, and favorable effects on insulin/glucose profile [34].

α-/β-blockers

Currently there are two agents which have both α- and β-blockade capability, which offsets the reduction in cardiac output with less reflex vasoconstriction (carvedilol and labetalol). However, the relative potency of these effects is largely in favor of β-blockade effects with less afterload reduction and greater negative chronotropic and inotropic effects. These features are particularly relevent in heart failure patients [34]. In heart failure studies with carvedilol, in addition to the standard treatment for heart failure, patients on carvedilol had improved survival. This study utilized lower doses than those required to treat hypertension and to achieve better BP reduction, it is often necessary to use higher doses. These agents are also useful in labile hypertensives as the source of lability may be the sympathetic nervous system. Also, in states of excess catecholamines, these agents may be very useful. Labetalol given orally or intravenously is a very effective treatment for hypertensive urgency or emergency. Oral doses of 100 mg or 200 mg in hypertensive urgency or emergency lower BP well in 1–2 h. Initial parenteral doses of 10–40 mg, with doubling of the dose every 10 min until BP is lowered is appropriate in treating hypertensive emergencies. The most common side-effects of these agents are orthostatic hypotension, dizziness and fatigue which are dose-dependent effects.

Centrally acting drugs

This class of antihypertensives, most notably represented by clonidine, lowers BP through central α-blockade reducing the release of catecholamines to the peripheral circulation.

Generally these agents are reserved as add-on therapy in the most resistant hypertensives. They are not recommended as initial therapy in hypertension. The side-effect profile of these agents includes significant fatigue, sleepiness, and sexual dysfunction, in addition to the same side-effects experienced with peripheral β-blockers and α-blockers. One advantage of clonidine is the transdermal delivery system in patients who have oral intake limitations. These agents may be used in the treatment of hypertensive urgency although after a few days patients may experience withdrawal side-effects with acute discontinuation. Therefore, these drugs should be weaned rather than abruptly discontinued. In hypertensive urgency oral clonidine may be given at doses of 0.1–0.2 mg initially, then additional doses of 0.1 mg hourly to reduce BP to <180/110 mmHg.

Aldosterone blockade

Aldosterone blockade offers an additional mechanism for reducing BP in hyperaldosteronism, difficult to treat hypertensives, heart failure and patients with concurrent low potassium. These drugs have demonstrated additional survival and morbidity benefits in heart failure [35, 36]. Patients in these trials were not all hypertensive yet these drugs may be used in higher doses to lower BP. The primary action of this class of agents is to block the effects of aldosterone at the receptor level which leads to diuresis through the distal renal tubule with reabsorption of potassium. In addition, these agents block the myocardial fibrosis effects of aldosterone. Although the potency of the BP response is most robust in hyperaldosteronism patients, recent studies show that BP reduction is not dependent on baseline aldosterone levels [37]. Caution must be exercised when using these agents as they may result in hyperkalemia, particularly in renal insufficiency and diabetics. In general, potassium and serum creatinine levels should be checked at 1 week after initiating aldosterone blockers and periodically thereafter. In combination with ACE-Is and/or angiotensin receptor antagonist use, the risk of hyperkalemia is increased.

Direct vasodilators

Direct vasodilators such as hydralazine and minoxidil act by directly affecting vasoconstriction of the vascular smooth muscle cell. Hydralazine has been shown to increase the availability of nitric oxide, a naturally occurring endothelial vasodilator. These drugs are very effective in lowering BP although they are limited by the side-effects of reflex tachycardia, and peripheral edema due to strong vasodilation. Frequently, it is necessary to use additional concurrent treatment to limit tachycardia and reduce fluid retention. Hydralazine in combination with nitrates offers particular benefit in heart failure (described elsewhere in this text). These drugs are good add-on therapy in uncontrolled hypertension. The most concerning side-effects, although uncommon, are the development of lupus-like antibodies with hydralazine and pericardial effusion due to minoxidil. Minoxidil is not recommended in heart failure due to its effect on sodium retention. It is reasonable however to consider these drugs for resistant hypertensives.

Combination drugs

Recent clinical trials have clearly demonstrated that monotherapy in the treatment of hypertension is largely ineffective in reaching BP goals. In addition, patient adherence to therapy is improved with fewer pills per day, and fewer doses. Heart failure patients are commonly prescribed multiple drugs. This makes combination drugs particularly attractive in managing hypertension. Another rationale for combination therapy is the synergistic effects exerted by complementary drug mechanisms, as well as minimizing side-effects with complementary actions [38, 39].

Multiple combinations are available (see Table 1.3). There is an ongoing debate regarding the best combination option. The only completed trial addressing combination therapy is the Anglo-Scandinavian Cardiac Outcomes Study (ASCOT). This trial compared atenolol + bendroflumethiazide to amlodipine + perindopril treatment in hypertensives at high risk for cardiovascular disease. The trial was discontinued early due to results favoring amlodipine + perindopril with a 15% reduction in all-cause mortality ($P \le 0.005$); a 15% reduction in all coronary events ($P \le 0.005$); 25% reduction in all fatal and non-fatal stroke ($P \le 0.001$); and a 25% reduction in CV mortality ($P \le 0.005$). However, the primary endpoint of non-fatal MI and fatal coronary heart disease (CHD) was not reached and only demonstrated a non-significant reduction of about 10% [40]. After adjustments for BP, these differences in outcomes were further attenuated [41]. Currently, the Avoiding Cardiovascular Events through COMBination Therapy in Patients Living with Systolic Hypertension (ACCOMPLISH Study) is comparing cardiovascular outcomes with amlodipine/benazepril vs. benazepril/ hydrochlorothiazide and is scheduled to be completed in 2008. These data will be helpful in making the best combination choices for individual patients.

Paradigms for treatment

Most paradigms for the treatment of hypertension were previously based on β-blockade and diuretic therapy in uncomplicated hypertension. New data such as the findings from the ASCOT study as well as meta-analyses suggest that this approach may not be the best initial therapy for all hypertensives. The ALLHAT study demonstrates that diuretics, dihydropyridine CCBs, and ACE-Is are equal in their effect on cardiovascular events [33]. Recommendations from both the JNC 7 report and the Hypertension in African-Americans Working Guidelines (HAAWG) suggest that BP treatment should always include lifestyle modifications alone or in combination with drugs [42]. The high fiber, low fat, and low sodium diet used in the Dietary Approaches to Stop Hypertension (DASH) demonstrated significant BP reduction in blacks and whites [43]. The difficulty with lifestyle modifications is not efficacy, but rather long-term maintenance. Nevertheless, the message should be reinforced regularly. Drug treatment may be initiated with ACE-I, ARB, β-blockade, CCB, or diuretics in patients who have uncomplicated hypertension. However, both guidelines recommend combination therapy as the starting point for more severe hypertension. The major difference in these guidelines is the BP threshold for initiating combination treatment; in the HAAWG guidelines, combination therapy is prescribed initially when the BP exceeds 15 mmHg and/or 10 mmHg above systolic and diastolic goals respectively, while the JNC 7 reserves combination therapy until the BP exceeds 20 mmHg and/or 10 mmHg above the systolic and diastolic goals.

According to JNC 7, normal BP is <120/80 mmHg based on epidemiologic data, however treatment goals are based on clinical trial experience which suggests that BP should be reduced to <140/90 mmHg in uncomplicated hypertension. The Hypertension Optimal Treatment (HOT) study demonstrated that the optimal reduction in cardiovascular disease (CVD) occurred at 138/83 mmHg. More recently, the TROPHY study showed that BP was safely reduced by 10/7 mmHg in prehypertensives with BPs of 134/84 mmHg without increasing adverse events using low-dose candesartan treatment [44]. Guidelines have not yet incorporated these data into current recommendations; however, these new findings provide important safety data. Further study is warranted into treatment goals. Both guidelines support specific drug recommendations for renal disease, diabetes, and heart failure. ACE-I and ARB treatment reduces proteinuria and the rate of progression of renal disease in both diabetic and non-diabetics and thus should be included in first-line therapy. Furthermore, the goal of therapy for hypertension complicated by diabetes and/or renal disease is <130/80 mmHg. This is justified by the tight relationship between BP level and loss of glomerular filtration rate [11]. The treatment of BP in heart failure should follow similar treatment goals [1].

SUMMARY

Optimal treatment of hypertension is a key feature in the prevention and management of heart failure. The best opportunity to reduce the incidence of heart failure lies in targeted and sustained goal reduction of BP. Future studies of prehypertension may further improve strategies to prevent heart failure.

REFERENCES

1. Hunt SA, Abraham WT, Chin MH et al. ACC/AHA 2005 Guideline Update for the Diagnosis and Management of Chronic Heart Failure in the Adult: a report of the American College of Cardiology/American Heart Association Task Force on Practice Guidelines (Writing Committee to Update the 2001 Guidelines for the Evaluation and Management of Heart Failure): developed in collaboration with the American College of Chest Physicians and the International Society for Heart and Lung Transplantation: endorsed by the Heart Rhythm Society. Circulation 2005; 112:e154–e235.
2. Chobanian AV, Bakris GL, Black HR et al. The Seventh Report of the Joint National Committee on Prevention, Detection, Evaluation, and Treatment of High Blood Pressure: the JNC 7 report. JAMA 2003; 289:2560–2572.
3. Hajjar I, Kotchen TA. Trends in prevalence, awareness, treatment, and control of hypertension in the United States, 1988–2000. JAMA 2003; 290:199–206.
4. Vasan RS, Beiser A, Seshadri S et al. Residual lifetime risk for developing hypertension in middle-aged women and men: The Framingham Heart Study. JAMA 2002; 287:1003–1010.
5. Lewington S, Clarke R, Qizilbash N et al. Age-specific relevance of usual blood pressure to vascular mortality: a meta-analysis of individual data for one million adults in 61 prospective studies. Lancet 2002; 360:1903–1913.
6. Wang Y, Wang QJ. The prevalence of prehypertension and hypertension among US adults according to the new Joint National Committee guidelines: new challenges of the old problem. Arch Intern Med 2004; 164:2126–2134.
7. Thom T, Haase N, Rosamond W et al. Heart disease and stroke statistics – 2006 update: a report from the American Heart Association Statistics Committee and Stroke Statistics Subcommittee. Circulation 2006; 113:e85–e151.
8. Vasan RS, Levy D. The role of hypertension in the pathogenesis of heart failure. A clinical mechanistic overview. Arch Intern Med 1996; 156:1789–1796.
9. Levy D, Larson MG, Vasan RS et al. The progression from hypertension to congestive heart failure. JAMA 1996; 275:1557–1562.
10. Baker DW. Prevention of heart failure. J Card Fail 2002; 8:333–346.
11. Bakris GL, Williams M, Dworkin L et al. Preserving renal function in adults with hypertension and diabetes: a consensus approach. National Kidney Foundation Hypertension and Diabetes Executive Committees Working Group. Am J Kidney Dis 2000; 36:646–661.
12. Julius S, Nesbitt SD, Egan BM et al. Feasibility of treating prehypertension with an angiotensin-receptor blocker. N Engl J Med 2006; 354:1685–1697.
13. Dzau V, Braunwald E. Resolved and unresolved issues in the prevention and treatment of coronary artery disease: a workshop consensus statement. Am Heart J 1991; 121:1244–1263.
14. Alexander RW. Theodore Cooper Memorial Lecture. Hypertension and the pathogenesis of atherosclerosis. Oxidative stress and the mediation of arterial inflammatory response: a new perspective. Hypertension 1995; 25:155–161.
15. Folkow B. Physicological aspects of primary hypertension. Physiol Rev 1982; 62:347–503.
16. Chobanian AV. 1989 Corcoran lecture: adaptive and maladaptive responses of the arterial wall to hypertension. Hypertension 1990; 15:666–674.
17. Alexander RW, Dzau VJ. Vascular biology: the past 50 years. Circulation 2000; 102:IV112–IV116.
18. Weir MR, Dzau V. The renin-angiotensin-aldosterone system: a specific target for hypertension management. Am J Hypertens 1999; 12:205S–213S.
19. Staessen JA, Thijs L, Fagard R et al. Predicting cardiovascular risk using conventional vs ambulatory blood pressure in older patients with systolic hypertension. Systolic Hypertension in Europe Trial Investigators. JAMA 1999; 282:539–546.

20. Clement DL, De Buyzere ML, De Bacquer DA *et al.* Prognostic value of ambulatory blood pressure recordings in patients with treated hypertension. *N Engl J Med* 2003; 348:2407–2415.
21. Sega R, Facchetti R, Bombelli M *et al.* Prognostic value of ambulatory and home blood pressures compared with office blood pressure in the general population: follow-up results from the Pressioni Arteriose Monitorate e Loro Associazioni (PAMELA) study. *Circulation* 2005; 111:1777–1783.
22. Obara T, Ohkubo T, Kikuya M *et al.* Prevalence of masked uncontrolled and treated white-coat hypertension defined according to the average of morning and evening home blood pressure value: from the Japan Home versus Office Measurement Evaluation Study. *Blood Press Monit* 2005; 10:311–316.
23. Pickering TG, Shimbo D, Haas D. Ambulatory blood-pressure monitoring. *N Engl J Med* 2006; 354:2368–2374.
24. O'Brien E, Coats A, Owens P *et al.* Use and interpretation of ambulatory blood pressure monitoring: Recommendations of the British Hypertension Society. *BMJ* 2000; 320:1128–1134.
25. Carey RM, Wang ZQ, Siragy HM. Role of the angiotensin type 2 receptor in the regulation of blood pressure and renal function. *Hypertension* 2000; 35:155–163.
26. Israili ZH, Hall WD. Cough and angioneurotic edema associated with angiotensin-converting enzyme inhibitor therapy. A review of the literature and pathophysiology. *Ann Intern Med* 1992; 117:234–242.
27. Cohen HW, Hailpern SM, Fang J *et al.* Sodium intake and mortality in the NHANES II follow-up study. *Am J Med* 2006; 119:275.e7–e14.
28. Alderman M, Einstein A. Evidence relating dietary sodium to cardiovascular disease. *J Am Coll Nutr* 2006; 25:256S–261S.
29. Zillich AJ, Garg J, Basu S *et al.* Thiazide diuretics, potassium, and the development of diabetes: a quantitative review. *Hypertension* 2006; 48:219–224.
30. Palmer BF. Managing hyperkalemia caused by inhibitiors of the renin-angiotensin-aldosterone system. *N Engl J Med* 2004; 351:585–592.
31. Materson BJ, Reda DJ, Cushman WC. Department of Veterans Affairs single-drug therapy of hypertension study. Revised figures and new data. Department of Veterans Affairs Cooperative Study Group on Antihypertensive Agents. *Am J Hypertens* 1995; 8:189–192.
32. Fogari R, Zoppi A, Mugellini A *et al.* Effects of benazepril plus amlodipine vs benazepril alone on urinary albumin excretion in hypertensive patients with type II diabetes and microalbuminuria. *Clin Drug Invest* 1997; 13:50–55.
33. ALLHAT. Major outcomes in high-risk hypertensive patients randomized to angiotensin-converting enzyme inhibitor or calcium channel blocker vs diuretic: The Antihypertensive and Lipid-Lowering Treatment to Prevent Heart Attack Trial (ALLHAT). *JAMA* 2002; 288:2981–2997.
34. Oparil S, Weber M. *Pharmokinetics of Antihypertensive Drugs. Hypertension: Companion to Brenner & Rector's The Kidney*, 2nd edition. Elsevier Saunders, Philadelphia, 2005.
35. Pitt B, Zannad F, Remme WJ *et al.* The effect of spironolactone on morbidity and mortality in patients with severe heart failure. Randomized Aldactone Evaluation Study Investigators. *N Engl J Med* 1999; 341:709–717.
36. Pitt B, Remme W, Zannad F *et al.* Eplerenone, a selective aldosterone blocker, in patients with left ventricular dysfunction after myocardial infarction. *N Engl J Med* 2003; 348:1309–1321.
37. Calhoun DA. Use of aldosterone antagonists in resistant hypertension. *Prog Cardiovasc Dis* 2006; 48:387–396.
38. Weir MR. The rationale for combination versus single-entity therapy in hypertension. *Am J Hypertens* 1998; 11:163S–169S.
39. Messerli FH, Weir MR, Neutel JM. Combination therapy of amlodipine/benazepril versus monotherapy of amlodipine in a practice-based setting. *Am J Hypertens* 2002; 15:550–556.
40. Dahlof B, Sever PS, Poulter NR *et al.* Prevention of cardiovascular events with an antihypertensive regimen of amlodipine adding perindopril as required versus atenolol adding bendroflumethiazide as required, in the Anglo-Scandinavian Cardiac Outcomes Trial–Blood Pressure Lowering Arm (ASCOT-BPLA): a multicentre randomised controlled trial. *Lancet* 2005; 366:895–906.
41. Poulter NR, Wedel H, Dahlof B *et al.* Role of blood pressure and other variables in the differential cardiovascular event rates noted in the Anglo-Scandinavian Cardiac Outcomes Trial–Blood Pressure Lowering Arm (ASCOT-BPLA). *Lancet* 2005; 366:907–913.
42. Douglas JG, Bakris GL, Epstein M *et al.* Management of high blood pressure in African Americans: consensus statement of the Hypertension in African Americans Working Group of the International Society on Hypertension in Blacks. *Arch Intern Med* 2003; 163:525–541.

43. Sacks FM, Svetkey LP, Vollmer WM *et al*. Effects on blood pressure of reduced dietary sodium and the Dietary Approaches to Stop Hypertension (DASH) diet. DASH-Sodium Collaborative Research Group. *N Engl J Med* 2001; 344:3–10.

44. Hansson L, Zanchetti A, Carruthers SG *et al*. Effects of intensive blood-pressure lowering and low-dose aspirin in patients with hypertension: principal results of the Hypertension Optimal Treatment (HOT) randomised trial. HOT Study Group. *Lancet* 1998; 351:1755–1762.

45. Medical Research Council Working Party. Medical Research Council trial of treatment of hypertension in older adults: principal results. *BMJ* 1992; 304:405–412.

46. Wilhelmsen L, Berglund G, Elmfeld D. Beta-blockers versus diuretics in hypertensive men. Main results from the HAPPY trial. *J Hypertens* 1987; 5:561–576.

47. Hansson L, Lindholm L, Niskanen L *et al*. Effect of angiotensin converting enzyme inhibition compared with conventional therapy on cardiovascular morbidity and mortality in hypertension: the Captopril Prevention Project (CAPP) randomised trial. *Lancet* 1999; 353:611–616.

48. UK Prospective Diabetes Study Group. Efficacy of atenolol and captropril in reducing risk of macrovascular and microvascular complication in type 2 diabetes. *BMJ* 1998; 317:713–720.

49. Staessen J, Fagard R, Thijs L *et al* Randomised double-blind comparison of placebo and active treatment for older patients with isolated systolic hypertension. *Lancet* 1997; 350:757–764.

50. Cohn J, Ziesche S, Loss L *et al*. Effects of felodipine on short-term exercise and neurohormone and long-term mortality in heart failure: results of V-Heft III. *Circulation* 1995; 92:1–143.

51. Liu L, Wang JG, Gong L *et al*. Comparison of active treatment and placebo in older Chinese patients with isolated systolic hypertension. Systolic Hypertension in China (Syst-China) Collaborative Group. *J Hypertens* 1998; 16:1823–1829.

52. Estacio RO, Jeffers BW, Hiatt WR *et al*. The effect of nisoldipine as compared with enalapril on cardiovascular outcomes in patients with non-insulin-dependent diabetes and hypertension. *N Engl J Med* 1998; 338:645–652.

53. Lubsen J, Wagener G, Kirwan BA *et al*. Effect of long-acting nifedipine on mortality and cardiovascular morbidity in patients with symptomatic stable angina and hypertension: the ACTION trial. *J Hypertens* 2005; 23:641–648.

54. Wing LM, Reid CM, Ryan P *et al*. A comparison of outcomes with angiotensin-converting enzyme inhibitors and diuretics for hypertension in the elderly. *N Engl J Med* 2003; 348:583–592.

55. Brown MJ, Palmer CR, Castaigne A *et al*. Morbidity and mortality in patients randomised to double-blind treatment with a long-acting calcium-channel blocker or diuretic in the International Nifedipine GITS study: Intervention as a Goal in Hypertension Treatment (INSIGHT). *Lancet* 2000; 356:366–372.

56. Bakris GL, Gaxiola E, Messerli FH *et al*. Clinical outcomes in the diabetes cohort of the INternational VErapamil SR-Trandolapril study. *Hypertension* 2004; 44:637–642.

57. Kuwajima I, Kuramoto K, Ogihara T *et al*. Tolerability and safety of a calcium channel blocker in comparison with a diuretic in the treatment of elderly patients with hypertension: secondary analysis of the NICS-EH. *Hypertens Res* 2001; 24:475–480.

58. Hansson L, Hedner T, Lund-Johansen P *et al*. Randomised trials of effects of calcium antagonist compared with diuretics and β-blockers on cardiovascular morbidity and mortality in hypertension: the Nordic Diltiazem (NORDIL) study. *Lancet* 2000; 356:359–365.

59. PROGRESS Collaborative Group. Randomised trial of perindopril-based blood-pressure-lowering regimen among 6,105 individuals with previous stroke or transient ischaemic attack. *Lancet* 2001; 358:1033–1041.

60. Rosei EA, Dal PC, Leonetti G *et al*. Clinical results of the Verapamil in Hypertension and Atherosclerosis Study. VHAS Investigators. *J Hypertens* 1997; 15:1337–1344.

61. Yancy CW, Fowler MB, Colucci WS *et al*. Race and the response to adrenergic blockade with carvedilol in patients with chronic heart failure. *N Engl J Med* 2001; 344:1358–1365.

62. Dens JA, Desmet WJ, Coussement P *et al*. Long term effects of nisoldipine on the progression of coronary atherosclerosis and the occurrence of clinical events: the NICOLE study. *Heart* 2003; 89:887–892.

63. Wright JT Jr, Bakris G, Greene T *et al*. Effect of blood pressure lowering and antihypertensive drug class on progression of hypertensive kidney disease: results from the AASK trial. *JAMA* 2006; 295:2726.

64. Tatti P, Pahor M, Byington RP *et al*. Outcome results of Fosinopril Versus Amlodipine Cardiovascular Events Randomised Trial (FACET) in patients with hypertension and NIDDM. *Diabetes Care* 1998; 4:597–603.

65. Ferrari R. Perindopril and Remodeling in Elderly with Acute Myocardial Infarction Investigators. Effects of angiotensin-converting enzyme inhibition with perindopril on left ventricular remodeling

and clinical outcome: results of the randomized Perindopril and Remodeling in Elderly with Acute Myocardial Infarction (PREAMI) Study. *Arch Intern Med* 2006; 166:659–666.

66.   Ruggenenti P, Fassi A, Ilieva AP *et al.* Preventing microalbuminuria in type 2 diabetes. *N Engl J Med* 2004; 351:1941–1951.

67.   Fox KM. EURopean Trial On Reduction of Cardiac Events with Perindopril in Stable Coronary Artery Disease Investigators. Efficacy of perindopril in reduction of cardiovascular events among patients with stable coronary artery disease: randomised, double-blind, placebo-controlled, multicentre trial (the EUROPA study). *Lancet* 2003; 362:782–788.

68.   Pitt B, O'Neill B, Feldman R *et al.* The QUinapril Ischemic Event Trial (QUIET): evaluation of chronic ACE inhibitor therapy in patients with ischemic heart disease and preserved left ventricular function. *Am J Cardiol* 2001; 87:1058–1063.

69.   Hansson L, Lindholm LH, Ekbom T *et al.* Randomised trial of old and new antihypertensive drugs in elderly patients: cardiovascular mortality and morbidity the Swedish Trial in Old Patients with Hypertension-2 study. *Lancet* 1999; 354:1751–1756.

70.   Black HR, Elliott WJ, Grandits G *et al.* Principal results of the Controlled Onset Verapamil Investigation of Cardiovascular End Points (CONVINCE) trial. *JAMA* 2003; 289:2073–2082.

71.   Lithell H, Hansson L, Skoog I *et al.* The Study on Cognition and Prognosis in the Elderly (SCOPE): principal results of a randomized double-blind intervention trial. *J Hypertens* 2003; 21:875–886.

72.   Zanchetti A, Rosei EA, Dal PC *et al.* The Verapamil in Hypertension and Atherosclerosis Study (VHAS): results of long-term randomized treatment with either verapamil or chlorthalidone on carotid intima-media thickness. *J Hypertens* 1998; 16:1667–1676.

73.   Braunwald E, Domanski MJ, Fowler SE *et al.* Angiotensin-converting-enzyme inhibition in stable coronary artery disease. *N Engl J Med* 2004; 351:2058–2068.

74.   Viberti G, Wheeldon NM. Microalbuminuria reduction with valsartan in patients with type 2 diabetes mellitus: a blood pressure-independent effect. *Circulation* 2002; 106:672–678.

75.   Yusuf S, Sleight P, Pogue J *et al.* Effects of an angiotensin-converting-enzyme inhibitor, ramipril, on cardiovascular events in high-risk patients. The Heart Outcomes Prevention Evaluation Study Investigators. *N Engl J Med* 2000; 342:145–153.

76.   Dahlof B, Devereux RB, Kjeldsen SE *et al.* Cardiovascular morbidity and mortality in the Losartan Intervention For Endpoint reduction in hypertension study (LIFE): a randomised trial against atenolol. *Lancet* 2002; 359:995–1003.

77.   Brenner BM, Cooper ME, de Zeeuw D *et al.* Effects of losartan on renal and cardiovascular outcomes in patients with type 2 diabetes and nephropathy. *N Engl J Med* 2001; 345:861–869.

78.   Lewis EJ, Hunsicker LG, Clarke WR *et al.* Renoprotective effect of the angiotensin-receptor antagonist irbesartan in patients with nephropathy due to type 2 diabetes. *N Engl J Med* 2001; 345:851–860.

79.   Packer M, O'Connor CM, Ghali JK *et al.* Effect of amlodipine on morbidity and mortality in severe chronic heart failure. Prospective Randomized Amlodipine Survival Evaluation Study Group. *N Engl J Med* 1996; 335:1107–1114.

80.   Julius S, Kjeldsen SE, Weber M *et al.* Outcomes in hypertensive patients at high cardiovascular risk treated with regimens based on valsartan or amlodipine: the VALUE randomised trial. *Lancet* 2004; 363:2022–2031.

81.   Jamerson KA, Bakris GL, Wun CC *et al.* Rationale and design of the avoiding cardiovascular events through combination therapy in patients living with systolic hypertension (ACCOMPLISH) trial: the first randomized controlled trial to compare the clinical outcome effects of first-line combination therapies in hypertension. *Am J Hypertens* 2004; 17:793–801.

82.   Pfeffer MA, Braunwald E, Moye LA *et al.* Effect of captopril on mortality and morbidity in patients with left ventricular dysfunction after myocardial infarction. Results of the survival and ventricular enlargement trial. The SAVE Investigators. *N Engl J Med* 1992; 327:669–677.

83.   Kostis JB. The effect of enalapril on mortal and morbid events in patients with hypertension and left ventricular dysfunction. *Am J Hypertens* 1995; 8:909–914.

84.   Kostis JB, Davis BR, Cutler J *et al.* Prevention of heart failure by antihypertensive drug treatment in older persons with isolated systolic hypertension. SHEP Cooperative Research Group. *JAMA* 1997; 278:212–216.

85.   Neaton JD, Grimm RH Jr, Prineas RJ, *et al.* Treatment of Mild Hypertension Study. Final results. Treatment of Mild Hypertension Study Research Group. *JAMA* 1993; 270:713–724.

86. Konstam MA, Neaton JD, Poole-Wilson PA *et al*. Comparison of losartan and captopril on heart failure-related outcomes and symptoms from the losartan heart failure survival study (ELITE II). *Am Heart J* 2005; 150:123–131.

87. Young JB, Dunlap ME, Pfeffer MA *et al*. Mortality and morbidity reduction with Candesartan in patients with chronic heart failure and left ventricular systolic dysfunction: results of the CHARM low-left ventricular ejection fraction trials. *Circulation* 2004; 110:2618–2626.

88. McMurray J, Solomon S, Pieper K *et al*. The effect of valsartan, captopril, or both on atherosclerotic events after acute myocardial infarction: an analysis of the Valsartan in Acute Myocardial Infarction Trial (VALIANT). *J Am Coll Cardiol* 2006; 47:726–733.

89. Maggioni AP, Anand I, Gottlieb SO, Latini R, Tognoni G, Cohn JN. Effects of valsartan on morbidity and mortality in patients with heart failure not receiving angiotensin-converting enzyme inhibitors. *J Am Coll Cardiol* 2002; 40:1414–1421.

90. Five-year findings of the hypertension detection and follow-up program. III. Reduction in stroke incidence among persons with high blood pressure. Hypertension Detection and Follow-up Program Cooperative Group. *JAMA* 1982; 247:633–638.

91. Dahlof B, Lindholm LH, Hansson L *et al*. Morbidity and mortality in the Swedish trial in Old Patients with Hypertension (STOP-Hypertension). *Lancet* 1991; 338:1281–1285.

92. Wikstrand J, Warnold I, Tuomilehto J *et al*. Metoprolol versus thiazide diuretics in hypertension. Morbidity results from the MAPHY Study. *Hypertension* 1991; 17:579–588.

93. Staessen J, Bulpitt C, Clement D *et al*. Relation between mortality and treated blood pressure in elderly patients with hypertension: report of the European Working Party on High Blood Pressure in the Elderly. *BMJ* 1989; 298:1552–1556.

94. Pitt B, Byington RP, Furberg CD *et al*. Effect of amlodipine on the progression of atherosclerosis and the occurrence of clinical events. PREVENT Investigators. *Circulation* 2000; 102:1503–1510.

95. Black H. *Clinical Trials in Hypertension*. Marcel Dekker, Inc., New York, 2001.

2

Insulin resistance: implications for the failing heart

B. Drabicki, S. Carr, R. P. Shannon

INTRODUCTION

Insulin resistance forms the mechanistic basis for both the metabolic syndrome and eventually Type 2 diabetes. Left ventricular (LV) systolic dysfunction is a newly recognized clinical state characterized by both myocardial and eventually whole body insulin resistance, even in the absence of conventional risk factors for the development of insulin resistance, such as obesity. The consequences of impaired insulin-mediated glucose uptake (IMGU) for the failing heart are considerable and contribute to the progression of myocardial energetic failure, leading to clinical decompensation and end-stage disease. Importantly, both the renin–angiotensin and sympathetic nervous systems are now recognized to contribute and exacerbate insulin resistance in heart failure. However, conventional neurohormonal blockade, while necessary, is insufficient to overcome myocardial insulin resistance in advanced heart failure. In general, there remains a paucity of therapies available to treat insulin resistance before it progresses to frank diabetes or before it leads to myocardial energetic failure in patients with advanced heart failure. Furthermore, many of the newer agents employed to treat Type 2 diabetes carry warnings or are contraindicated in heart failure, leaving the issue of myocardial insulin resistance unattended. There are several new therapeutic approaches under development that are designed to modulate myocardial substrate choice or enhance myocardial insulin action which offer promise in the treatment of the myocardial metabolic derangements in patients with LV systolic dysfunction.

With the abundance of available food sources in our modern society, humans no longer need to 'expend calories to attain calories' and, as a result, the western world faces an epidemic of obesity. Recent estimates suggest that a majority (>56%) of adults are overweight, 1 in 5 are obese, and 7.3% have diabetes [1]. In 2000, the prevalence of obesity (body mass index ≥30) was 19.8% among US adults, which reflects a 61% increase since 1991 [1]. As such, obesity has become a major health problem associated with increased risk of diabetes and cardiovascular disease, leading to a significant impairment of quality of life. In the last decade, there was a doubling of the number of US adults who were both obese and diabetic, such that the two conditions account for nearly 10% of overall healthcare expenditure in the

Brandy Drabicki, MD, Department of Medicine, Allegheny General Hospital, Drexel University College of Medicine, Pittsburgh, Pennsylvania, USA.

Steven J. Carr, MD, Department of Medicine, Allegheny General Hospital, Drexel University College of Medicine, Pittsburgh, Pennsylvania, USA.

Richard P. Shannon, MD, Interim Chairman, Department of Medicine, University of Pennsylvania School of Medicine, Hospital of the University of Pennsylvania, Philadelphia, Pennsylvania, USA.

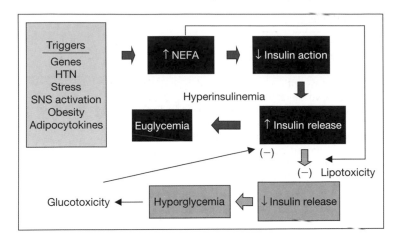

Figure 2.1 Distinguishing insulin resistance from diabetes: insulin resistance is mediated by increases in NEFA and the ecoptic accumulation of NEFA called lipotoxicity. Initially, plasma glucose is normal due to compensatory hyperinsulinemia. Diabetes occurs when pancreatic reserves become limited, hyperinsulinemia is reduced and hyperglycemia develops. Glucose-mediated tissue injury is called glucotoxicity (HTN, hypertension; NEFA, non-esterified fatty acids).

US [1, 2]. Not surprisingly, obesity alone may result in a reduction in life expectancy of up to 3 years [3].

The epidemic of obesity and the accompanying increase in Type 2 diabetes have focused renewed attention on the pathogenic links between these conditions. The central theme linking these common metabolic disorders, including hypertension, obesity, the metabolic syndrome and eventually diabetes, involve altered cellular insulin action or 'insulin resistance' [4, 5]. Insulin governs numerous metabolic processes including glucose uptake by insulin-responsive tissues, the suppression of lipolysis and the stimulation of lipogenesis in adipose tissue. In addition to its recognized metabolic actions, insulin also governs aspects of cellular growth and survival as well as possessing vascular actions [6]. As such, resistance to insulin can be selective to one or several of its regulatory actions and can also be tissue specific, being evident in some but not all insulin-responsive tissues. It is now recognized that both circulating and ectopic deposition of non-esterified fatty acids (NEFA) plays an important pathophysiologic role in the development of resistance to the cellular actions of insulin [7, 8].

Figure 2.1 illustrates a conceptual framework useful in understanding the relationship between increases in NEFA, insulin resistance and the subsequent development of Type 2 diabetes. Increases in circulating NEFA lead to altered insulin action particularly in skeletal muscle, adipose tissue and the liver, and require compensatory increases in circulating insulin to maintain plasma glucose levels at or near normal. The compensatory response can be maintained for a decade or more, but exacts the price of ultimate pancreatic β-cell failure, such that as many as 70% of the β-cells are exhausted by the time hyperglycemia emerges. The loss of β-cell function is not simply due to physiologic overdrive, but is related to apoptotic cell death mediated in large measure by the accumulation of NEFA in the pancreas. Recent evidence [7, 8] suggests that the β-cells of the pancreas are not the only target of ectopic accumulation NEFA, but similar processes occur in the liver (hepatic steatosis) and the heart (cardiac steatosis). Thus, it is now accepted that insulin resistance is mediated by NEFA accumulation in target tissues and that this process can itself lead to end organ injury, now referred to as 'lipotoxicity' [9, 10]. While compensatory hyperinsulinemia helps to counteract the effects of insulin resistance on glucose homeostasis, the response over many years takes its toll, leading to the exhaustion of pancreatic β-cells. Eventually, insulin

Table 2.1 Summary of UKPDS trial

Background	Improved glycemic control has been shown to decrease microvascular complications.
Objectives	Does improved glycemic control prevent macrovascular changes? What is the best way to achieve glycemic control?
Study design	3867 patients with newly diagnosed Type 2 diabetes mellitus were randomly assigned to intensive therapy with either a sulfonylurea or insulin, or conventional therapy with diet. A composite endpoint including (a) any diabetes-related endpoint, (b) diabetes-related death, and (c) all-cause mortality was assessed. Patients were followed over a mean interval of 10 years.
Results	HgbA$_1$C improved significantly in intense vs conventional therapy (7.0 vs 7.9). The intensive group had 12% lower incidence of any diabetes-related endpoint ($P = 0.029$), 10% lower for any diabetes-related death ($P = 0.34$) and 6% lower all-cause mortality, but did not reach statistical significance ($P = 0.44$). There was a 25% reduction in microvascular endpoints ($P = 0.0099$) in the intensive vs conventional therapy, but there was no difference in macrovascular events.
Conclusions	Intense glycemic control decreases microvascular changes, but not macrovascular changes, diabetes-related death or all-cause mortality.

resistance gives way to impaired fasting and postprandial glucose levels, ushering in the onset of Type 2 diabetes. The signature feature of Type 2 diabetes is hyperglycemia and the mechanism of end organ injury is referred to as 'glucotoxicity'.

Thus, insulin resistance can be considered as a disorder of NEFA while Type 2 diabetes is a disorder of glucose homeostasis as a consequence of years of insulin resistance. The additive effects of increased NEFA, compensatory hyperinsulinemia, and eventually hyperglycemia lead to progressive microvascular (retinopathy, neuropathy, nephropathy) and macrovascular (stroke and myocardial infarction [MI]) complications that are the hallmarks of Type 2 diabetes [11]. In turn, the macrovascular and microvascular complications of diabetes are now believed to be a result, not only of glucotoxity, but also lipotoxicity and hyperinsulinemia that herald and accompany the development of diabetes. The therapeutic implications of these pathophysiologic relationships were defined in the UK Prospective Diabetes Study (UKPDS) trial (Table 2.1, [12]). Type 2 diabetics were randomized to dietary intervention, insulin or sulfonylureas to attain tight glycemic control. While insulin and sulfonylureas were associated with better glycemic control and a lower incidence of microvascular complications, there were no differences in macrovascular complications compared to diet alone. Notably, both pharmacologic strategies achieved glycemic control by augmenting plasma insulin levels as opposed to restoring insulin responsiveness. These findings are consistent with the emerging notion that microvascular complications are attributable mostly to glucotoxicity while macrovascular complications may be more a consequence of the interaction of hyperinsulinemia and lipotoxicity. This thinking was further supported by a small subset of patients who received metformin, an insulin-sensitizing agent, in whom macrovascular events were reduced. The observations from UKPDS have led to a change in therapeutic approach from augmenting insulin levels to augmenting insulin action. It may not simply be a matter of achieving glycemic control, but rather how it is achieved.

What then is the metabolic syndrome [13, 14]? As with neurohormonal activation in LV systolic dysfunction, there are no readily available screening tests to identify insulin resistance. Routine measurements of plasma insulin and NEFA, like norepinephrine and angiotensin, are largely research tools and not readily available clinically. The metabolic syndrome is therefore a collection of clinical manifestations of insulin resistance that allow for the identification of patients with this increasingly common metabolic disorder. In this

New feature of NCEP ATP III*
Identification of the metabolic syndrome
Positive diagnosis based on the presence of three or
more of the following:

Risk factor	Defining level
Abdominal obesity (waist circumference**)	
Men	>102 cm (>40 in)
Women	>88 cm (>35 in)
Triglycerides	150 mg/dl
HDL-cholesterol	
Men	<40 mg/dl
Women	<50 mg/dl
Blood pressure	130/85 mmHg
Fasting glucose	110 mg/dl

Figure 2.2 The clinical determinants of the metabolic syndrome. *NCEP ATP III = National Cholesterol Education Program Adult Treatment Panel III; **Some male patients can develop multiple metabolic risk factors when waist circumference is only marginally increased (e.g. 94–102 cm [37–40 in). With permission [15].

sense, the metabolic syndrome is a clinical marker for insulin resistance just as LV systolic dysfunction is a clinical marker for activation of the sympathetic nervous system and the renin–angiotensin system in heart failure. Figure 2.2 lists the ATP III criteria for diagnosing the metabolic syndrome[15]. Patients with three of these features are considered to have the metabolic syndrome. However, the presence of these recognizable phenotypes does not identify all patients with insulin resistance. While obesity, particularly visceral obesity as evidenced by increased waist circumference, are considered the hallmark of the metabolic syndrome, it is important to remember that not all obese patients are insulin resistant and not all insulin resistance patients are obese. The most sensitive and readily available method for identifying insulin resistance is to consider the ratio of triglycerides to high-density lipoprotein (HDL)-cholesterol. When the ratio is >4, insulin resistance is common [13].

Are there increased cardiovascular risks associated with insulin resistance in general or the metabolic syndrome more specifically? Lakka *et al*. [16] demonstrated that patients with the metabolic syndrome were five times more likely to die of a MI and ten times more likely to die from other cardiovascular disease over a 10-year period of follow-up compared to age-matched controls without the metabolic syndrome. Such epidemiologic evidence has led to the recognition that increased NEFA and compensatory hyperinsulinemia seen in the metabolic syndrome are markedly pro-thrombotic (increases in plasminogen activator inhibitor-1 (PAI-1) and endothelial dysfunction [6]) and pro-inflammatory (macrophage activation and increased adhesion molecule expression [6]) in addition to promoting a unique dyslipidemia characterized by normal total and low-density lipoprotein (LDL) but increased triglycerides and reduced HDL-cholesterol [17]. In addition, insulin resistance and the accompanying hyperinsulinemia lead to activation of the sympathetic nervous system, contributing to the development of hypertension and LV hypertrophy [18]. Taken together, it is clear that insulin resistance is not only the pathophysiologic link between obesity and diabetes, but is itself a pathologic condition clinically manifest in the metabolic syndrome and associated with an increased risk of adverse cardiac events. As with the activation of the neurohormonal cascade in heart failure, acute increases in plasma insulin may be compensatory, but chronic activation is maladaptive.

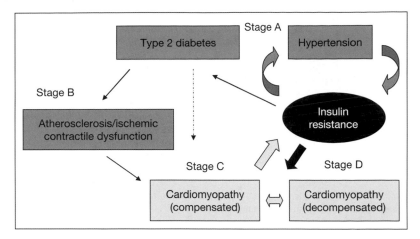

Figure 2.3 Relationship between insulin resistance and dilated cardiomyopathy: insulin resistance mediates several of the risk factors for developing heart failure. There is increasing evidence that insulin resistance also plays a role in the progression to end-stage heart failure.

IS INSULIN RESISTANCE OF CLINICAL IMPORTANCE TO THE FAILING HEART?

The intimate relationship between insulin resistant states – the metabolic syndrome, hypertension, Type 2 diabetes – and coronary atherosclerosis are now well-established and accepted clinically. But what role does insulin resistance play in the pathogenesis of LV systolic dysfunction? Our current understanding of the role of insulin resistance in heart failure is summarized in Figure 2.3. Hypertension and diabetes and the associated coronary atherosclerosis remain the most common antecedents to the development of LV systolic dysfunction, now recognized in the new American College of Cardiology/American Heart Association (ACC/AHA) guideline as Stage A and B cardiomyopathy [19]. However, less well-appreciated is the role that organ-specific insulin resistance, particularly myocardial insulin resistance, plays in the progression of heart failure, particularly from a compensated (Stage C) to a decompensated or end-stage condition (Stage D). Furthermore, it is now apparent that advanced heart failure may itself trigger tissue-specific insulin resistance [20, 21].

To understand the putative role of myocardial insulin resistance in the progression from compensated to decompensated heart failure requires an understanding of the critical role of myocardial substrate metabolism in cardiac function. The studies of 'myocardial energy deprivation' as a sentinel event in the progression to end-stage heart failure have largely been carried out in experimental models, including work from our laboratory [22]. The continuous contractile performance of the heart carries an obligatory requirement for high-energy phosphate synthesis as the heart has limited capacity to store ATP. This requires continuous oxidative phosphorylation of both NEFA and glucose to maintain the supply of high-energy phosphates needed to perform mechanical work and to maintain vital electrochemical balance within the cellular milieu. The concept of impaired ATP synthesis and ultimate energetic failure [23, 24] contributing to the progression to end-stage cardiomyopathy is an appealing hypothesis, but how does the heart develop energetic failure?

Under normal circumstances, the heart prefers and derives the majority of its energy from the β-oxidation of fatty acids [25]. Under circumstances in which the myocardium has been injured, the failing heart shifts its preference from NEFA to glucose given the greater efficiency of glucose oxidation with respect to oxygen consumption in generating ATP [24].

> **Why is myocardial insulin resistance of clinical importance in DCM?**
>
> - The failing heart has limited energy reserves and has a continuous requirement for ATP.
> - The failing heart becomes increasingly dependent on glucose as its preferred substrate.
> - Insulin is required for efficient glucose uptake and oxidation by the heart.
> - Impaired myocardial insulin action may limit the ability of the failing heart to acquire and utilize its preferred substrate.

Figure 2.4 Summary of the rationale as to why myocardial insulin resistance is important in the progression to end-stage heart failure (DCM, dilated cardiomyopathy).

While the shift in substrate preference is relative, it is critical to the maintenance of energetic balance. In turn, myocardial glucose uptake is dependent on the integrity of cellular insulin action [25]. Increasing evidence suggests that advanced heart failure is associated with mitochondrial dysfunction, limiting oxidative phosphorylation [23] and leaving the failing heart with a greater dependence on glycolysis as its source of high-energy phosphates [26, 27]. Under these circumstances, insulin-mediated myocardial glucose uptake becomes critical. Therefore, as heart failure progresses, the development of myocardial insulin resistance may constitute a critical limit on myocardial glucose uptake and glycolysis, limiting the heart's last line of defense in generating ATP (Figure 2.4). The progressive development of myocardial insulin resistance in dilated cardiomyopathy is accompanied by changes in plasma hormones that provide important mechanistic information. In particular, the increase in plasma insulin despite normal fasting glucose levels as heart failure progresses occurs in parallel with a rise in plasma NEFA levels. In turn, the associated increase in plasma NEFA occurs in parallel with the increase in plasma norepinephrine that accompanies the development of progressive LV contractile dysfunction. These events culminate in progressive myocardial insulin resistance and impaired ATP production [27, 28].

These experimental observations have been recapitulated in clinical trials in patients with cardiomyopathy and severe LV systolic dysfunction. In particular, the work of Paolisso *et al.* [29–31] and others [32] demonstrated a similar correlation between LV systolic dysfunction, plasma norepinephrine levels, and significant increases in plasma NEFA. This group also studied over 200 patients with heart failure and classified them based on their IMGU. They demonstrated that the two groups with lower IMGU had a lower probability of survival than the patients in the group with the higher IMGU. This study demonstrates that insulin resistance is a negative prognostic indicator in patients with CHF [31]. Taken together, these findings suggest that insulin may play a critical role in the maintenance of energetic balance that sustains myocardial function in advanced heart failure and prevents the progression to a decompensated state. Thus, overcoming insulin resistance in general and myocardial insulin resistance specifically may constitute an important new therapeutic target in LV systolic dysfunction.

THE ROLE OF THE RENIN–ANGIOTENSIN AND SYMPATHETIC NERVOUS SYSTEMS IN INSULIN RESISTANCE IN HEART FAILURE

The sympathetic nervous system and the renin–angiotensin system have been found to play a fundamental role in the progression of heart failure. Both neurohormonal cascades contribute to progressive ventricular remodeling, and attenuation of the cellular effects through neurohormonal blockade has contributed greatly to the improvement in clinical outcomes in patients with LV systolic dysfunction. With increasing evidence that advanced heart failure is an insulin-resistant state, what is the role of conventional neurohormonal activation in mediating insulin resistance?

The sympathetic nervous system and its two major neotransmitters – norepinephrine and epinephrine – are known to be potent counter-regulatory hormones to the action of insulin [33]. In contrast to what has been a predominant focus on β_1 adrenergic effects in heart failure, all three adrenergic receptor subtypes contribute to altered insulin action [33]. Specifically, β_1 adrenergic stimulation increases myocardial ATP requirements by increasing heart rate and contractility, stretching the heart's limited energy reserves. In contrast, the effect of β_1 adrenergic receptor stimulation on pancreatic β-cells is to suppress insulin release, although the effect is modest [33]. As such, the overall influence of β_1 adrenergic receptor stimulation is to increase myocardial oxygen demand. However, β_2 adrenergic receptors play a significant role in modulating myocardial substrate preference and insulin action [33]. In particular, myocardial β_2 adrenergic receptor stimulation increases NEFA uptake and oxidation by decreasing malonyl CoA and thereby increasing carnitine-palmitoyltransferase-1 (CPT-1) expression, a rate-limiting step in fatty acid oxidation. β_2 adrenergic receptor stimulation also impairs glycolysis by decreasing phosphofructokinase 2, 6 biphosphate and thereby inhibiting phosphofructokinase, the rate-limiting step in glycolysis [33]. Finally, β_2 adrenergic receptor stimulation impairs insulin signaling by chronically activating Akt-1, which in turn phosphorylates serine residues in the docking protein insulin receptor substrate-1 (IRS-1), altering insulin action [33]. Thus, myocardial β_2 adrenergic stimulation shifts preference toward fatty acid oxidation and alters both IMGU and glycolysis. Finally, α_1 adrenergic receptor stimulation contributes to systemic insulin resistance in heart failure by inhibiting insulin secretion and limiting glucose uptake by skeletal muscle by reducing blood flow [33]. Taken together, the combined effects of adrenergic stimulation in heart failure affect both myocardial substrate preference as well as alter insulin action. All three adrenergic receptor subtypes participate in the process.

Both combined and selective β_1 adrenergic receptor blockade have been shown to be effective in reducing morbidity and mortality in LV dysfunction [34]. Whether there is an advantage of one class of agents over another remains controversial despite the superiority of carvedilol over metoprolol succinate in the Carvedilol versus Metoprolol European Trial (COMET) trial [35]. Notably, not only was carvediolol associated with a 17% greater reduction in mortality, but there was also a 23% reduction in new onset diabetes in the groups treated with combined adrenergic blockade compared to β_1 blockade [35]. The relative advantage of combined vs selective adrenergic blockade on glycemic control was recently examined in the GEMINI trial (Table 2.2, [36]). The GEMINI trial is a randomized trial comparing the effects of two different β-blockers, carvedilol vs metoprolol (a β_1 selective blocker), on glycemic control in hypertensive patients on background angiotensin-converting enzyme inhibitor (ACE-I) therapy. The study demonstrated that carvedilol stabilized HbA$_1$C, improved insulin resistance, and slowed development of microalbuminuria compared to metoprolol [36]. Taken together, these data suggest that combined adrenergic blockade has greater metabolic advantages over selective blockade, consistent with our understanding of adrenergic pharmacology as it pertains to insulin action as well as myocardial substrate preference. The extent to which these metabolic advantages contribute to the relative benefits of carvedilol over metoprolol in human heart failure [34] remains to be determined.

There is similar evidence supporting a role for angiotensin II in predisposing to insulin resistance and diabetes [37]. There is a compelling body of evidence that suggests that angiotensin II stimulates the serine phosphorylation and inactivation of IRS-1, a docking protein required for binding and activation of phosphatidylinositol-3 (PI-3) kinase, the rate-limiting step in insulin signaling [38]. Carvalho et al. [39] attempted to determine whether

Table 2.2 Summary of GEMINI trial

Background	β-blockers have been shown to improve cardiovascular risk in patients with hypertension and Type 2 diabetes mellitus. They have also been shown to increase fasting plasma glucose.
Objectives	Is there a difference between selective and non-selective β-blockers on glycemic and metabolic control in patients with hypertension who are already receiving ACE-I or ARB?
Study design	A randomized, double-blind, parallel-group trial containing 1235 diabetic patients. Patients were randomized to receive either carvedilol or metoprolol titrated to blood pressure control. All patients were already receiving either an ACE-I or an ARB. They were followed over 35 weeks. Primary outcome was change in HgbA$_1$C from baseline between the two groups.
Results	The difference in mean change in HgbA$_1$C was 13% ($P = 0.004$) in the two groups. Mean HgbA$_1$C increased by 15% in the metoprolol group ($P < 0.001$), not in the carvedilol group. Progression to microalbuminuria was less frequent with carvedilol (6.4%) than metoprolol (10.3%; $P = 0.04$). There was decreased insulin resistance in the carvedilol group, with the between-group difference -7.2% ($P = 0.004$). Carvedilol showed a 16% relative reduction ($P = 0.003$) in the albumin/creatinine ratio when compared to metoprolol.
Conclusions	In the presence of renin–angiotensin systems blockade, carvedilol had no effect on glycemic control, whereas metoprolol worsened it. Carvedilol showed improvement in other metabolic derangements when compared to metoprolol, such as microalbuminuria, insulin resistance, and albumin/creatinine ratio.

the improvement in insulin sensitivity induced by captopril is related to modulation of the early steps of insulin action. Captopril significantly increased the insulin-induced insulin receptor and IRS-1 phosphorylation and was accompanied by an increase in IRS-1/PI-3 kinase association [39]. They also showed that the angiotensin receptor blocker (ARB) losartan and AT1 receptor blocker did not significantly affect the insulin-stimulated IRS-1 association with PI 3-kinase [40]. A major target of angiotensin-induced alterations in insulin signaling is the effect on endothelial cells and vascular smooth muscle. Folli *et al.* [40] pretreated aortic smooth muscle cells with angiotensin II and showed a decrease in insulin-stimulated phosphorylation of IRS-1 and inhibition in insulin-stimulated IRS-1/PI 3-kinase association. Rett *et al.* [41] also showed that bradykinin at a concentration not affecting coronary flow, mimics the insulin-induced translocation of both GLUT4 and GLUT1 in isolated rat hearts. The finding that bradykinin improves insulin sensitivity may account for the difference seen between treatment with an ACE-I and ARB. Recent evidence suggests an alternative mechanism by which newer generations of tissue-specific ACE-Is may restore insulin action by acting as partial agonists to peroxisome proliferative activated receptor γ (PPARγ) [42]. The relative difference in metabolic profiles of ACE-Is compared to ARBs may serve to explain the relative benefits of ACE-Is over ARBs in heart failure. Thus, both the renin–angiotensin system and the sympathetic nervous system play important roles in promoting insulin resistance and predisposing to new onset Type 2 diabetes in heart failure.

ARE THERE SPECIFIC THERAPEUTIC APPROACHES TO OVERCOMING INSULIN RESISTANCE?

Despite the fundamental role that myocardial metabolism plays in the ultimate fate of the failing heart, therapeutic strategies targeting metabolic abnormalities in heart failure have not been studied extensively. For that matter, there are no pharmacologic strategies yet developed that specifically target systemic insulin resistance, despite the critical role that it

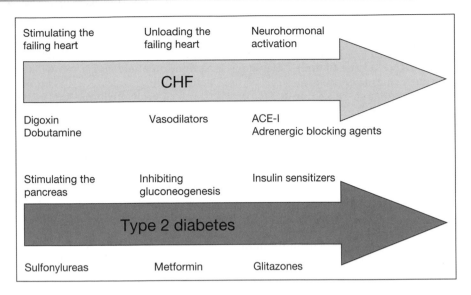

Figure 2.5 Evolving therapies in CHF and diabetes: the shift in the therapeutic paradigm for treating Type 2 diabetes parallels the evolution in approach seen in heart failure.

plays in the pathogenesis of metabolic syndrome and Type 2 diabetes [43, 44]. Weight reduction and exercise [43, 45] remain the cornerstones of management of systemic insulin resistance, although their efficacy is limited.

By contrast, there have been significant advances in the therapeutic approach to Type 2 diabetes. The evolution closely mirrors the evolution in the treatment of LV systolic dysfunction. Figure 2.5 illustrates the paradigm shift. In heart failure, treatment has evolved from 'whipping' the failing heart with inotropic agents to unloading the failing heart with non-specific vasodilators to the current approach in which specific neurohormonal antagonists are employed to prevent ventricular remodeling. In Type 2 diabetes, the paradigm is shifting from exclusive reliance on sulfonylureas to stimulate pancreatic insulin release, to agents such as metformin that inhibit gluconeogenesis, to the use of insulin sensitizers, the thiazolidinediones (TZDs) targeting insulin resistance, as the recognized pathophysiologic abnormality in Type 2 diabetes. The thinking with respect to the treatment in Type 2 diabetes has been shaped in large measure by the results of UKPDS [12] where insulinotropic therapies achieved glycemic control, but did not impact cardiovascular outcomes.

Despite the promise of these new therapeutic approaches in Type 2 diabetes, they offer little direct benefit in states of insulin resistance alone where hyperglycemia is absent. Furthermore, the most promising approaches using metformin and TZDs are of limited utility in Type 2 diabetes with heart failure [46]. Metformin is contraindicated for the treatment of diabetes in heart failure due to concerns regarding the risks of lactic acidosis, particularly in patients with renal insufficiency [47]. The TZDs carry a warning in patients with heart failure due to the increased risk of edema, precipitating decompensation in heart failure [48]. However, despite early concerns that TZDs may have direct negative effects on myocardial performance in heart failure [49], it is now clear that this is not the case. The mechanism of increased peripheral edema is uncertain, but concomitant use of insulin and pre-existing renal insufficiency seem to constitute risk factors for TZD-induced edema in heart failure [50]. Furthermore, the development of edema can be checked through the use of diuretics or by reducing the dose of the TZDs. The beneficial effects of tight glycemic control mediated through improved insulin action as opposed to creating additional hyper-insulinemia likely outweigh the risks of edema in heart failure, although this remains to be proven. The increased use of both TZDs and metformin in patients with heart failure suggests that these important therapies can be used safely in heart failure with careful monitoring [48]. Nonetheless, these important clinical concerns underscore the fact that there is a paucity of therapeutic options available to treat diabetics with LV systolic dysfunction and no available agents targeting insulin resistance alone in the absence of hyperglycemia.

TREATING MYOCARDIAL INSULIN RESISTANCE AS A NEW THERAPEUTIC TARGET IN CARDIOMYOPATHY

If insulin resistance predisposes to the progression of heart failure by limiting myocardial glucose uptake and glycolysis, then therapeutic strategies designed to overcome myocardial insulin resistance and restore energetic balance should have favorable clinical effects. Several classes of agents are currently under development to target energetic balance in heart failure by stimulating glucose as opposed to fatty acid oxidation. These agents fall into two broad categories: agents that inhibit fatty acid oxidation and insulinomimetic agents.

There are several classes of agents under development or available that alter the heart's use of fatty acids and thereby favor glucose oxidation [51]. These include inhibitors of CPT-1 (etomoxir, oxfenicine, and perhexiline), inhibitors of pyruvate dehydrogenase kinase-4 (ranolazine), and inhibitors of β-oxidation (trimetazidine). Ranolazine, a partial fatty acid oxidation inhibitor acting at PDK-4, has been studied extensively for the treatment of chronic angina [51]. Limited experimental studies in heart failure have demonstrated that intravenous ranolazine improves LV function acutely in dogs with cardiomyopathy [52], but did not improve exercise capacity chronically in rats with heart failure following MI [53]. Trimetazidine is a 3-ketoacyl-CoA thiolase inhibitor that has also been studied extensively in chronic angina. Results in heart failure have been controversial with some studies showing improvement in LV function in patients with ischemic cardiomyopathy after 15 days of treatment [54], while others showed no effect on exercise performance or LV function in diabetics with heart failure [55]. The most encouraging evidence of the efficacy of CPT-1 inhibition in chronic heart failure comes from the recent studies of Lee *et al.* [56] in which perhexiline treatment in addition to standard therapy improved functional outcomes and quality of life. Additional studies are needed to determine the populations likely to receive the greatest benefit from attenuation of fatty acid oxidation by these mechanisms. Notably, these agents may be of limited utility in advanced heart failure where mitochondrial dysfunction may preclude oxidative phosphorylation of TCA intermediates derived from either glucose or fatty acids.

Alternatively, there is emerging experimental and clinical evidence that the naturally occurring incretin hormone, glucagon like peptide-1 (GLP-1), has potent effects to stimulate myocardial glucose uptake and glycolysis in the failing heart [57–59]. GLP-1 has insulinotropic effects that are predicated on the ambient glucose concentration, thereby mitigating the risk of hypoglycemia. Most importantly, GLP-1 possesses insulin-sensitizing properties that enhance myocardial glucose uptake without requiring an increase in insulin. These properties make GLP-1 an attractive agent in insulin-resistant states, such as advanced heart failure. Experimental studies in conscious dogs have shown that GLP-1 stimulates myocardial glucose uptake in an insulin-independent fashion and improves LV function and mechanical efficiency [58]. GLP-1 infusion has also been shown to improve functional recovery following brief periods of myocardial ischemia [57] or large MIs in patients with LV systolic dysfunction undergoing emergent percutaneous coronary intervention [59]. Finally, studies in humans with Class III and IV heart failure treated with a

3-week subcutaneous infusion of GLP-1 demonstrated significant improvement in LV function, exercise capacity, and quality of life [60]. Additional studies are needed to determine whether these benefits are enduring with prolonged administration and whether the active moiety is GLP-1 (7–36) amide or its active metabolite GLP-1 (9–36) amide.

SUMMARY

The epidemic of obesity and the accompanying epidemic of insulin resistance and diabetes require new therapeutic approaches based upon our emerging understanding of the underlying pathogenesis. Importantly, the development and progression of LV systolic dysfunction create an insulin-resistant state that is most evident in the myocardium, but also observed in skeletal muscle. This realization has led to renewed interest in myocardial metabolism as a therapeutic target, particularly in advanced stages of dilated cardiomyopathy. Both the renin–angiotensin system and the sympathetic nervous system play important pathophysiologic roles in facilitating myocardial insulin resistance through distinct receptor-mediated mechanisms. Understanding these cellular effects may help to explain the relative advantage of one class of agents (combined vs selective adrenergic blockade or ACE-I vs ARB) in the treatment of heart failure.

Current strategies to treat insulin resistance in general and myocardial insulin resistance in particular are lacking. The evolution in the treatment of Type 2 diabetes is encouraging, but insufficient to deal with antecedent insulin resistance selectively. However, there are promising new developments with respect to altering myocardial substrate choice and overcoming myocardial insulin resistance that offer new therapeutic approaches for treating heart failure by preserving energetic balance.

- Insulin resistance is mediated by increases in NEFA and the ectopic accumulation of NEFA called lipotoxicity. Initially, plasma glucose is normal due to compensatory hyperinsulinemia. Diabetes occurs when pancreatic reserves become limited, hyperinsulinemia is reduced and hyperglycemia develops. Glucose-mediated tissue injury is called glucotoxicity.

The clinical determinants of the metabolic syndrome:

- Insulin resistance mediates several of the risk factors for developing heart failure. There is increasing evidence that insulin resistance also plays a role in the progression to end-stage heart failure.
- Figure 2.4 summarizes the rationale as to why myocardial insulin resistance is important in the progression to end-stage heart failure.
- The shift in the therapeutic paradigm for treating Type 2 diabetes parallels the evolution in approach seen in heart failure.

REFERENCES

1. Mokdad AH, Bowman BA, Ford ES, Vinicor F, Marks JS, Koplan JP. The continuing epidemics of obesity and diabetes in the United States. *JAMA* 2001; 286:1195–1200.
2. Mokdad AH, Serdula MK, Dietz WH, Bowman BA, Marks JS, Koplan JP. The spread of the obesity epidemic in the United States, 1991–1998. *JAMA* 1999; 282:1519–1522.
3. Allison DB, Fontaine KR, Manson JE, Stevens J, VanItallie TB. Annual deaths attributable to obesity in the United States. *JAMA* 1999; 282:1530–1538.
4. Reaven GM. The insulin resistance syndrome: definition and dietary approaches to treatment. *Annu Rev Nutr* 2005; 25:391–406.

5. Reaven G, Abbasi F, McLaughlin T. Obesity, insulin resistance, and cardiovascular disease. *Recent Prog Horm Res* 2004; 59:207–223.

6. Bloomgarden ZT. Inflammation, atherosclerosis, and aspects of insulin action. *Diabetes Care* 2005; 28:2312–2319.

7. Raz I, Eldor R, Cernea S, Shafrir E. Diabetes: insulin resistance and derangements in lipid metabolism. Cure through intervention in fat transport and storage. *Diabetes Metab Res Rev* 2005; 21:3–14.

8. Garg A. Regional adiposity and insulin resistance. *J Clin Endocrinol Metab* 2004; 89:4206–4210.

9. Lelliott C, Vidal-Puig AJ. Lipotoxicity, an imbalance between lipogenesis de novo and fatty acid oxidation. *Int J Obes Relat Metab Disord* 2004; 28(suppl 4):S22–S28.

10. Robertson RP, Harmon J, Tran PO, Poitout V. Beta-cell glucose toxicity, lipotoxicity, and chronic oxidative stress in type 2 diabetes. *Diabetes* 2004; 53(suppl 1):S119–S124.

11. Clark MG, Barrett EJ, Wallis MG, Vincent MA, Rattigan S. The microvasculature in insulin resistance and type 2 diabetes. *Semin Vasc Med* 2002; 2:21–31.

12. UK Prospective Diabetes Study (UKPDS) Group. Intensive blood-glucose control with sulphonylureas or insulin compared with conventional treatment and risk of complications in patients with type 2 diabetes (UKPDS 33). *Lancet* 1998; 352:837–853.

13. Reaven G. The metabolic syndrome or the insulin resistance syndrome? Different names, different concepts, and different goals. *Endocrinol Metab Clin North Am* 2004; 33:283–303.

14. Sorrentino MJ. Implications of the metabolic syndrome: the new epidemic. *Am J Cardiol* 2005; 96:3E–7E.

15. Executive Summary of The Third Report of The National Cholesterol Education Program (NCEP) Expert Panel on Detection, Evaluation, And Treatment of High Blood Cholesterol In Adults (Adult Treatment Panel III). *JAMA* 2001; 285:2486–2497.

16. Lakka HM, Laaksonen DE, Lakka TA *et al.* The metabolic syndrome and total and cardiovascular disease mortality in middle-aged men. *JAMA* 2002; 288:2709–2716.

17. DeFronzo RA. Dysfunctional fat cells, lipotoxicity and type 2 diabetes. *Int J Clin Pract Suppl* 2004; 143:9–21.

18. Manrique C, Lastra G, Whaley-Connell A, Sowers JR. Hypertension and the cardiometabolic syndrome. *J Clin Hypertens (Greenwich)* 2005; 7:471–476.

19. Hunt SA, Abraham WT, Chin MH *et al.* ACC/AHA 2005 Guideline Update for the Diagnosis and Management of Chronic Heart Failure in the Adult—Summary Article. A Report of the American College of Cardiology/American Heart Association Task Force on Practice Guidelines (Writing Committee to Update the 2001 Guidelines for the Evaluation and Management of Heart Failure). *J Am Coll Cardiol* 2005; 46:1116–1143.

20. Abel ED. Myocardial insulin resistance and cardiac complications of diabetes. *Curr Drug Targets Immune Endocr Metabol Disord* 2005; 5:219–226.

21. Kostis JB, Sanders M. The association of heart failure with insulin resistance and the development of type 2 diabetes. *Am J Hypertens* 2005; 18(pt 1):731–737.

22. Nikolaidis LA, Sturzu A, Stolarski C, Elahi D, Shen YT, Shannon RP. The development of myocardial insulin resistance in conscious dogs with advanced dilated cardiomyopathy. *Cardiovasc Res* 2004; 61:297–306.

23. Schrauwen P, Hesselink MK. Oxidative capacity, lipotoxicity, and mitochondrial damage in type 2 diabetes. *Diabetes* 2004; 53:1412–1417.

24. Morgan HE. Fueling the heart. *Circ Res* 2003; 92:1276–1278.

25. Depre C, Rider MH, Hue L. Mechanisms of control of heart glycolysis. *Eur J Biochem* 1998; 258:277–290.

26. Lopaschuk GD, Rebeyka IM, Allard MF. Metabolic modulation: a means to mend a broken heart. *Circulation* 2002; 105:140–142.

27. Taegtmeyer H. Energy metabolism of the heart: from basic concepts to clinical applications. *Curr Probl Cardiol* 1994; 19:59–113.

28. Goodwin GW, Taylor CS, Taegtmeyer H. Regulation of energy metabolism of the heart during acute increase in heart work. *J Biol Chem* 1998; 273:29530–29539.

29. Paolisso G, De Riu S, Marrazzo G, Verza M, Varricchio M, D'Onofrio F. Insulin resistance and hyperinsulinemia in patients with chronic congestive heart failure. *Metabolism* 1991; 40:972–977.

30. Amato L, Paolisso G, Cacciatore F *et al.* Congestive heart failure predicts the development of non-insulin-dependent diabetes mellitus in the elderly. The Osservatorio Geriatrico Regione Campania Group. *Diabetes Metab* 1997; 23:213–218.

31. Paolisso G, Tagliamonte MR, Rizzo MR *et al.* Prognostic importance of insulin-mediated glucose uptake in aged patients with congestive heart failure secondary to mitral and/or aortic valve disease. *Am J Cardiol* 1999; 83:1338–1344.

32. Coats AJ, Anker SD. Insulin resistance in chronic heart failure. *J Cardiovasc Pharmacol* 2000; 35(suppl 4): S9–S14.
33. Nonogaki K. New insights into sympathetic regulation of glucose and fat metabolism. *Diabetologia* 2000; 43:533–549.
34. Metra M, Nodari S, Dei CL. Beta-blockade in heart failure: selective versus nonselective agents. *Am J Cardiovasc Drugs* 2001; 1:3–14.
35. Poole-Wilson PA, Swedberg K, Cleland JG et al. Comparison of carvedilol and metoprolol on clinical outcomes in patients with chronic heart failure in the Carvedilol Or Metoprolol European Trial (COMET): randomised controlled trial. *Lancet* 2003; 362:7–13.
36. Bakris GL, Fonseca V, Katholi RE et al. Metabolic effects of carvedilol vs metoprolol in patients with type 2 diabetes mellitus and hypertension: a randomized controlled trial. *JAMA* 2004; 292:2227–2236.
37. Bernobich E, de Angelis L, Lerin C, Bellini G. The role of the angiotensin system in cardiac glucose homeostasis: therapeutic implications. *Drugs* 2002; 62:1295–1314.
38. Nawano M, Anai M, Funaki M et al. Imidapril, an angiotensin-converting enzyme inhibitor, improves insulin sensitivity by enhancing signal transduction via insulin receptor substrate proteins and improving vascular resistance in the Zucker fatty rat. *Metabolism* 1999; 48:1248–1255.
39. Carvalho CR, Thirone AC, Gontijo JA, Velloso LA, Saad MJ. Effect of captopril, losartan, and bradykinin on early steps of insulin action. *Diabetes* 1997; 46:1950–1957.
40. Folli F, Kahn CR, Hansen H, Bouchie JL, Feener EP. Angiotensin II inhibits insulin signaling in aortic smooth muscle cells at multiple levels. A potential role for serine phosphorylation in insulin/angiotensin II crosstalk. *J Clin Invest* 1997; 100:2158–2169.
41. Rett K, Maerker E, Renn W, van Gilst W, Haering HU. Perfusion-independent effect of bradykinin and fosinoprilate on glucose transport in Langendorff rat hearts. *Am J Cardiol* 1997; 80:143A–147A.
42. Kurtz TW. Treating the metabolic syndrome: telmisartan as a peroxisome proliferator-activated receptor-gamma activator. *Acta Diabetol* 2005; 42(suppl 1):S9–S16.
43. Goodpaster BH, Brown NF. Skeletal muscle lipid and its association with insulin resistance: what is the role for exercise? *Exerc Sport Sci Rev* 2005; 33:150–154.
44. Flordellis CS, Ilias I, Papavassiliou AG. New therapeutic options for the metabolic syndrome: what's next? *Trends Endocrinol Metab* 2005; 16:254–260.
45. Stone NJ, Saxon D. Approach to treatment of the patient with metabolic syndrome: lifestyle therapy. *Am J Cardiol* 2005; 96:15E–21E.
46. Giles TD. The patient with diabetes mellitus and heart failure: at-risk issues. *Am J Med* 2003; 115 (suppl 8A): 107S–110S.
47. Masoudi FA, Wang Y, Inzucchi SE et al. Metformin and thiazolidinedione use in Medicare patients with heart failure. *JAMA* 2003; 290:81–85.
48. Nesto RW, Bell D, Bonow RO et al. Thiazolidinedione use, fluid retention, and congestive heart failure: a consensus statement from the American Heart Association and American Diabetes Association. October 7, 2003. *Circulation* 2003; 108:2941–2948.
49. Kermani A, Garg A. Thiazolidinedione-associated congestive heart failure and pulmonary edema. *Mayo Clin Proc* 2003; 78:1088–1091.
50. Nikolaidis LA, Elahi D, Hentosz T et al. Recombinant glucagon-like peptide-1 increases myocardial glucose uptake and improves left ventricular performance in conscious dogs with pacing-induced dilated cardiomyopathy. *Circulation* 2004; 110:955–961.
51. Taegtmeyer H. Cardiac metabolism as a target for the treatment of heart failure. *Circulation* 2004; 110:894–896.
52. Sabbah HN, Chandler MP, Mishima T et al. Ranolazine, a partial fatty acid oxidation (pFOX) inhibitor, improves left ventricular function in dogs with chronic heart failure. *J Card Fail* 2002; 8:416–422.
53. Aaker A, McCormack JG, Hirai T, Musch TI. Effects of ranolazine on the exercise capacity of rats with chronic heart failure induced by myocardial infarction. *J Cardiovasc Pharmacol* 1996; 28:353–362.
54. Fragasso G, Piatti PM, Monti L et al. Short- and long-term beneficial effects of trimetazidine in patients with diabetes and ischemic cardiomyopathy. *Am Heart J* 2003; 146:E18.
55. Thrainsdottir IS, von Bibra H, Malmberg K, Ryden L. Effects of trimetazidine on left ventricular function in patients with type 2 diabetes and heart failure. *J Cardiovasc Pharmacol* 2004; 44:101–108.
56. Lee L, Campbell R, Scheuermann-Freestone M et al. Metabolic modulation with perhexiline in chronic heart failure: a randomized, controlled trial of short-term use of a novel treatment. *Circulation* 2005; 112:3280–3288.

57. Nikolaidis LA, Doverspike A, Hentosz T *et al*. Glucagon-like peptide-1 limits myocardial stunning following brief coronary occlusion and reperfusion in conscious canines. *J Pharmacol Exp Ther* 2005; 312:303–308.

58. Tang WH, Francis GS, Hoogwerf BJ, Young JB. Fluid retention after initiation of thiazolidinedione therapy in diabetic patients with established chronic heart failure. *J Am Coll Cardiol* 2003; 41:1394–1398.

59. Nikolaidis LA, Mankad S, Sokos GG *et al*. Effects of glucagon-like peptide-1 in patients with acute myocardial infarction and left ventricular dysfunction after successful reperfusion. *Circulation* 2004; 109:962–965.

60. Sokos GG, Nikolaidis LA, Mankad S, Elahi D, Shannon RP. Glucagon-like peptide-1 improves left ventricular ejection fraction and functional status in patients with chronic heart failure. *J Card Fail* 2006; 12:694–699.

Section II

Established pharmacologic therapies for chronic heart failure

3

Digoxin therapy: does it still have a role in the management of heart failure?

J. Kalman

INTRODUCTION

Digitalis glycosides have been used to treat heart failure (HF) for more than two centuries. During a period in which most inotropic agents have been shown to worsen mortality in HF [1–3], it has become apparent that digitalis acts in HF primarily by attenuating the activation of neurohormonal systems and not as a positive inotropic agent [4]. Digoxin, the most commonly used digitalis preparation, has been shown in several placebo-controlled trials to improve symptoms, quality of life and exercise tolerance in patients with HF [5–7]. These benefits have been shown regardless of the underlying rhythm, cause of HF, or concomitant therapy. Digoxin has been shown to reduce hospitalizations as well, but there is no effect on long-term mortality [8]. The effect of digoxin therapy may differ between men and women [9], and serum digoxin levels do not correlate with clinical efficacy. Higher levels are associated with an increase in adjusted mortality rates from retrospective analyses [10, 11]. Interestingly, since 2001 there have been no new data or trials using digoxin therapy in the treatment of HF. Thus, a critical review of the existing randomized trials of digoxin therapy in chronic HF is of significant importance.

MECHANISM OF ACTION

The mechanism of action of digitalis glycosides in patients with HF is typically noted by their ability to inhibit sodium–potassium (Na^+–K^+) adenosine triphosphatase (ATPase), which leads to an increase in the contractility of the heart, otherwise known as a positive inotropic action. Unfortunately, improvement in hemodynamics in response to an inotropic agent may occur at the expense of increased activation of neuroendocrine systems and may adversely affect prognosis. Thus, current clinical data suggest that an agent to treat HF which improves hemodynamics must do so without further activation of neurohormonal systems. In addition to its ability to affect contractility, observations have revealed that digitalis also exerts its actions by turning down the activation of neurohormonal systems. Digitalis glycosides can produce sympathoinhibitory, sympathoexcitatory and direct vasoconstricting effects, with a net sympathoinhibitory effect. HF, while certainly associated with neurohormonal activation, is also associated with blunting of baroreceptor mechanisms which may contribute to excessive sympathetic activation [12]. Digitalis glycosides act

Jill Kalman, MD, Associate Professor of Medicine, New York University Medical Center, Director, Cardiomyopathy Program, Chief, Cardiac Service, Tisch Hospital, New York, USA.

to sensitize cardiac baroreceptors and thereby reduce sympathetic outflow and restore baroreceptor mechanisms in HF [13, 14]. They increase cardiac contractility but not at the expense of enhancing levels of circulatory vasoactive hormones that are noted with other inotropic agents. Thus, digitalis glycosides, as well as exerting inotropic effects, have potentially beneficial neurohormonal modulating effects by mediating baroreceptor reflex mechanisms. The most commonly used digitalis glycoside preparation used in the US is digoxin.

CLINICAL TRIALS

In spite of the widespread use of digoxin over the past 200 years, it was not until the more recent era that double-blind, randomized, placebo-controlled trials of digoxin therapy in moderate HF were conducted. Early small, short-term studies showed that treatment with digoxin improved symptoms of HF, quality of life, and improved exercise tolerance in patients with mild-to-moderate HF [15–18]. In addition, two prospective, double-blind studies in patients with systolic dysfunction and sinus rhythm, revealed the interesting fact that withdrawal of digoxin therapy led to worsening HF and worsening functional capacity [6, 7]. It was not until the Digitalis Investigation Group (DIG) study, that the effects of digoxin were tested on mortality in a long-term trial (Table 3.1).

In 1988, the Captopril-Digoxin Multicenter Study [19] compared the effects of digoxin, captopril and placebo with background therapy of diuretics in patients with symptomatic HF. The 6-month effects of digoxin on 300 patients with mild-to-moderate HF, maintained on diuretics, demonstrated that compared to placebo + diuretics, patients taking digoxin + diuretics required fewer hospitalizations and emergency room visits, showed fewer treatment failures, and revealed an increase in ejection fraction (EF).

In 1989, the Milrinone-Digoxin Study [20], a large, double-blind, randomized placebo-controlled parallel group trial, demonstrated that continued treatment with digoxin resulted in improved exercise capacity, reduced need for co-intervention, reduced incidence of treatment failures, and a higher rate of study completion and improvement in EF in the group treated with digoxin compared to the group treated with oral milrinone. This provided additional evidence that digoxin is clinically effective in patients with chronic HF and normal sinus rhythm.

Two trials have assessed the effect of withdrawal of digoxin from patients with chronic HF, one trial with only background diuretic treatment and a companion trial in the presence of anogiotensin-converting enzyme inhibitors (ACE-Is). The Prospective Randomized Study of Ventricular Failure and the Efficacy of Digoxin (PROVED) study [6] assessed the effects of digoxin withdrawal in 88 patients with stable HF and EF ≤35%, not treated with an ACE-I. In this study, digoxin withdrawal resulted in a significant worsening of exercise performance and an increased incidence of, and a decreased time to, treatment failure. Additional evidence of clinical efficacy was an increase in EF and a decrease in body weight and heart rate in the digoxin group. However, it was still not clear regarding the benefits of digoxin therapy in the presence of ACE-I, which had become universally used in patients with HF. The RADIANCE study or the withdrawal of digoxin from patients with chronic HF treated with ACE-I [7] evaluated the role of digoxin in patients with moderate HF, already receiving ACE-I. The study once again found that in patients withdrawn from digoxin, there was a higher risk of worsening HF throughout the 12-week study period, a greater deterioration in functional capacity, and a lower quality of life. Therefore, the use of ACE-I does not obviate the need for digoxin in patients with chronic HF.

The DIG trial [8] was a randomized, double-blind, placebo-controlled trial of the effects of digoxin, in addition to diuretics and ACE-I, on rates of mortality and hospitalization in 6800 patients with systolic HF, and left ventricular EF ≤ 45%. Patients with HF and a left ventricular EF ≥45% were enrolled in an ancillary trial conducted parallel to the main study. It is the only mortality trial of digoxin in HF. The overall mortality rate over 3 years

Table 3.1 Major trials

Trial	Design	Inclusion/exclusion	Endpoints	Results
PROVED	Prospective, randomized, placebo-controlled digoxin withdrawal trial	NYHA II–III, NSR, on digoxin and diuretics, EF ≤35%. Patients excluded with MI within 3 months, acute ischemia, atrial fibrillation	1.Treadmill time on maximal exercise testing; 2. distance covered during a 6-min walk; 3. incidence of treatment failure	Patients withdrawn from digoxin showed worsened maximal exercise capacity, increased incidence of treatment failures, and a decreased time to treatment failure
RADIANCE	Prospective, randomized, placebo-controlled digoxin withdrawal trial	NYHA II–III, NSR, on digoxin, diuretics, and ACE-I, EF ≤35%. Patients excluded with MI within 3 months, acute ischemia, atrial fibrillation	1. Rates of withdrawal from study due to worsening HF; 2. time to withdrawal; 3. changes in exercise tolerance	Patients withdrawn from digoxin were withdrawn from study more frequently for worsening HF, had a greater incidence of worsening HF, and had worse measures of exercise endurance
DIG	Prospective, randomized, double-blind, placebo-controlled trial	NYHA II–III, on diuretics and ACE-I, EF ≤45%	1. Mortality; 2. hospitalization	Digoxin did not reduce overall mortality, but reduced the rate of hospitalization both overall and for worsening HF

ACE = angiotensin-converting enzyme inhibitor; EF = ejection fraction; HF = heart failure; MI = myocardial infarction; NSR = normal sinus rhythm; NYHA = New York Heart Association

did not differ between the two groups. While digoxin did slightly reduce the risk of death from worsening HF, an excess of deaths was observed, seemingly secondary to arrhythmic deaths. There was a modest reduction in hospitalizations due to worsening HF in the patients treated with digoxin. Thus, we learned from the DIG trial that digoxin therapy does not decrease overall mortality, while maintaining an effect of decreasing hospitalizations.

Cardiac glycosides represent the only available positive inotropic agent for long-term oral treatment of HF. Prior to the neurohormonal theories, chronic HF was regarded primarily as a disease of abnormal cardiac contractility in the traditional hemodynamic model, and, therefore, positive inotropic agents represented an appealing treatment. Thus far, however, other inotropic agents have failed to be safe in areas proven to be safe with digoxin. Milrinone, for example, has been shown to have a deleterious effect on survival in patients with severe chronic HF as evidenced in the PROMISE study or effect of oral milrinone on mortality in severe chronic HF [1]. Milrinone, a phosphodiesterase inhibitor, enhances cardiac contractility by increasing intracellular levels of cyclic AMP. In an earlier study [18], milrinone significantly increased exercise tolerance and reduced the frequency of worsening HF, but with a suggestion that the drug might aggravate ventricular arrhythmias. The PROMISE trial revealed that milirinone adversely affected survival in all subgroups, failed to improve functional capacity, and was associated with an increased risk of hospitalization and serious adverse cardiovascular reactions. The results of the PROMISE trial are highly consistent with results from studies of other inotropic agents: enoximone, vesnarinone, flosequinan, and others, with all revealing an increase in mortality rates. It should be noted that digoxin, in addition to its inotropic effects, may modulate the neurohormonal abnormalities in HF, perhaps by changes in baroreceptor function, and exert its effects without the expense of increase sympathetic stimulation, thus creating a safer treatment than traditional inotropes. Indeed, the benefit of digoxin may be unrelated to its inotropic properties and more aligned with its neurohormonal modulatory properties.

The effect of digoxin therapy may differ between men and women. A retrospective subgroup analysis of data from the Digitalis Investigation Group trial indicated that there is a gender difference in the effect of digoxin in the treatment of patients with chronic HF [9]. Men and women differ with respect to their risk, etiology and prognosis of HF. The DIG trial did not prespecify or report sex-specific subgroup analyses, perhaps because the trial included almost four times the number of men then women. In addition, current HF guidelines do not differentiate the use of treatments based on sex. Nevertheless, in this *post hoc* analysis, digoxin therapy was associated with an increased risk of death from any cause among women, but not men with HF and low EF. Among women, digoxin was also associated with an increased risk of death from cardiovascular causes and death from worsening HF. There are no additional published analyses of the interaction between sex and digoxin. In addition, this is a retrospective, subgroup analysis, and needs to be interpreted with the understanding of the pitfalls of this type of assessment. However, this analysis does raise concerns of an interaction between sex and digoxin therapy and suggests an increased risk of death among women with HF treated with digoxin. The newest American College of Cardiology/American Heart Association (ACC/AHA) Practice Guidelines for HF suggest that if digoxin is prescribed in women, particular attention should be paid to dosing and renal function [21].

PRACTICAL CONSIDERATIONS

In patients with HF, digoxin can be added to the treatment regimen if the patient remains symptomatic in spite of therapy with diuretics and neurohormonal antagonists: ACE-I (or ARB), and β-blockers. In more severe symptoms of HF, consider adding digoxin to the initial regimen before awaiting a response from the above medications. In these severe patients, one also has the option of adding an aldosterone antagonist before digoxin.

Importantly, if a patient is already taking digoxin, before an ACE-I and β-blocker has been added, digoxin treatment should not be withdrawn, but the neurohormonal antagonists should be added. In atrial fibrillation, digoxin, which is often prescribed routinely, can be considered as adjunctive therapy for rate control in addition to β-blockers, and may be more effective in rate control during exercise [22].

In patients with acute decompensated HF, digoxin is not indicated as primary treatment, not indicated for hypotension and not indicated for fluid overload. It may be started after stabilization, as part of the chronic treatment regimen.

The most common doses for chronic digoxin therapy are between 0.125–0.25 mg/day, for both initiation and maintenance. There is no need to utilize loading doses of digoxin when initiating chronic treatment. The low dose, 0.125 mg daily, should be used in patients over the age of 70, those with impaired renal function, and patients with low body mass [23] with an option of every other day dosing as age advances or renal function further deteriorates. Doses > 0.25 mg each day are rarely needed in the treatment of chronic HF.

In the past, there was little attention paid to serum digoxin levels. However, two retrospective analyses of serum digoxin levels have re-emphasized both the importance of the lower dose regimen and new attention to serum levels [10, 11]. A retrospective analysis of the DIG trial suggested that higher serum digoxin levels, i.e. >1.0 ng/dl, were associated with increased mortality and that the effectiveness of digoxin therapy in men may very well be optimized in a range of 0.5–0.8 ng/dl. A retrospective analysis of the PROVED and the RADIANCE trials found beneficial effects of digoxin regardless of serum digoxin levels, specifically, patients with low-serum digoxin levels were also less likely than placebo to experience worsening HF during follow-up. Essentially, levels of digoxin >1.0 ng/dl are not associated with a superior outcome.

How does one assess the risk–benefit ratio of the utilization of digoxin? We should consider the adverse reactions and established side-effects, as well as the potential long-term deleterious cardiovascular effects of digoxin. In the short term, when attention is paid to dose, age, renal function, and body mass, digoxin is well tolerated. The major adverse reactions are ectopic atrial arrhythmias, heart block, re-entrant cardiac rhythms, nausea, vomiting, anorexia, visual disturbances, confusion, and disorientation. Digoxin toxicity most commonly occurs with serum digoxin levels >2 ng/dl, but may occur at lower levels in the presence of hypokalemia, hypomagnesemia, or hypothyroidism [24, 25]. Concomitant use of certain medications may increase the likelihood of digoxin toxicity and the dose of digoxin should be reduced when these medications are initiated: erythromycin, clarithromycin, cyclosporine, itraconazole, amiodarone, quinidine, and verapamil. When either of these drugs is combined with digoxin, careful subsequent monitoring of serum digoxin levels should follow. Beyond short-term adverse effects, there appears to be some concern that levels of digoxin even in the therapeutic range, >1 ng/dl and up to 2 ng/dl, may exert deleterious cardiovascular effects. In this range the data are discordant. A large meta-analysis of the effect of digoxin on mortality [26], which is mostly based on the DIG trial, demonstrated that digoxin has no effect on mortality. However, a subsequent analysis of only the DIG trial raised a concern that higher serum digoxin levels, in ranges thought to be therapeutic, were associated with higher rates of mortality and hospitalization. The best summary of these data is that perhaps a level <1.0 ng/dl represents an optimal range for efficacy and safety. In addition, digoxin should be used with caution or not at all in post-MI patients or in patients with ongoing ischemia [27].

The traditional view of digoxin as an inotropic agent needs to be expanded to one that has neurohormonal and baroreceptor modulating actions. While digoxin therapy has failed to reduce mortality, it should be used in symptomatic patients receiving neurohormonal antagonists, with the expectation of improving symptoms, exercise abilities, quality of life, and reducing hospitalizations, with attention to dosage and levels. The ACC/AHA 2005 guidelines for the care of adults with chronic HF give digoxin therapy a class IIA recommendation acknowledging reasonable benefit but also highlighting the presence of some risk with this therapy.

SUMMARY

Does digoxin still have a role in the management of HF?

- Digoxin's mechanism as an inotrope and a neurohormonal modulator creates a safe and effective therapy for HF.
- Digoxin improves symptoms, quality of life, and exercise tolerance in patients with mild-to-moderate HF.
- Digoxin has no effect on mortality but can decrease hospitalizations.
- An interaction exists between sex and digoxin therapy and analyses suggest an increased risk of death among women with HF treated with digoxin.

Therapeutic strategies:

- Add digoxin to treatment regimens in patients who remain symptomatic in spite of treatment with ACE-Is and β-blockers.
- Initiate and maintain digoxin in low doses of 0.125–0.25 mg each day without loading, as higher serum levels may be associated with adverse cardiovascular outcomes.
- Careful attention must be paid to the use of concomitant medications that may increase the serum digoxin level.

REFERENCES

1. Packer M, Carver JR, Rodeheffer RJ et al. The PROMISE Study Research Group. Effect of oral milrinone on mortality in severe chronic heart failure. N Engl J Med 1991; 325:1468–1475.
2. Cohn JN, Goldstein SO, Greenberg BH et al. A Dose-Dependent Increase in Mortality with Vesnarinone among Patients with Severe Heart Failure. Vesnarinone Trial Investigators. N Engl J Med 1998; 339:1810–1816.
3. Cowley AJ, Skene AM. Treatment of severe heart failure: quantity or quality of life? A trial of enoximone. Enoximone Investigators. Br Heart J 1994; 72:226–230.
4. Gheorghiade M, Ferguson D. Digoxin: a neurohormonal modulation in heart failure? Circulation 1991; 84:2181–2186.
5. The Captopril-Digoxin Multicenter Research Group. Comparative effects of therapy with captopril and digoxin in patients with mild to moderate heart failure. JAMA 1988; 259:539–544.
6. Uretsky BF, Young JB, Shahidi FE, Yellen LG, Harrison MC, Jolly MK, for the PROVED trial. Randomised study assessing the effect of digoxin withdrawal in patients with mild to moderate chronic congestive heart failure. J Am Coll Cardiol 1993; 22:955–962.
7. Packer M, Gheorghiade M, Young JB et al. Withdrawal of digoxin in patients with chronic heart failure treated with angiotensin-converting-enzyme inhibitors: RADIANCE Study. N Engl J Med 1993; 329:1–7.
8. The Digitalis Investigation Group. The effect of digoxin on mortality and morbidity in patients with heart failure. N Engl J Med 1997; 336:525–533.
9. Rathore S, Wang Y, Krumholz H. Sex-based differences in the effect of digoxin for the treatment of heart failure. N Engl J Med 2002; 347:1403–1411.
10. Adams KF Jr, Gheorghiade M, Uretsky BF et al. Clinical benefits of low serum digoxin concentrations in heart failure. J Am Coll Cardiol 2002; 39:946–953.
11. Rathore SS, Curtis JP, Wang Y, Bristow MR, Krumholz HM. Association of serum digoxin concentration and outcomes in patients with heart failure. JAMA 2003; 289:871–878.
12. Hirsch AT, Dzau VJ, Creager MA. Baroreceptor function in congestive heart failure: Effect on neurohumoral activation and regional vascular resistance. Circulation 1987; 75(suppl IV): IV36–48.

13. Thames MD. Acetylstrophanthidin-induced reflex inhibition of receptors with vagal afferents. *Circ Res* 1979; 44:8–15.
14. Ferguson DW, Berg WJ, Sanders JS, Roach PJ, Kempf JS, Kienzle MG. Sympathoinhibitory responses to digitalis glycosides in heart failure patients: direct evidence from sympathetic neural recordings. *Circulation* 1989; 80:65–77.
15. Dobbs SM, Kenyon WI, Dobbs RJ. Maintenance digoxin after an episode of heart failure: placebo controlled trial in outpatients. *Br Med J* 1977; 1:749–752.
16. Lee DC, Johnson RA, Bingham JB *et al.* Heart failure in outpatients: a randomized trial of digoxin versus placebo. *N Engl J Med* 1982; 306:699–705.
17. Guyatt GH, Sullivan MJ, Fallen EL *et al.* A controlled trial of digoxin in congestive heart failure. *Am J Cardiol* 1988; 61:371–375.
18. DiBianco R, Shabetai R, Kostuk W, Moran J, Schlant RC, Wright R. A comparison of oral milrinone, digoxin, and their combination in the treatment of patients with chronic heart failure. *N Engl J Med* 1989; 320:677–683.
19. Captopril Multicenter Research Group. Comparative effects of therapy with captopril and digoxin in patients with mild to moderate heart failure. *JAMA* 1988; 259:539–544.
20. DiBianco R, Shabetai R, Kostuk W, Moran J, Schlant RC, Wright R, for the Milrinone Multicenter Trial Group. Oral milrinone and digoxin in heart failure: results of a placebo controlled prospective trial of each agent and the combination. *N Engl J Med* 1989; 320:677–683.
21. Hunt SA, Abraham WT, Chin MH *et al.* ACC/AHA 2005 Guideline Update for the Diagnosis and Management of Chronic Heart Failure in the Adult. A Report of the American College of Cardiology/American Heart Association Task Force on Practice Guidelines (Writing Committee to Update the 2001 Guidelines for the Evaluation and Management of Heart Failure). *Circulation* 2005; 112:1825.
22. David D, Segni ED, Klein HO, Kaplinsky E. Inefficacy of digitalis in the control of heart rate in patients with chronic atrial fibrillation: beneficial effect of an added beta adrenergic blocking agent. *Am J Cardiol* 1979; 44:1378–1382.
23. Jelliffe RW, Brooker G. A nomogram for digoxin therapy. *Am J Med* 1974; 57:63–68.
24. Fogelman AM, La Mont JT, Finkelstein S, Rado E, Pearce ML. Fallibility of plasma-digoxin in differentiating toxic from nontoxic patients. *Lancet* 1971; 2:727–729.
25. Ingelfinger JA, Goldman P. The serum digitalis concentration: does it diagnose digitalis toxicity? *N Engl J Med* 1976; 294:867–870.
26. Hood WB, Dans AL, Guyatt GH, Jaeschke R, McMurray JJ. Digitalis for treatment of congestive heart failure in patients in sinus rhythm: a systematic review and meta-analysis. *J Card Fail* 2004; 10:155–164.
27. Eichhorn EJ, Gheorghiade M. Digoxin. *Prog Cardiovasc Dis* 2002; 44:251–266.

4

Neurohormonal activation in heart failure: ACE inhibitors

D. W. Markham

INTRODUCTION

Angiotensin-converting enzyme (ACE) inhibitors remain the best studied class of drugs for the treatment of heart failure (HF). Numerous clinical trials since the late 1980s have established the essential role of ACE inhibitors (ACE-Is) in reducing mortality and major non-fatal events. ACE inhibitors are now recommended for all patients with HF, unless there is a significant contraindication, and multiple hemodynamic and cardiovascular benefits can be achieved through appropriate administration. The positive effects of ACE inhibitors are many, but administration should be followed by careful monitoring and follow-up. This review details the current evidence and recommendations for ACE inhibitors in the treatment of HF.

The efficacy of ACE inhibitors is currently established in the treatment of hypertension, coronary artery disease, diabetes mellitus, renal disease, and left ventricular (LV) dysfunction [1]. Clinical trials of ACE inhibitors have included thousands of patients with LV dysfunction, and the reduction of major clinical events in HF is firmly established. These include improvement in mortality, hospitalization rates, clinical status, and symptoms.

The clinical studies of ACE inhibitors in patients with LV dysfunction began in 1987 with the publication of the Cooperative North Scandinavian Enalapril Study (CONSENSUS) [2]. Now, after nearly 20 years, the latest American College of Cardiology/American Heart Association (ACC/AHA) Guideline Update for the Diagnosis and Management of Chronic Heart Failure in the Adult [3] and the Heart Failure Society of America (HFSA) Comprehensive Heart Failure Practice Guideline [4], published in 2005 and 2006 respectively, clearly affirm the place of ACE inhibitors in treating HF and recommend that all HF patients receive these drugs unless clearly contraindicated or if there is a significant intolerance. Furthermore, administration of an ACE inhibitor or angiotensin receptor blocker (ARB) is recommended in the ACC/AHA Clinical Performance Measures [5]. This positions the use of ACE inhibitors in the highest tier of recommended interventions for HF. These guidelines were developed to provide continued assessment and improvement in the care of patients with HF. ACE inhibitors should be considered fundamental in the treatment of HF for patients with mild, moderate, or severe symptoms. They are also appropriate in selected patients (as studied in the Heart Outcomes Prevention Evaluation trial [HOPE]), at high risk for the development of HF [6].

David W. Markham, MD, Assistant Professor of Medicine, Department of Internal Medicine, Division of Cardiology, Heart Failure/Transplant Program, University of Texas Southwestern Medical Center, Dallas, Texas, USA.

THE CLINICAL EFFECTS OF ACE INHIBITORS

ACE inhibitors are in a general class of pharmacologic agents that have vasodilatory effects. In HF, as myocardial performance deteriorates, there is compensatory peripheral vasoconstriction. This physiologic response functions to maintain systemic perfusion pressure *via* activation of the sympathetic nervous system, the renin–angiotensin system, and multiple endogenous vasoconstrictive/vasodilatory factors. However, in chronic HF these responses lead to decreased cardiac output, increased myocardial oxygen consumption, decreased coronary perfusion, and increased cell death [7, 8].

The wide-ranging effectiveness of ACE inhibitor therapy is not only due to the inhibition of the renin–aldosterone system (i.e. angiotensin II production), but also the increase in bradykinin due to inhibition of degradation. ACE inhibitors are balanced arterial and venous vasodilators that also have numerous non-hemodynamic effects on the vascular endothelium and the cardiac myocyte. These include plaque stabilization, regression of ventricular hypertrophy, regression of vascular smooth muscle proliferation, decreased formation of superoxide anions, decreased coronary vasoconstriction, and anti-macrophage effects. Two clinical examples of these positive effects are the regression of LV hypertrophy in patients with hypertension [9] and the prevention of remodeling. The effect on remodeling is evident in several clinical scenarios, including elderly patients with HF [10], patients with symptomatic HF (New York Heart Association [NYHA] class II–IV) [11], and patients' status post-myocardial infarction (MI) [12]. Following an acute MI, ACE inhibitors lessen myocardial damage, and increase endothelial dilatory capacity [13, 14].

Although not known to be clinically important at this time, some ACE inhibitors have greater inhibition of tissue ACE [15]. Further studies are needed to investigate whether these drugs (i.e. trandolapril, quinapril, benazapril, and ramipril, listed in order of lipophilicity) have greater clinical benefits compared to other ACE inhibitors. Preliminary data suggest that tissue-specific ACE inhibitors may have the following benefits: (1) inhibition of formation of angiotensin II in cardiac and vascular smooth muscle cells, (2) additional benefits on regression of hypertrophy and ventricular remodeling, (3) improvement in plaque instability, and (4) improvement of the effects of nitric oxide on the endothelium.

Another pharmacologic issue with ACE inhibitors involves the concept of 'escape'. With chronic therapy, many patients experience near normalization of angiotensin levels due to the up-regulation of secondary pathways that convert angiotensin I to angiotensin II [16, 17]. This issue of escape led to the consideration of the addition of ARBs to ACE inhibitors, which was tested in the Candesartan Cilexitil in Heart Failure Assessment of Reduction in Mortality and Morbidity (CHARM) trial and proven to be beneficial [18] (discussed in more detail in chapter 5).

There is no ACE inhibitor deemed to be preferred over any other and the practitioner should be guided by Food and Drug Administration (FDA) approved indications, clinical experience and especially clinical trial data. A general recommendation is that the choice of an ACE inhibitor should be based on the particular agents tested in clinical studies. Further, the ACE inhibitor should be titrated up to the target dose used in the clinical trials or the highest dose tolerated by the patient.

CLINICAL STUDIES OF ACE INHIBITORS IN CHRONIC HEART FAILURE

ACE inhibitors have been extensively tested in clinical trials of HF. Selected results of these trials are shown in Table 4.1. The first trial showing benefit was the CONSENSUS, which compared enalapril (2.5–40 mg) with placebo in patients with advanced HF, i.e. NYHA class IV HF [2]. There was a 40% reduction in mortality in the enalapril-treated patients ($P = 0.002$), and NYHA classification significantly improved.

Table 4.1 Selected results of major clinical trials

Trial	Design	Inclusion/ exclusion	Primary endpoint	Results
CONSENSUS	Placebo vs enalapril 253 patients	NYHA class IV	Mortality	40% mortality reduction ($P = 0.002$) at 6 months No difference in sudden death Trial stopped early
SOLVD Treatment	Placebo vs enalapril 2569 patients	NYHA class II–IV (90% were II or III) LVEF ≤35%	Mortality	16% decrease in mortality ($P = 0.0036$) Fewer hospitalizations ($P = 0.0001$)
SOLVD Prevention	Placebo vs enalapril 4228 patients	Asymptomatic HF LVEF ≤35%	Mortality	12% insignificant trend for reduction in CV mortality ($P = 0.12$) Fewer hospitalizations ($P = 0.001$) and less incidence of HF ($P = 0.001$)
AIRE	Placebo vs ramapril 2006 patients	Post-MI with clinical HF	Mortality	27% reduction in overall mortality ($P = 0.002$)
TRACE	Placebo vs trandolapril 1749 patients	Post-MI LVEF ≤35%	Mortality	Significant reduction in mortality ($P = 0.001$) and CV death ($P = 0.001$)
ATLAS	Low-dose vs high-dose lisinopril 3164 patients	NYHA class II–IV	Mortality	No significant difference in death Fewer hospitalizations ($P = 0.002$) in high dose

The relatively short CONSENSUS trial (average follow-up 188 days) was followed by the much longer and larger Studies of Left Ventricular Dysfunction (SOLVD) Treatment trial (average follow-up 41 months), which also showed statistically significant benefit in a less ill patient population, i.e. symptomatic NYHA class II–IV patients with EF ≤35% [19]. Treatment with an ACE inhibitor in this study (enalapril 2.5–20 mg vs placebo) reduced mortality from 39.7% to 35% ($P = 0.0036$), and there were fewer hospitalizations with ACE inhibitor therapy ($P = 0.0001$). This translated into a 16% relative risk reduction in death and 26% reduction in hospitalization.

The SOLVD Prevention trial included asymptomatic patients with an EF ≤35% randomized to either enalapril (2.5–20 mg) or placebo. This trial included over 4000 patients with a follow-up average of over 37 months [20]. All-cause mortality was not significantly reduced ($P = 0.30$), although there was a trend for mortality reduction (8% reduction in death) with ACE inhibitor therapy. Cardiovascular mortality was also not reduced significantly. When the combined endpoint of hospitalization and death was analyzed, there was a statistically significant reduction of 20% ($P = 0.001$).

More recent trials using ACE inhibitors in HF include Acute Infarction Ramipril Efficacy (AIRE), Trandolopril Cardiac Evaluation (TRACE), and Assessment of Treatment with Lisinopril and Survival (ATLAS). AIRE randomized post-MI patients with clinical HF to ramipril (2.5–5 mg) or placebo. Follow-up ranged from 6 to 30 months. There was a

Table 4.2 Recommended doses of ACE inhibitors

ACE inhibitor	Minimum dose	Target dose*
Captopril	6.25 mg TID	50 mg TID
Enalapril	2.5 mg BID	10–20 mg BID
Fosinopril	5 mg QD	40 mg QD
Lisinopril	2.5–5 mg QD	20–40 mg QD
Perindopril	2 mg QD	8–16 mg QD
Quinapril	5 mg BID	20 mg BID
Ramipril	1.25–2.5 mg QD	10 mg QD
Trandolapril	1 mg QD	4 mg QD

*Based on clinical trials in HF.

significant 27% reduction in mortality ($P = 0.002$) [21]. There was also a significant reduction in the incidence of HF, stroke, and MI. The benefit of ramipril occurred early, even at the 30 day time-point. The TRACE study also evaluated patients in the post-MI setting. Trandolapril (1–4 mg) was compared to placebo in post-MI patients with decreased LV function (EF ≤35%) [22]. Although risk of recurrent MI was not reduced ($P = 0.29$), all-cause mortality ($P = 0.001$) and cardiovascular death ($P = 0.001$) were significantly decreased. Sudden death was also significantly decreased ($P = 0.03$). Interestingly, data from the TRACE study suggest that trandolapril may reduce the incidence of diabetes. It may also diminish the incidence of atrial fibrillation. These findings have occurred in several ACE inhibitor and ARB trials and are not necessarily limited to trandolapril.

The ATLAS trial was quite interesting in its design and outcomes [23, 24]. The trial was performed to test the difference between low- and high-dose ACE inhibitor in HF. NYHA class II–IV patients with EF ≤30% were randomized to either low-dose (2.5–5 mg) or high-dose (32.5–35 mg) lisinopril. Patients were followed for 39–58 months. High-dose lisinopril reduced hospitalization by 24% ($P = 0.002$) compared to low-dose. The results on mortality were not significantly different between the two groups ($P = 0.128$), but the higher-dose group had an 8% lower risk of death. In another study, high-dose enalapril (42 mg/day) was compared to a standard dose (18 mg/day) [25]. No significant difference was noted in survival, but there was limited tolerability and an increased withdrawal rate with the higher-dose ACE inhibitor. Because there was no demonstration of difference in mortality in these studies, recommendations currently advocate the up-titration of ACE inhibitors to either a dose tested in clinical trials or the highest tolerated dose. Minimum and target doses are shown in Table 4.2.

In summary, ACE inhibitors reduce mortality, hospitalization, and clinical symptoms in HF. Recommended target doses should be the goal, but lower doses are certainly warranted if dosing limitations occur, and similar mortality reduction and symptom improvement can be expected. On average, ACE inhibitors reduce mortality from HF by approximately 16% at 12 months. This is compared to 36% for β-blockers. It is important to note that each of the ACE inhibitor studies mentioned did not include patients with preserved systolic function, renal insufficiency (e.g. creatinine >2.5–3.0), or hypotension.

INITIATION AND CHRONIC ADMINISTRATION OF ACE INHIBITORS TO HF PATIENTS

The general recommendation for the initiation of ACE inhibitors is to begin at a low dose and slowly increase in steady increments as tolerated to the target dose (Table 4.2). Usually this involves doubling the dose of the chosen agent and checking serum potassium and creatinine levels 1–2 weeks after each dose adjustment. Based on clinical studies, particularly the ATLAS trial [24], low and intermediate doses should be maintained if higher doses cannot be tolerated due to side-effects, e.g. hypotension, renal insufficiency, or hyperkalemia. As mentioned, based on current clinical data, the difference in mortality between low and high doses is insignificant. Thus, the minor differences in efficacy between low and high doses should generally lead to continued administration of the highest dose tolerated by the individual patient, even if it is only a low dose. This approach relies on the overwhelming evidence that ACE inhibitors should be administered to all HF patients. Care should be given to an appropriate diuretic dose in order to maintain proper fluid balance. Over-diuresis compromises renal function and minimizes the attainment of optimal doses of ACE inhibitors. After symptomatic improvement with chronic ACE inhibitor therapy occurs, down-titration or even discontinuation of diuretics is occasionally possible.

Most often, treatment with an ACE inhibitor is given concurrently with both β-blockers and diuretics. ACE inhibitors should not be deferred in the setting of HF. The recent Cardiac Insufficiency Bisoprolol Study (CIBIS) III trial studied whether an ACE inhibitor-first (enalapril) or a β-blocker-first (bisoprolol) regimen should be chosen in patients with mild-to-moderate HF [26]. The trial failed to show that the bispoprolol-first regimen was non-inferior to the enalapril group, at least by the per-protocol analysis, but the data did suggest that they were similar in the intention-to-treat analysis. Thus, it may be safe and efficacious to start either an ACE inhibitor or β-blocker first; however, titration of medications in HF patients needs to be individualized based on comorbidities, hemodynamics, and clinical symptoms.

Diuretics prevent fluid retention and maintain sodium balance, and represent an important complement to ACE inhibitor therapy. In the decompensated patient with volume overload, it is often useful to reduce or temporarily discontinue the ACE inhibitor while stability is achieved, especially if hypotension or renal insufficiency are present. Over-diuresis can lead to electrolyte abnormalities, hypotension, and renal insufficiency, which increases the risk associated with ACE inhibitor therapy. Thus, volume-depleted patients receiving ACE inhibitors can have an acute decrease in angiotensin II and subsequent hypotension. Special attention should be paid to these situations, and it may be necessary to discontinue ACE inhibitors in the setting of volume depletion. On similar grounds, non-steroidal anti-inflammatory drugs (NSAIDs) should not be prescribed for HF patients. Also, it is often feasible to reduce potassium supplementation following the initiation of ACE inhibitors.

The combination of aspirin and ACE inhibitors has received much examination. Because aspirin decreases prostaglandins and ACE inhibitors increase prostaglandins, studies have evaluated whether this interaction is clinically important. A recent meta-analysis of several ACE inhibitor trials showed that aspirin use was associated with a 20% reduction in major events, whereas those who did not take aspirin had a 29% reduction [27]. This difference was not statistically significant. Another retrospective review also failed to demonstrate a difference in outcomes with aspirin use in HF patients also on ACE inhibitors [28]. Theoretically, the aspirin/ACE inhibitor interaction may be significant, but it may also vary according to the etiology of LV dysfunction, i.e. ischemic vs non-ischemic HF and may be dose related. The clinical importance of the aspirin/ACE inhibitor interaction has yet to be fully elucidated. Certainly, more data are needed before clinical practice is altered.

Lastly, one of the largest hurdles in HF treatment involves the underutilization of ACE inhibitors and other proven therapies. Patients at the highest risk for death from HF are the least likely to receive ACE inhibitors [29] perhaps because of intolerance. Elderly patients also have a much lower utilization of ACE inhibitors [30]. A review of national data of outpatient drug usage revealed that ACE inhibitor use for HF patients has increased very slowly: 24% in 1990, 36% in 1996, and 39% in 2001 [31]. These data from 2004 show that approximately 63% of patients hospitalized for HF and discharged on an ACE inhibitor remain on this medication at one year. There is also underutilization in women compared

Table 4.3 Potential adverse reactions of ACE inhibitors

Hypotension
Renal insufficiency
Cough
Angioedema
Hyperkalemia
Rash
Fetal abnormalities
Taste disturbances
Neutropenia

to men [32] and in patients with asymptomatic LV dysfunction [33]. It is much more likely for a patient to continue on an ACE inhibitor if the medication is initiated as an inpatient, but utilization as an outpatient is proven to be vastly deficient [34].

ADVERSE EFFECTS OF ACE INHIBITORS

ACE inhibitors are generally well-tolerated by most HF patients. A summary of potential adverse reactions is shown in Table 4.3. Hypotension, particularly symptomatic postural hypotension, occasionally warrants decreasing or discontinuing the drug. However, if hypotension occurs with initiation there may not be a necessity to abandon ACE inhibitor therapy. If this occurs, volume status should be reassessed, and down-titration of other blood pressure medications can be considered.

Hyperkalemia also should be carefully monitored, especially in patients who have the following risk factors: renal insufficiency, diabetes, and the use of drugs such as potassium supplements, potassium-sparing diuretics, ARBs, or aldosterone antagonists. Some patients may also develop hyperkalemia with the use of high potassium foods or salt substitutes. A mild increase in serum potassium levels can be tolerated and carefully followed without a change in dose, since these mild fluctuations are often self-limited.

The incidence and risk of renal insufficiency with ACE inhibitor therapy increase with NYHA class. As with hypotension, azotemia does not always mean that therapy must be discontinued, and often a decreased diuretic dose permits stabilization of renal function. Also, many HF patients will have persistently tolerated mild azotemia with chronic ACE inhibitor therapy. A common principle involves consideration of dosage adjustment if the creatinine increases by more than 50%. If the creatinine increases by more than 100%, ACE inhibitor therapy should probably be discontinued. Bilateral renal artery stenosis is a contraindication of ACE inhibitor therapy. Likewise, a significant increase in creatinine following the initiation of therapy may warrant further evaluation for this condition. Also, in patients who develop the cardiorenal syndrome, permanent discontinuation of ACE inhibitors may be necessary.

Other adverse reactions include cough and angioedema. The dry, persistent cough of ACE inhibitor therapy can occur in up to 40–50% of patients, particularly in the Asian population and among women. The cough dissipates on cessation of the medication and will recur on re-challenge [35]. A mild cough often warrants at least temporary perseverance with therapy and monitoring of progressive symptoms, particularly since a cough can signify volume overload necessitating intensification rather than withdrawal of therapy. Angioedema is a rare event, occurring in only 0.1–0.2% of patients. It is more frequent in African-Americans and may develop early or late in the course of therapy [36, 37]. Angioedema always necessitates immediate discontinuation of the drug and permanent avoidance of ACE inhibitors. ARBs may be used in patients who experience angioedema with ACE inhibitors [36, 37].

ETHNIC, AGE, AND GENDER CONSIDERATIONS IN ACE INHIBITOR TREATMENT

Data from the Vasodilator Heart Failure Trial (V-HeFT) II demonstrated that African-Americans had no greater benefit from ACE inhibitors when compared to the isosorbide dinitrate and hydralazine combination [38]. These data may mean that the ACE inhibitor had limited efficacy in African-Americans or that the combination of isosorbide dinitrate and hydralazine was uniquely beneficial. This is discussed in chapter 8. Non-African-Americans did benefit from ACE inhibitor treatment in this study. It is important to state, however, that African-Americans in V-HeFT II had a much better response to either therapy (ACE inhibitor or isordil/hydralazine) than the placebo group in V-HeFT I (a trial comparing isordil/hydralazine vs prazosin vs placebo) [39]. These observations led to the African-American Heart Failure Trial (A-HeFT), a study that compared isosorbide dinitrate/hydralazine vs placebo in African-American patients on standard therapy [40]. Additional data on the use of ACE inhibitors in African-Americans came from a matched reanalysis of the SOLVD data, including patients from both the prevention and treatment trials [41]. African-Americans had similar mortality outcomes compared to whites, but African-Americans had an increased risk for hospitalization for HF. Notably, the blood pressure response in non-African-Americans averaged 6/3 mmHg on enalapril, while it was 0/0 mmHg in African-Americans. Thus, there may be a greater need in African-Americans to fully titrate ACE inhibitors to high doses. Indeed, ACE inhibitors should be used in this patient population as standard therapy along with β-blockers and diuretics. It is reasonable to consider ARBs in African-Americans if they are ACE-intolerant [42, 43].

There are also special considerations when using ACE inhibitors in the elderly. HF in the elderly population is common, and often misdiagnosed and under-treated. Older patients have been starkly under-represented in clinical trials, and they commonly have multiple comorbidities that make HF treatment more complex (e.g. renal insufficiency and other comorbidities). They are also known to be less responsive to ACE inhibitor therapy and more likely to be on other medications that may exacerbate HF symptoms (e.g. non-steroidal anti-inflammatory drugs [NSAIDs]) [44]. There is a higher risk of side-effects and adverse reactions with ACE inhibitors. Therefore, special care should be taken with regard to frequent electrolyte, renal, and hemodynamic monitoring in the elderly.

Women, also, have been under-represented in clinical trials. Large HF trials have included approximately only 20% women. There are several important differences between men and women with HF. Some studies suggest that survival is much better for women than men, possibly because diastolic dysfunction is much more common in women. The efficacy of ACE inhibitors in women has largely been extrapolated from studies containing mostly men, and there are conflicting reports on the beneficial effects in women compared to men [45, 46]. Some studies, in fact, show no mortality benefit of ACE inhibitors in women. Women have higher rates of side-effects from ACE inhibitors, including an increased risk for creatinine elevation [19, 20, 47]. Women also have higher rates of ACE inhibitor-induced cough. There is now an increased emphasis to enroll more women [and minorities] in clinical trials. This much needed directive will allow improvement in delivery of care and will greatly increase clinical data on the efficacy of current and future therapies.

CONCLUSION

ACE inhibitors are a mainstay of HF treatment and should be given to all patients unless there is a significant contraindication or intolerance. ACE inhibitors have been proven effective in numerous, large-scale clinical studies to reduce mortality, hospitalization, and symptoms. With careful dosing and monitoring for side-effects, most patients can take ACE inhibitors safely.

SUMMARY

- ACE inhibitors are well-studied and proven in the therapy of HF. They continue to be the mainstay of the typical HF regimen.
- ACE inhibitors should be utilized in all HF patients unless there is a significant contraindication or intolerance.
- Appropriate therapy is not delayed upon discovery of asymptomatic left ventricular dysfunction or symptomatic HF.
- Patients should be monitored closely for the most common side-effects of ACE inhibitors. These include hypotension, hyperkalemia, renal insufficiency, cough, and angioedema.

Therapeutic strategies:

- ACE inhibitors should be considered first-line therapy for HF, along with β-blockers and diuretics.
- Monitor serum potassium and renal function frequently during ACE inhibitor therapy, particularly after each dosing increase.
- Hypotension, hyperkalemia, cough, and renal insufficiency may require dose adjustment or discontinuation of ACE inhibitors.
- Angioedema is a rare side-effect of ACE inhibitors and requires discontinuation of therapy for life. However, ARBs may be substituted in the setting of this side-effect or other significant intolerances.

REFERENCES

1. Wong J, Patel R, Kowey P. The clinical use of angiotensin-converting enzyme inhibitors. *Prog Cardiovasc Dis* 2004; 47:116–130.
2. The CONSENSUS Trial Study Group. Effects of enalapril on mortality in severe congestive heart failure. Results of the Cooperative North Scandinavian Enalapril Survival Study (CONSENSUS). *N Engl J Med* 1987; 316:1429–1435.
3. Hunt SA, Abraham WT, Chin MH *et al*. ACC/AHA 2005 Guideline Update for the Diagnosis and Management of Chronic Heart Failure in the Adult. *Circulation* 2005; 112:e154–e235.
4. Heart Failure Society of America Executive Summary: HFSA 2006 Comprehensive Heart Failure Practice Guideline. *J Card Fail* 2006; 12:10–38.
5. Bonow RO, Bennett S, Casey JDE *et al*. ACC/AHA Clinical Performance Measures for Adults With Chronic Heart Failure: A Report of the American College of Cardiology/American Heart Association Task Force on Performance Measures. *J Am Coll Cardiol* 2005; 46:1144–1178.
6. The Heart Outcomes Prevention Evaluation Study I. Effects of an angiotensin-converting-enzyme inhibitor, ramipril, on cardiovascular events in high-risk patients. *N Engl J Med* 2000; 342:145–153.
7. McEwan PE, Gray GA, Sherry L, Webb DJ, Kenyon CJ. Differential effects of angiotensin II on cardiac cell proliferation and intramyocardial perivascular fibrosis in vivo. *Circulation* 1998; 98:2765–2773.
8. Creager MA, Faxon DP, Cutler SS, Kohlmann O, Ryan TJ, Gavras H. Contribution of vasopressin to vasoconstriction in patients with congestive heart failure: comparison with the renin-angiotensin system and the sympathetic nervous system. *J Am Coll Cardiol* 1986; 7:758–765.
9. Pitt B, Reichek N, Willenbrock R *et al*. Effects of eplerenone, enalapril, and eplerenone/enalapril in patients with essential hypertension and left ventricular hypertrophy: The 4E-Left Ventricular Hypertrophy Study. *Circulation* 2003; 108:1831–1838.
10. Konstam MA, Patten RD, Thomas I *et al*. Effects of losartan and captopril on left ventricular volumes in elderly patients with heart failure: Results of the ELITE ventricular function substudy. *Am Heart J* 2000; 139:1081–1087.
11. McKelvie RS, Yusuf S, Pericak D *et al*. Comparison of candesartan, enalapril, and their combination in congestive heart failure: randomized evaluation of strategies for left ventricular dysfunction (RESOLVD). *Circulation* 1999; 100:1056–1064.

12. Foster RE, Johnson DB, Barilla F *et al*. Changes in left ventricular mass and volumes in patients receiving angiotensin-converting enzyme inhibitor therapy for left ventricular dysfunction after Q-wave myocardial infarction. *Am Heart J* 1998; 136:269–275.

13. Vaughan DE. Endothelial function, fibrinolysis, and angiotensin-converting enzyme inhibition. *Clin Cardiol* 1997; 20(suppl 2):II-34–II-37.

14. Adams KF Jr. Angiotensin-converting enzyme inhibition and vascular remodeling in coronary artery disease. *Coron Artery Dis* 1998; 9:675–684.

15. Dzau VJ, Bernstein K, Celermajer D *et al*. The relevance of tissue angiotensin-converting enzyme: manifestations in mechanistic and endpoint data. *Am J Cardiol* 2001; 88:1L–20L.

16. van de Wal RMA, Plokker HWM, Lok DJA *et al*. Determinants of increased angiotensin II levels in severe chronic heart failure patients despite ACE inhibition. *Int J Cardiol* 2006; 106:367–372.

17. Ennezat PV, Berlowitz M, Sonnenblick EH, Le Jemtel TH. Therapeutic implications of escape from angiotensin-converting enzyme inhibition in patients with chronic heart failure. *Curr Cardiol Rep* 2000; 2:258–262.

18. McMurray JJV, Ostergren J, Swedberg K *et al*. Effects of candesartan in patients with chronic heart failure and reduced left-ventricular systolic function taking angiotensin-converting-enzyme inhibitors: the CHARM-Added trial. *Lancet* 2003; 362:767–771.

19. Effect of enalapril on survival in patients with reduced left ventricular ejection fractions and congestive heart failure. The SOLVD Investigators. *N Engl J Med* 1991; 325:293–302.

20. The SOLVD Investigators. Effect of enalapril on mortality and the development of heart failure in asymptomatic patients with reduced left ventricular ejection fractions. *N Engl J Med* 1992; 327:685–691.

21. The Acute Infarction Ramipril Efficacy Study I. Effect of ramipril on mortality and morbidity of survivors of acute myocardial infarction with clinical evidence of heart failure. *Lancet* 1993; 342:821–828.

22. Kober L, Torp-Pedersen C, Carlsen JE *et al*. A clinical trial of the angiotensin-converting-enzyme inhibitor trandolapril in patients with left ventricular dysfunction after myocardial infarction. *N Engl J Med* 1995; 333:1670–1676.

23. Massie BM, Armstrong PW, Cleland JGF *et al*. Toleration of high doses of angiotensin-converting enzyme inhibitors in patients with chronic heart failure: Results from the ATLAS Trial. *Arch Intern Med* 2001; 161:165–171.

24. Packer M, Poole-Wilson PA, Armstrong PW *et al*. Comparative effects of low and high doses of the angiotensin-converting enzyme inhibitor, lisinopril, on morbidity and mortality in chronic heart failure. *Circulation* 1999; 100:2312–2318.

25. Nanas JN, Alexopoulos G, Anastasiou-Nana MI *et al*. Outcome of patients with congestive heart failure treated with standard versus high doses of enalapril: a multicenter study. *J Am Coll Cardiol* 2000; 36:2090–2095.

26. Willenheimer R, van Veldhuisen DJ, Silke B *et al*. Effect on survival and hospitalization of initiating treatment for chronic heart failure with bisoprolol followed by enalapril, as compared with the opposite sequence: Results of the Randomized Cardiac Insufficiency Bisoprolol Study (CIBIS) III. *Circulation* 2005; 112:2426–2435.

27. Tea KK, Yusuf S, Pfeffer M *et al*. Effects of long-term treatment with angiotensin-converting-enzyme inhibitors in the presence or absence of aspirin: a systematic review. *Lancet* 2002; 360:1037–1043.

28. Harjai KJ, Solis S, Prasad A, Loupe J. Use of aspirin in conjunction with angiotensin-converting enzyme inhibitors does not worsen long-term survival in heart failure. *Int J Cardiol* 2003; 88:207–214.

29. Lee DS, Tu JV, Juurlink DN *et al*. Risk-treatment mismatch in the pharmacotherapy of heart failure. *JAMA* 2005; 294:1240–1247.

30. Ahmed A, Allman RM, DeLong JF, Bodner EV, Howard G. Age-related underutilization of angiotensin-converting enzyme inhibitors in older hospitalized heart failure patients. *South Med J* 2002; 95:703–710.

31. Koelling TM, Eagle KA. Measuring quality of outpatient cardiovascular care. *J Am Coll Cardiol* 2003; 41:69–72.

32. Mortality risk and patterns of practice in 4606 acute care patients with congestive heart failure. The relative importance of age, sex, and medical therapy. Clinical Quality Improvement Network Investigators. *Arch Intern Med* 1996; 156:1669–1673.

33. Kermani M, Dua A, Gradman AH. Underutilization and clinical benefits of angiotensin-converting enzyme inhibitors in patients with asymptomatic left ventricular dysfunction. *Am J Cardiol* 2000; 86:644–648.

34. Butler J, Arbogast PG, Daugherty J, Jain MK, Ray WA, Griffin MR. Outpatient utilization of angiotensin-converting enzyme inhibitors among heart failure patients after hospital discharge. *J Am Coll Cardiol* 2004; 43:2036–2043.

35. Dicpinigaitis PV. Angiotensin-converting enzyme inhibitor-induced cough: ACCP evidence-based clinical practice guidelines. *Chest* 2006; 129(suppl):169S–173S.

36. Sondhi D, Lippmann M, Murali G. Airway compromise due to angiotensin-converting enzyme inhibitor-induced angioedema: clinical experience at a large community teaching hospital. *Chest* 2004; 126:400–404.

37. Sica DA. The African American Study of Kidney Disease and Hypertension (AASK) trial: what more have we learned? *J Clin Hypertens* 2003; 5:159–167.

38. Carson P, Ziesche S, Johnson G, Cohn JN. Racial differences in response to therapy for heart failure: analysis of the vasodilator-heart failure trials. *J Card Fail* 1999; 5:178–187.

39. Cohn JN, Archibald DG, Ziesche S *et al.* Effect of vasodilator therapy on mortality in chronic congestive heart failure. Results of a Veterans Administration Cooperative Study. *N Engl J Med* 1986; 314:1547–1552.

40. Taylor AL, Ziesche S, Yancy C *et al.* Combination of isosorbide dinitrate and hydralazine in blacks with heart failure. *N Engl J Med* 2004; 351:2049–2057.

41. Exner DV, Dries DL, Domanski MJ, Cohn JN. Lesser response to angiotensin-converting-enzyme inhibitor therapy in black as compared with white patients with left ventricular dysfunction. *N Engl J Med* 2001; 344:1351–1357.

42. Cohn JN, Tognoni G, the Valsartan Heart Failure Trial I. A randomized trial of the angiotensin-receptor blocker valsartan in chronic heart failure. *N Engl J Med* 2001; 345:1667–1675.

43. Granger CB, McMurray JJV, Yusuf S *et al.* Effects of candesartan in patients with chronic heart failure and reduced left-ventricular systolic function intolerant to angiotensin-converting-enzyme inhibitors: the CHARM-Alternative trial. *Lancet* 2003; 362:772–776.

44. Aronow WS, Ahn C, Kronzon I. Prognosis of congestive heart failure in elderly patients with normal versus abnormal left ventricular systolic function associated with coronary artery disease. *Am J Cardiol* 1990; 66:1257–1259.

45. Wenger NK, Speroff L, Packard B. Cardiovascular health and disease in women. *N Engl J Med* 1993; 329:247–256.

46. Garg R, Yusuf S. Overview of randomized trials of angiotensin-converting enzyme inhibitors on mortality and morbidity in patients with heart failure. Collaborative Group on ACE Inhibitor Trials. *JAMA* 1995; 273:1450–1456.

47. Petrie MC, Dawson NF, Murdoch DR, Davie AP, McMurray JJV. Failure of women's hearts. *Circulation* 1999; 99:2334–2341.

5

Neurohormonal activation in heart failure: angiotensin receptor antagonists

A. E. Atchley, G. Michael Felker

INTRODUCTION

Modulation of the renin–angiotensin–aldosterone system (RAAS) with angiotensin-converting enzyme (ACE) inhibitors is a cornerstone of therapy for chronic heart failure (HF), with proven mortality benefit in multiple clinical trials. The development of angiotensin receptor blockers (ARBs) has provided an alternate means for RAAS inhibition. ARBs have several pharmacologic differences that distinguish them from ACE inhibitors and may lead to differential clinical effects and a lower incidence of side-effects such as cough and angioedema. Multiple clinical trials over the last decade have attempted to define the role of ARBs, whether as an alternative to ACE inhibitors or as an additional neurohormonal blocker. The available evidence does not fully support the concept that ARBs are equivalent to ACE inhibitors for chronic HF therapy. In patients who are intolerant of ACE inhibitors, however, ARBs are associated with a clear mortality benefit and should be considered standard of care. In patients already taking ACE inhibitors and β-blockers, the addition of ARBs may provide modest reduction in non-fatal endpoints such as HF hospitalization. Finally, ARBs may have modest beneficial effects in patients with HF and preserved systolic function.

Neurohormonal activation is a hallmark of the HF syndrome. Over the last three decades, pharmacologic interventions aimed at modulating various aspects of the neurohormonal milieu have led to significant improvements in survival for patients with chronic HF. As discussed in detail elsewhere, ACE inhibitor therapy has been demonstrated to have a substantial impact on long-term survival in chronic HF, and has become a cornerstone of the pharmacologic treatment of this syndrome. In the last decade, the development of ARBs has created an alternative to ACE inhibitors for modulation of the RAAS, with several potentially important differences when compared to ACE inhibitors. In this chapter, we will outline the pharmacologic differences between ACE inhibitors and ARBs, and review the clinical trial data supporting the use of ARBs in the treatment of chronic HF, whether in place of or in addition to ACE inhibitors.

PHARMACOLOGY OF ANGIOTENSIN RECEPTOR BLOCKERS

Activation of the RAAS is central to the pathophysiology of chronic HF. RAAS activation leads to sodium retention and vasoconstriction, which are adaptive in the short term during

Allen E. Atchley, MD, Cardiology Fellow, Division of Cardiovascular Medicine, Duke University Medical Center, Durham, North Carolina, USA.

G. Michael Felker, MD, MHS, FACC, Assistant Professor of Medicine, Division of Cardiovascular Medicine, Duke University Medical Center, Durham, North Carolina, USA.

acute hemodynamic stress (such as acute blood loss) but prove maladaptive when chronic-ally activated, as is the case in patients with HF. The biologically active end-product of the RAAS cascade is angiotensin II, which in addition to causing sodium retention and vasocon-striction has been found to have direct adverse effects on the structure and function of both the myocardium and the vascular endothelium [1, 2]. The biologic actions of angiotensin II are mediated by two distinct cellular receptors with opposing effects, the AT1 receptor (which mediates vasoconstriction and is the most widely expressed) and the AT2 receptor (which mediates vasodilation) [3]. Pharmacologic approaches to blocking the adverse biologic effects of angiotensin II have focused on inhibition of its production through blockade of the ACE or, alternatively, direct blockade of its biologic effects at the level of the AT1 receptor using selective AT1 receptor blockers (ARBs). Although both ACE inhibitors and ARBs decrease the biologic activity of angiotensin II, there are important differences in their mechanisms of action that may lead to differences in clinical efficacy. While ACE inhibitor therapy is associ-ated with initial rapid decrease in circulating angiotensin II, during chronic ACE inhibitor therapy circulating levels of angiotensin II gradually return towards pre-treatment values. This phenomenon has been termed 'ACE escape', and appears to be due to the conversion of angiotensin I to angiotensin II by non-specific circulating chymases, bypassing the ACE sys-tem [4]. Since ARBs do not depend on inhibition of angiotensin II production for their phar-macologic activity, these agents theoretically provide more complete antagonism of the effects of angiotensin II. Additionally, the selective blockade of the AT1 receptor by ARBs may lead to greater activation of AT2 receptors, which may potentially lead to beneficial car-diovascular effects [5]. Additionally, some evidence does suggest that other molecules may play a role in mediating the favorable effects of RAAS inhibition, specifically bradykinin. Bradykinin has potentially favorable effects in HF, promoting nitric oxide release and lead-ing to vasodilation [6]. Since bradykinin is a substrate for ACE, inhibition of ACE activity (such as with an ACE inhibitor) leads to an increase in circulating levels of bradykinin. This elevation in bradykinin levels with ACE inhibitors is responsible for some ACE inhibitor-related side-effects (such as cough and angioedema), but may also mediate some of the benefit of ACE inhibitor therapy. Although traditionally ARBs were not thought to elevate bradykinin levels, more recent data suggest that therapy with the ARB losartan may also increase bradykinin levels in patients with hypertension (potentially mediated through the increased activation of the AT2 receptor) [7]. The relative importance of these mechanistic differences in the overall clinical efficacy of these drug classes remains uncertain.

CLINICAL TRIALS OF ARBS IN HEART FAILURE

PRELIMINARY STUDIES: ELITE AND RESOLVD

With the development of clinically available ARBs in the 1990s, several preliminary trials sought to evaluate the efficacy of this class in chronic HF. The Evaluation of Losartan in the Elderly (ELITE) study was a preliminary randomized trial of 722 patients with age >65, designed to test the tolerability of the ARB losartan compared to captopril, with a primary endpoint of worsening renal function (increase in serum creatinine ≥0.3 mg/dl). ELITE found no difference in this primary endpoint between losartan and captopril, but did demonstrate an unexpected decrease in mortality in the losartan-treated patients (4.8% for losartan vs 8.7% for captopril; $P = 0.035$) [8]. Given that ELITE was not powered to detect a mortality difference, this finding was further evaluated in the ELITE II study, as detailed below.

The Randomized Evaluation of Strategies for Left Ventricular Dysfunction (RESOLVD) was a pilot study looking at the effects of candesartan, enalapril, or their combination in those with HF [9]. This study differed from the ELITE trial in that it included a combination therapy arm with both an ACE inhibitor and an ARB. RESOLVD enrolled 768 patients with New York

Heart Association (NYHA) class II–IV HF, a left ventricular ejection fraction (LVEF) <40%, and a 6-minute walk test <500 ms in a 3:3:1 fashion to the ARB candesartan (4 mg, 8 mg or 16 mg), candesartan (4 mg or 8 mg) plus addition to 10 mg enalapril twice daily, or enalapril 10 mg twice daily alone. Outcome measures for the study were exercise tolerance, ventricular function, quality of life (QOL), and measures of neurohormonal activation. Outcomes were assessed at 17–18 weeks and again at 43 weeks with a total follow-up of 47 weeks.

There was no difference between the three groups in 6-minute walk distance, NYHA functional class, or QOL as measure by the Minnesota Living with Heart Failure questionnaire. Ventricular volumes increased in all three groups, but to a lesser degree with combination therapy. There was also a non-significant increase in LVEF in all three groups that was most pronounced with combination therapy. A transient decrease in aldosterone concentration was noted with combination therapy at 17 weeks that was statistically significant compared to either therapy alone, but this difference was not observed at 43 weeks. Plasma brain natriuretic peptide (BNP) concentrations decreased more with combination therapy than with either therapy alone ($P < 0.01$). No statistical difference was noted in the change in serum concentrations of other neurohormones between the three groups. Although not powered to evaluate mortality or hospitalization, there was a statistically significant difference in the rate of HF hospitalization (3.7% with enalapril alone vs 10.7% with candesartan vs 7.2% with combination therapy ($P = 0.048$). Mortality for the 43-week period was 3.7% for enalapril alone vs 6.1% with candesartan and 8.7% with combination therapy, but the small number of patients (particularly in the enalapril arm) and unequal β-blocker utilization between the study arms prevented definitive conclusions about the relative mortality effects of the three treatments. Candesartan alone was well-tolerated and in combination with enalapril, with no significant differences in the rates of clinically significant hyperkalemia or creatinine increase. RESOLVD demonstrated that combination therapy with ACE inhibitor and ARB was well-tolerated and may improve some underlying pathophysiologic mechanisms with greater decreases in plasma BNP, less ventricular remodeling, and a trend toward increased LVEF.

MAJOR OUTCOME TRIALS

In light of the inconsistent results from the early trials of ARBs in chronic HF, several large clinical trials powered to definitively address the mortality benefit of ARBs, alone or in combination with ACE inhibitors, were undertaken.

ELITE II

The unexpected mortality benefit seen in the ELITE study led to the larger ELITE II study, which was formally statistically powered to detect a difference in all-cause mortality in a similar study population to that studied in ELITE. Enrollment criteria for ELITE II included age over 60, NYHA class II–IV HF, and a LVEF <40%. A total of 3152 patients were randomized to losartan or captopril. Randomization was stratified by baseline β-blocker use, and most patients had not received any previous therapy with ACE inhibitors or ARBs. The primary endpoint of the trial was all-cause mortality and the secondary endpoint was a composite of sudden cardiac death or resuscitated cardiac arrest.

After a median follow-up of 18 months, there was no statistically significant difference in the primary endpoint. There were 280 deaths (17.7%) in those treated with losartan compared to 250 deaths (15.9%) in those treated with captopril (hazard ratio [HR] 1.13; $P = 0.16$). There was also no statistically significant difference in the secondary outcomes of sudden cardiac death/resuscitated cardiac arrest or all-cause hospitalization. Importantly, the ELITE II trial was not statistically powered to demonstrate equivalence between losartan and captopril, and should not be interpreted as suggesting equivalence between these two agents.

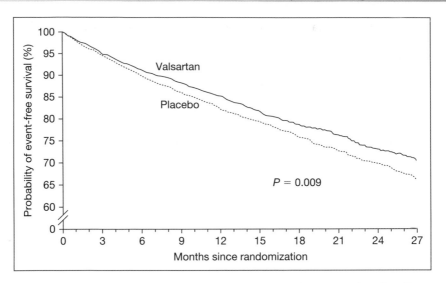

Figure 5.1 Kaplan-Meier curves for probability of combined endpoint (death, resuscitated cardiac arrest, HF hospitalization, or need for intravenous inotropes or vasodilators) in the VAL-HeFT study [10]. Copyright © 2001, Massachusetts Medical Society. All rights reserved.

Overall, ELITE II showed no significant clinical benefit of losartan over captopril, and suggested that the more favorable survival observed with losartan in the initial ELITE study may have been spurious due to small sample size. ELITE II remains the only large mortality trial to directly compare an ACE inhibitor vs an ARB in patients with chronic HF.

VAL-HEFT

The Valsartan Heart Failure Trial (VAL-HeFT) was a randomized, double-blind, placebo-controlled trial designed to assess the use of the ARB valsartan in 5010 patients with systolic HF who were already receiving background therapy with ACE inhibitors and/or β-blockers [10]. This trial had two primary endpoints – all-cause mortality and a combined endpoint of mortality and morbidity. For the purposes of the trial, morbidity was defined as cardiac arrest with resuscitation, HF hospitalization, or HF exacerbation necessitating 4 h of therapy with intravenous inotropic or vasodilator therapy. Other secondary outcome measures included change in baseline ejection fraction, NYHA functional class, QOL scores, and reported signs or symptoms of HF.

Approximately 93% of the patients in the trial were on background treatment with ACE inhibitors, 35% were on β-blockers, and 85% were on diuretics. Randomization was stratified by β-blocker use. The starting dose of valsartan was 40 mg twice daily with upward titration every 2 weeks to a goal of 160 mg twice daily as tolerated. The mean dose of valsartan achieved was 254 mg daily and this was well-tolerated with a discontinuation rate of 10% compared to 7.2% in placebo. The most common reasons for study drug discontinuation were dizziness (1.6%), hypotension (1.3%), and renal impairment (1.1%), all of which were statistically significant vs placebo.

The mean follow-up duration was approximately 2 years (0–38 months) during which 495 patients on valsartan and 484 patients on placebo died. This represented a non-significant difference in the primary endpoint of all-cause mortality (HR 1.02; $P = 0.8$). The combined endpoint of mortality and morbidity was significantly different in those taking valsartan with a 13% relative risk reduction (HR 0.87; $P = 0.009$; Figure 5.1). This risk reduction was primarily driven by a substantial difference in the rate of hospitalization for HF in those taking valsartan. There were 346/2511 (13.8%) patients hospitalized for worsening HF with valsartan vs 455/2499 (18.2%) with placebo which resulted in a 24% risk reduction for this endpoint. Other secondary endpoints such as change in ejection fraction, NYHA class, and QOL generally favored valsartan when compared to placebo.

Several subgroup analyses of VAL-HeFT suggested potentially important differential effects based on background therapy. As anticipated, in the 366 patients (7%) who were not taking ACE inhibitors, the use of valsartan was associated with 33% reduction in mortality (95% confidence interval [CI] 0.42–1.06) and a 44% reduction in the combined endpoint of mortality and morbidity (95% CI 0.39–0.81), suggesting that ARBs are highly beneficial in patients intolerant of ACE inhibitors [11]. In patients who were receiving an ACE inhibitor but not a β-blocker, the use of valsartan was associated with a statistically significant reduction in the combined endpoint ($P = 0.002$) and a trend toward benefit in mortality. Conversely, in patients taking both a β-blocker and an ACE inhibitor, there was a significant increase in mortality in patients assigned to valsartan compared to placebo. Although potentially suggestive that too great a degree of neurohormonal blockade (i.e. the combination of β-blocker, ACE inhibitor and an ARB) may be harmful, this finding has not been confirmed in other large ARB studies and is likely due to chance alone [12, 13]. Overall, VAl-HeFT demonstrated no significant benefit on mortality but a modest effect on morbidity endpoints with the addition of valsartan to standard therapy in chronic HF.

CHARM PROGRAM

The Candesartan in Heart failure Assessment of Reduction in Mortality and Morbidity program (CHARM) represents the most comprehensive evaluation of the clinical efficacy of ARBs in chronic HF. This program consisted of three separate randomized, double-blind, placebo-controlled trials conducted in parallel. CHARM was designed to evaluate the ARB candesartan vs placebo in patients intolerant to ACE inhibitors (CHARM-Alternative), in patients already receiving background ACE inhibitor therapy (CHARM-Added), and in patients with signs or symptoms of HF and preserved systolic function (CHARM-Preserved). The primary outcome of the overall program was all-cause mortality and the primary outcome for each constituent trial was a composite of cardiovascular death or hospital admission for HF.

The CHARM-Alternative trial randomized 2028 patients to candesartan or placebo who were greater than 18 years of age, had chronic NYHA class II–IV HF, had an LVEF of 40% or less, and who were defined as intolerant to ACE inhibitor therapy [14]. The most common reasons cited for ACE inhibitor intolerance were cough (72%), hypotension (13%), renal dysfunction (12%), and angioedema (approximately 3%). The initial dose of candesartan was 4–8 mg daily with a mean daily dose of 23 mg achieved at 6 months. Candesartan was generally well-tolerated with a 30% rate of permanent discontinuation throughout the study compared to 29% for placebo ($P = 0.53$), although there were statistically significant rates of discontinuation for hypotension, increased creatinine, and hyperkalemia in those randomized to candesartan. The median follow-up time was 33.7 months where 334/1013 (33%) of those taking candesartan and 406/1015 (40%) of those taking placebo experienced one of the primary outcome measures. This resulted in a 23% relative risk reduction for cardiovascular death or HF hospitalization in those taking candesartan (unadjusted HR 0.77; $P = 0.0004$; Figure 5.2). This finding underscored subgroup analyses of the VAL-HeFT trial, demonstrating definitively that ARB therapy has a significant benefit on mortality and morbidity in patients with chronic HF who are intolerant of ACE inhibitors.

The CHARM-Added trial randomized 2548 patients to candesartan or placebo who were greater than 18 years of age, had chronic NYHA class II–IV HF, had a LVEF of 40% or less, and who were currently taking ACE inhibitor therapy at a stable dose for longer than

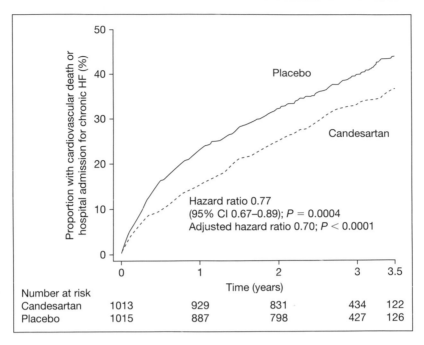

Figure 5.2 Kaplan-Meier curves for probability of cardiovascular death or HF hospitalization in patients intolerant of ACE inhibitors from the CHARM-Alternative trial. With permission from Elsevier [14].

30 days [12]. At enrollment, 55% of patients were being treated with β-blockers, 17% were being treated with spironolactone, and ACE inhibitor therapy was being used in 100% of those randomized to candesartan and 99.8% of those randomized to placebo. The starting dose of candesartan was 4 or 8 mg daily with a mean daily dose of 24 mg daily achieved at 6 months. Overall, there was a 24% rate of discontinuation for candesartan and an 18% rate of discontinuation for placebo ($P = 0.0003$). The most common reasons for discontinuation of candesartan were increased creatinine and hyperkalemia. Of note, the rates of discontinuation due to creatinine elevation more than double the baseline value, serum potassium elevation to a value greater than 6 mmol/l, and for hypotension did not differ significantly between candesartan and placebo. The median follow-up time was 41 months where 483/1276 (38%) of those taking candesartan and 538/1272 (42%) of those taking placebo experienced one of the primary outcomes. This resulted in a relative risk reduction of 15% for cardiovascular death or HF hospitalization for those taking candesartan (unadjusted HR 0.85; $P = 0.011$). Additionally, both cardiovascular mortality (HR 0.84; $P = 0.029$) and time to first HF hospitalization (HR 0.83; $P = 0.014$) were significantly decreased by treatment with candesartan. Unlike what was seen in the subgroup analyses of the VAL-HeFT trial, there was clear benefit from candesartan in patients already being treated with both a β-blocker and an ACE inhibitor. When combined with the results from VAL-HeFT, the CHARM-Added trial suggests that the addition of an ARB to contemporary background pharmacotherapy is associated with a modest improvement in clinical endpoints, including a reduction in hospitalizations (seen in both VAL-HeFT and CHARM-Added) and potentially a mortality benefit as well (seen only in CHARM-Added).

HF with preserved systolic function is an important clinical problem, and constitutes up to one-half of the 500 000 new diagnoses of HF annually [15]. Despite the magnitude of the

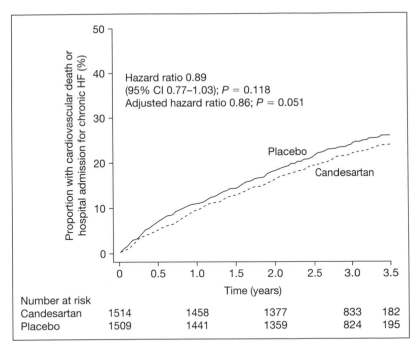

Figure 5.3 Kaplan-Meier curves for probability of cardiovascular death or HF hospitalization in patients with HF and preserved systolic function from the CHARM-Preserved Study. With permission from Elsevier [17].

problem, evidence to guide therapy is sparse, and current recommendations have focused on control of blood pressure, heart rate, and volume status as the fundamental aspects of treatment [16]. The CHARM-Preserved trial was the first large-scale, randomized controlled clinical trial to specifically evaluate pharmacotherapy in this population. CHARM-Preserved randomized 3023 patients who were greater than 18 years of age, had NYHA class II–IV HF, had a history of hospitalization for a cardiac reason, and had a LVEF >40% to candesartan or placebo [17]. The initial dose of candesartan was 4–8 mg daily with a mean daily dose of 25 mg achieved at 6 months. The permanent rates of therapy discontinuation for the study were 18% in those treated with candesartan and 14% for those assigned to placebo ($P = 0.001$). The most common causes of study drug discontinuation were increased creatinine, hypotension, and hyperkalemia, all of which were more common in those treated with candesartan. The median follow-up time was 36.6 months, during which 333/1514 (22%) in those treated with candesartan and 366/1509 (24%) experienced one of the primary outcome measures. This resulted in a relative risk reduction of 11% for cardio-vascular death or HF hospitalization that failed to reach statistical significance (unadjusted HR 0.89; $P = 0.118$; Figure 5.3). However, when the primary outcome was adjusted for pre-specified covariates, the treatment benefit increased to a relative risk reduction of 14% ($P = 0.051$). When the two components of the composite primary endpoint were analyzed separately, there was no difference in cardiovascular death but there was a statistically significant difference in the rate of HF hospitalization ($P = 0.017$). Although marginally statistically significant, the risk reduction seen in CHARM-Preserved was consistent with that seen in the other constituent trials in the CHARM program, and suggests that the addition of candesartan may have a favorable effect on clinical outcomes in patients with HF and preserved systolic function. Further clarification of the role of ARBs in the therapy of HF with preserved systolic function will be provided by ongoing trials such as Irbesartan in Heart Failure with Preserved Systolic Function (I-PRESERVE) trial [18].

The CHARM-Overall program was designed to look at various outcome measures across the spectrum of the 7599 patients in the three component trials [19]. Although the primary outcome of all three CHARM trials was cardiovascular death or HF hospitalization, the primary outcome measure in the overall program was all-cause mortality. The median follow-up time for the program was 37.7 months where 886/3803 (23%) of those treated with candesartan and 945/3796 (25%) of those treated with placebo died. This resulted in a relative risk reduction of all-cause mortality of 9% in the candesartan treated group (HR 0.91; $P = 0.055$). The treatment effect increased to a relative risk reduction of 10% when controlled for potentially confounding factors (adjusted HR 0.90; $P = 0.032$). These data were primarily driven by a reduction in cardiovascular death of 12% ($P = 0.012$) which was most pronounced in those with LVEF of 40% or less. The combined endpoint of cardiovascular mortality and hospital admission for HF was reduced by 16% ($P < 0.0001$) in those randomized to candesartan. Furthermore, more recently published data from further analysis of the overall program revealed a statistically significant 13% relative risk reduction in the composite endpoint of cardiovascular death and non-fatal MI ($P = 0.004$) in patients randomized to candesartan [20].

PRACTICAL ISSUES IN THE USE OF ARBS IN HEART FAILURE

Despite the clinical trial data summarized above, uncertainty remains regarding the appropriate role for ARBs in the armamentarium of contemporary HF therapy. Given the increasing complexity of evidence-based pharmacotherapy, patient tolerability is an important concern that may significantly influence compliance with therapy. Overall, ARBs appear to be better tolerated with a lower incidence of adverse effects than ACE inhibitors. Approximately 10% of patients treated with ACE inhibitors experience side-effects requiring discontinuation of therapy. The most common of these adverse effects are cough, renal insufficiency, systemic hypotension, and hyperkalemia. Angioedema is a rare but potentially life-threatening side-effect of ACE inhibitors. Of these side-effects, some are general to vasodilators (hypotension, renal insufficiency) while others are specific to the mechanism of action of ACE inhibitors (cough, hyperkalemia, angioedema). A frequent practical issue in the use of ARBs concerns the likelihood of adverse effects with ARB therapy in patients who were previously intolerant of ACE inhibitors. Data from a randomized 12-week trial of candesartan in patients deemed intolerant of ACE inhibitors suggest that candesartan is well-tolerated in these patients, with a rate of discontinuation (17%) not significantly greater than placebo (13%) [21]. Similarly, in the CHARM-Alternative study, the rate of discontinuation of therapy did not differ between those assigned to candesartan (30%) and those taking placebo (29%). Angioedema, which had been the cause of ACE intolerance in 39 patients in the CHARM-Alternative study, recurred in three patients treated with candesartan, and in only one case required permanent discontinuation of the drug. Even with the addition of ARBs to patients already taking ACE inhibitors (as in VAL-HeFT and CHARM-Added), the rate of adverse events requiring discontinuation of therapy was relatively low (a few percent greater than placebo in each trial). In all the major trials, rates of hypotension, renal insufficiency, and hyperkalemia were higher in ARB treated patients than in those treated with placebo, underscoring the need for careful laboratory monitoring of patients treated with ARBs for HF (Table 5.1).

CONCLUSIONS

Based on the currently available evidence from randomized clinical trials, ACE inhibitors should remain the foundation of chronic medical therapy for patients with systolic dysfunction and HF. There are no compelling data to suggest that ARBs are superior or

Table 5.1 Major clinical trials

Trial	Design	Inclusion criteria	Endpoints	Results
RESOLVD	RCT Captopril vs candesartan vs both	768 patients, LVEF <40%, NYHA II–IV, and 6-MWD <500 m	6-MWD, LVEF, ESV, EDV, QOL, neurohormone concentrations	Lower BP, less increase in ESV/EDV, and lower aldosterone concentrations with combination compared to either therapy alone. Others – difference NS
ELITE II	RCT Losartan vs placebo	3152 patients, age >60, LVEF <40%, NYHA II–IV	1 – all-cause mortality; 2 – SCD or resuscitated cardiac arrest	1 – difference NS; 2 – difference NS; Trend toward fewer HF hospitalizations with ARB
VAL-HeFT	RCT Valsartan vs placebo	5010 patients, age >18, LVEF <40%, NYHA II–IV *93% of patients were on stable ACE inhibitor dose	1 – all-cause mortality; 2 – mortality + morbidity (see text); Other – LVEF, NYHA class, and QOL	1 – difference NS; 2 – 13% RRR with ARB, (24% RRR in HF hospitalization) Improved EF (mild) and NYHA class
CHARM Overall program	RCT Candesartan vs placebo	7599 patients, age >18, NYHA II–IV	1 – all-cause mortality; 2 – cardiovascular death or HF hospitalization	1 – RRR 10% with ARB; 2 – RRR 16% with ARB
CHARM Preserved	RCT Candesartan vs placebo	3023 patients, age >18, LVEF >40% + history of/or current NYHA II–IV	Cardiovascular death or HF hospitalization	NS RRR 14% with ARB. Fewer HF hospitalizations with ARB
CHARM Added	RCT Candesartan vs placebo	2548 patients, age >18, LVEF <40%, NYHA II–IV, stable ACE inhibitor dose >30 days	Cardiovascular death or HF hospitalization	RRR 15% with ARB. Benefit seen in those with BB + ACE inhibitor + ARB
CHARM Alternative	RCT Candesartan vs placebo	2028 patients, age >18, LVEF <40%, NYHA II–IV, ACE inhibitor-intolerance	Cardiovascular death or HF hospitalization	RRR 23% with ARB

BB = beta-blockade; EDV = end-diastolic volume; EF = ejection fraction; ESV = end-systolic volume; LVEF = left ventricular ejection fraction; MWD = minute walking distance; QOL = quality of life; RRR = relative risk reduction; SCD = sudden cardiac death

even equivalent to ACE inhibitors in preventing mortality in patients with chronic HF. The largest head-to-head comparison, the ELITE II study, showed a hazard ratio of 1.13 (95% CI 0.95–1.35) for losartan compared to captopril. In patients who are intolerant of ACE inhibitors, the data strongly support the mortality benefit of ARBs, and it appears that these agents are well-tolerated, with a low incidence of side-effects requiring discontinuation. Data also support a modest incremental benefit on morbidity endpoints from the addition of ARB therapy to patients already receiving ACE inhibitors and β-blockers. Finally, data from the CHARM-Preserved trial suggest the possibility of benefit from candesartan treatment in patients with HF and preserved systolic function.

As pharmacotherapy for chronic HF increases in complexity, the optimal regimen for a given patient will need to take into account the balance of risks and benefits for that individual. In patients taking ACE inhibitors and β-blockers, but who continue to have significant symptoms of HF, the clinician is faced with several choices for additional drug therapy, including aldosterone blockers, the combination of isosorbide dinitrate and hydralazine, or ARBs. Given the proven survival benefit of aldosterone antagonists (in NYHA class III–IV patients) [22] and the combination of nitrates and hydralazine (in African-American patients) [23], these agents would seem to be preferred over ARBs in patients who fit the profile of patients enrolled in the relevant clinical trials. Ongoing studies will continue to define the role of ARBs in the treatment of chronic HF.

Recommendations for the use of Angiotensin Receptor Antagonists from the 2005 ACC/AHA 2005 Guidelines for the Diagnosis and Management of Chronic Heart Failure in the Adult

- ARBs approved for the treatment of HF are recommended in patients with current or prior symptoms of HF and reduced LVEF who are ACE inhibitor-intolerant; class I, level of evidence A.
- An ARB should be administered to post-MI patients without HF who are ACE inhibitor-intolerant and have a low LVEF; class I, level of evidence B.
- Are reasonable to use as alternatives to ACE inhibitors as first-line therapy for patients with mild-to-moderate HF and reduced LVEF, especially for patients already taking ARBs for other indications; class IIa, level of evidence A.
- Can be beneficial in patients with low LVEF and no symptoms of HF who are ACE inhibitor-intolerant; class IIa, level of evidence C.
- Addition of an ARB may be considered in persistently symptomatic patients with reduced LVEF who are already being treated with conventional therapy; class IIb, level of evidence B.
  [Full copy available at: www.acc.org]

SUMMARY

Are ARBs reasonable alternatives to ACE inhibitors in patients with congestive HF?

- Available data do not support the broad utilization of ARBs in place of ACE inhibitors in patients with chronic HF.
- ARBs provide a clear mortality and morbidity benefit in HF patients not taking or intolerant of ACE inhibitors.
- ARBs result in a modest decrease on clinically relevant endpoints (particularly HF hospitalization) when added to background therapy with ACE inhibitors and/or β-blockers.

■ ARBs may decrease HF morbidity such as hospitalization in patients with HF and preserved systolic function.

Therapeutic strategies for the use of ARBs in HF:

■ ACE inhibitors should remain first-line therapy for HF in patients who tolerate them.
■ ARBs are usually well-tolerated in patients who have been intolerant of ACE inhibitors, and should be considered standard therapy in such patients.
■ ARBs are the only pharmacologic treatment with a proven benefit on clinical outcomes in patients with HF and preserved systolic function.

REFERENCES

1. Timmermans PB, Wong PC, Chiu AT *et al*. Angiotensin II receptors and angiotensin II receptor antagonists. *Pharmacol Rev* 1993; 45:205–251.
2. McEwan PE, Gray GA, Sherry L, Webb DJ, Kenyon CJ. Differential effects of angiotensin II on cardiac cell proliferation and intramyocardial perivascular fibrosis in vivo. *Circulation* 1998; 98:2765–2773.
3. Carey RM, Wang ZQ, Siragy HM. Role of the angiotensin type 2 receptor in the regulation of blood pressure and renal function. *Hypertension* 2000; 35:155–163.
4. Jorde UP, Ennezat PV, Lisker J *et al*. Maximally recommended doses of angiotensin-converting enzyme (ACE) inhibitors do not completely prevent ACE-mediated formation of angiotensin II in chronic heart failure. *Circulation* 2000; 101:844–846.
5. Batenburg WW, Garrelds IM, Bernasconi CC *et al*. Angiotensin II type 2 receptor-mediated vasodilation in human coronary microarteries. *Circulation* 2004; 109:2296–2301.
6. Cruden NL, Witherow FN, Webb DJ, Fox KA, Newby DE. Bradykinin contributes to the systemic hemodynamic effects of chronic angiotensin-converting enzyme inhibition in patients with heart failure. *Arterioscler Thromb Vasc Biol* 2004; 24:1043–1048.
7. Campbell DJ, Krum H, Esler MD. Losartan increases bradykinin levels in hypertensive humans. *Circulation* 2005; 111:315–320.
8. Pitt B, Martinez FA, Meurers G *et al*. Randomized trial of losartan versus captopril in patients over 65 with heart failure (Evaluation of Losartan in the Elderly Study, ELITE). *Lancet* 1997; 349:747–752.
9. McKelvie RS, Yusuf S, Pericak D *et al*. Comparison of candesartan, enalapril, and their combination in congestive heart failure: Randomized Evaluation of Strategies for Left Ventricular Dysfunction (RESOLVD) Pilot Study: The RESOLVD Pilot Study Investigators. *Circulation* 1999; 100:1056–1064.
10. Cohn JN, Tognoni G, for the Valsartan Heart Failure Trial Investigators. A randomized trial of the angiotensin receptor blocker valsartan in chronic heart failure. *N Engl J Med* 2001; 341:1675.
11. Maggioni AP, Anand I, Gottlieb SO, Latini R, Tognoni G, Cohn JN. Effects of valsartan on morbidity and mortality in patients with heart failure not receiving angiotensin-converting enzyme inhibitors. *J Am Coll Cardiol* 2002; 40:1414–1421.
12. McMurray JJV, Ostergren J, Swedberg K *et al*. Effects of candesartan in patients with chronic heart failure and reduced left-ventricular systolic function taking angiotensin-converting-enzyme inhibitors: the CHARM-Added trial. *Lancet* 2003; 362:767–771.
13. Pfeffer MA, McMurray JJV, Velazquez EJ *et al*. Valsartan, captopril, or both in myocardial infarction complicated by heart failure, left ventricular dysfunction, or both. *N Engl J Med* 2003; 349: 1893–1906.
14. Granger CB, McMurray JJ, Yusuf S *et al*. Effects of candesartan in patients with chronic heart failure and reduced left-ventricular systolic function intolerant to angiotensin-converting-enzyme inhibitors: the CHARM-Alternative trial. *Lancet* 2003; 362:772–776.
15. Hogg K, Swedberg K, McMurray J. Heart failure with preserved left ventricular systolic function: epidemiology, clinical characteristics, and prognosis. *J Am Coll Cardiol* 2004; 43:317–327.
16. Developed in Collaboration With the American College of Chest Physicians and the International Society for Heart and Lung Transplantation. ACC/AHA 2005 Guideline Update for the Diagnosis and Management of Chronic Heart Failure in the Adult–Summary Article: A Report of the American

College of Cardiology/American Heart Association Task Force on Practice Guidelines (Writing Committee to Update the 2001 Guidelines for the Evaluation and Management of Heart Failure). *J Am Coll Cardiol* 2005; 46:1116–1143.

17. Yusuf S, Pfeffer MA, Swedberg K *et al.* Effects of candesartan in patients with chronic heart failure and preserved left-ventricular ejection fraction: the CHARM-Preserved Trial. *Lancet* 2003; 362:777–781.

18. Carson P, Massie BM, McKelvie R *et al.* The irbesartan in heart failure with preserved systolic function (I-PRESERVE) trial: rationale and design. *J Card Fail* 2005; 11:576–585.

19. Pfeffer MA, Swedberg K, Granger CB *et al.* Effects of candesartan on mortality and morbidity in patients with chronic heart failure: the CHARM-Overall programme. *Lancet* 2003; 362:759–766.

20. Demers C, McMurray JJV, Swedberg K *et al.* Impact of candesartan on nonfatal myocardial infarction and cardiovascular death in patients with heart failure. *JAMA* 2005; 294:1794–1798.

21. Granger CB, Ertl G, Kuch J *et al.* Randomized trial of candesartan cilexetil in the treatment of patients with congestive heart failure and a history of intolerance to angiotensin-converting enzyme inhibitors. *Am Heart J* 2000; 139:609–617.

22. Pitt B, Zannad F, Remme WJ *et al.* The effect of spironolactone on morbidity and mortality in patients with severe heart failure. *N Engl J Med* 1999; 341:709–717.

23. Taylor AL, Ziesche S, Yancy C *et al.* Combination of isosorbide dinitrate and hydralazine in blacks with heart failure. *N Engl J Med* 2004; 351:2049–2057.

6

Neurohormonal activation in heart failure: β-blockers

S. A. Kamath, C. W. Yancy

INTRODUCTION

Blockade of the β-adrenergic receptor system may be the most efficacious therapeutic modality in the management of chronic heart failure (HF) with impaired systolic function. Earlier concerns that β-blockade would thwart compensatory mechanisms preserving myocardial function are no longer valid in the compensated state. Over the past two decades, a large body of evidence has accrued indicating marked benefits in symptoms and survival as well as favorable dose-dependent changes in myocardial architecture with β-blocker therapy, in addition to angiotensin-converting enzyme (ACE) inhibitors, in patients with compensated HF and impaired systolic function. There is also emerging evidence that β-blocker therapy may be efficacious when administered prior to an ACE inhibitor and when used in the management of HF with preserved systolic function. Despite the overwhelming evidence indicating the positive effects of β-blocker therapy, not all patients who are candidates for β-blocker therapy receive these medications. This chapter will outline the rationale for β-blocker therapy, examine both the early and large-scale clinical work with β-blocker therapy as a therapeutic imperative for congestive HF, and outline recommendations regarding the use of β-blockers in patients with systolic dysfunction.

NEUROHORMONAL PARADIGM

Classically, HF was considered primarily in terms of hemodynamic derangement with the focus of therapy being aimed at restoring normal hemodynamics. This led to the widespread use of diuretics, peripheral vasodilators, and positive inotropic agents, but long-term use of these drugs failed to improve mortality and the use of inotropes was accompanied by an increase in the risk of death [1]. Although this approach is still used in the treatment of HF in the acute setting (i.e. 'acute decompensated HF'), its utility in treating chronic HF and in representing effective therapy for preventing progression of chronic HF is minimal. The failure of the hemodynamic paradigm to yield effective long-term therapies for HF led to the development of alternative models of HF – most importantly, the neurohormonal paradigm [2]. According to this model, HF develops and progresses because of exuberant activation of endogenous neurohormonal systems in response to left ventricular dysfunction, primarily the sympathetic nervous system (SNS) and renin–angiotensin–aldosterone axis (RAAS).

Sandeep A. Kamath, MD, Cardiology Fellow, University of Texas Southwestern Medical Center, Dallas, Texas, USA.

Clyde W. Yancy, MD, FACC, FAHA, FACP, Medical Director and Chief, Cardiothoracic Transplantation, Baylor Heart and Vascular Institute, Baylor University Medical Center, Dallas, Texas, USA.

These neurohormonal systems are activated by an initial injury to the heart, which can be difficult to ascertain, particularly in idiopathic dilated cardiomyopathy. The injury is more evident in acute myocardial infarction. Continued neurohormonal activation exerts a deleterious effect on the circulation, leading to progression of HF *via* ventricular remodeling. At the level of the cardiomyocyte, this process is associated with hypertrophy, apoptosis, and fibrosis, all leading to progressively worsening pump dysfunction [3]. Continued neurohormonal activation also leads to the clinical manifestations of HF, *via* vasoconstriction, increased afterload, impaired cardiac output, sodium retention and congestion [4].

EXCESSIVE SYMPATHETIC STIMULATION IS DELETERIOUS TO THE HEART

It has long been known that the activity of the SNS is increased in patients with HF [5–7]. The bioavailability of norepinephrine to cardiac cells is increased both due to increased sympathetic nerve activity and a reduction in clearance of norepinephrine. In contrast to RAAS (the activation of which shows little or no relationship to the severity of hemodynamic dysfunction), SNS activity generally relates to the severity of hemodynamic dysfunction. The SNS tends to be activated earlier than RAAS, even in asymptomatic patients with left ventricular dysfunction [8]. The SNS also stimulates RAAS and thus activation of the SNS may be a primary disorder in HF. The heart also appears to be the first target of increased sympathetic activity in patients with HF [9].

Increased sympathetic activation may be both beneficial and detrimental in patients with HF. Increased SNS activity helps to support cardiovascular function by increasing heart rate, myocardial contractility, venous return to the heart, and systemic vascular resistance, all of which help to maintain the cardiac output and blood pressure and thus preserve flow to vital organs. Continued increased sympathetic discharge to the heart leads to downregulation of β-adrenergic receptors as well as uncoupling of the β-adrenergic receptor from adenylate cyclase [10], the result of which is that these initial compensatory mechanisms begin to fail. This decrease in responsiveness to adrenergic stimulation results in a further increase in the degree of sympathetic activation in order to overcome the decrease in cardiac output. This, in turn, increases the local concentration of norepinephrine to which the myocardium is exposed [11]. Prolonged exposure to elevated levels of norepinephrine from continued SNS activation results in deleterious effects on cardiovascular structure and function. Norepinephrine can directly affect the biology of cardiac cells leading to changes in the structure and function of the heart by the process of myocardial remodeling. At the molecular and cellular level, myocardial remodeling includes hypertrophy and apoptosis of myocytes, regression to a molecular phenotype characterized by the expression of fetal genes and proteins, and alterations in the quantity and composition of the extracellular matrix. Exposure to norepinephrine has been demonstrated to cause each of the above mentioned key aspects of myocardial remodeling in cultured myocytes *in vitro*, and β-adrenergic blockade has been demonstrated to blunt these responses [8].

EARLY EXPERIENCE WITH β-BLOCKERS

With preliminary data indicating that chronic exposure to norepinephrine resulted in deleterious effects on the heart and that blockade of the β-adrenergic receptor could ameliorate these effects, the potential of using β-adrenergic receptor antagonists as a therapeutic agent for chronic HF was investigated. However, strong opposition was opined as β-blockade was acknowledged to have a role in impeding the SNS which was deemed critical in support of the failing myocardium. Institution of β-adrenergic receptor antagonists (β-blockers) had been reported to produce serious adverse clinical reactions, with most of these being in patients with the most advanced disease who were likely decompensated patients.

In 1975, Swedish investigators noted that despite a lack of hemodynamic improvement with short-term therapy, long-term treatment with β-blockers could improve ventricular performance and symptoms in patients with idiopathic dilated cardiomyopathy [12]. In another similarly-sized study of about 20 patients with chronic HF, the use of β-blockers for extended duration (i.e. 10–12 months) was associated with improvements in functional class and ejection fraction as well as a decrease in left ventricular end-diastolic dimension [13]. Chronic therapy with β-blockers had thus shown promise in alleviating the symptoms of HF and improving myocardial performance, and it stood to reason that they would have a favorable impact on survival. However, no study was sufficiently powered to assess survival as an outcome measure, thus paving the way for the initiation of more definitive β-blocker efficacy trials.

MAJOR CLINICAL TRIALS WITH β-BLOCKERS

Table 6.1 summarizes the major clinical trials discussed below.

MILD–MODERATE HF: US CARVEDILOL TRIALS PROGRAM, MERIT-HF

The US Carvedilol Trials Program sought to determine the effect of long-term therapy with carvedilol in patients with New York Heart Association (NYHA) class II–III HF and left ventricular ejection fraction (LVEF) ≤35%. In this multicenter, randomized, double-blind, placebo-controlled trial, a total of 1094 patients were enrolled. The primary endpoint was a composite of all-cause mortality and hospitalization for cardiovascular causes. The trial was terminated early due to a significant effect of carvedilol on survival. At a mean follow-up of 6.5 months, patients treated with carvedilol had a 65% lower risk of death, a 26% lower risk of hospitalization for cardiovascular causes, and a 38% reduction in the composite endpoint. Mortality alone however was not a prespecified endpoint of the US Carvedilol Trials Program. To enhance the safety of patients, therapy with carvedilol was initiated in small doses that were gradually increased over a period of several weeks. Despite such care, however, the frequency of early side-effects was expected to be high enough potentially to unblind both the patient and the investigator as to the treatment-group assignment. To avoid this difficulty, it was required that patients complete a 2-week, open-label period before randomly assigning them to double-blind therapy. Events during this 2-week open-label period did occur, including mortality, but after much debate it was determined that the 'run-in' period did not compromise the results of the trial [14].

The Metoprolol CR/XL Randomized Intervention Trial in Congestive Heart Failure (MERIT-HF) evaluated the effect of extended-release metoprolol on all-cause mortality in 3991 patients with chronic HF (NYHA class II–IV and LVEF ≤40%). The majority of the patients enrolled in the trial were class II–III, with only 3% being class IV. Ninety-five percent of patients were receiving therapy with ACE inhibitor or angiotensin receptor blocker (ARB) prior to enrollment. Those patients in the metoprolol group with NYHA class II started at a dose of 25 mg once daily and those with NYHA class III–IV started at a dose of 12.5 mg once daily. The target dose was 200 mg once daily and doses were up-titrated over 8 weeks. The mean daily dose of study drug at the end of the study in the metoprolol CR/XL group was 159 mg once daily, with 87% patients receiving 100 mg or more, and 64% receiving the target dose of 200 mg once daily. Like the US Carvedilol Trials, MERIT-HF was terminated prematurely at the recommendation of the independent safety committee for a significant difference in mortality between the two groups. At a mean follow-up of 1 year, therapy with extended-release metoprolol (compared to placebo) lowered all-cause mortality by 34% (Figure 6.1), sudden death by 41%, and deaths from worsening HF by 49% [15]. With the results of the US Carvedilol Trials and MERIT-HF, β-blocker therapy for mild–moderate HF became standard of care.

Table 6.1 Major randomized, placebo-controlled trials of β-blockers in patients with HF

Study (References)	Patient population	No. enrolled	Drug regimen	Mean follow-up (months)	Primary outcome	Results
US Carvedilol Trials [14]	NHYA class II–III, LVEF ≤35%	1094	Carvedilol 25–50 mg BID vs placebo	6.5	All-cause mortality, exercise tolerance, quality of life	Significant mortality reduction (HR 0.65), reduced CV admissions
MERIT-HF [15]	NYHA class II–IV, LVEF ≤40%	3991	Metoprolol CR/XL 200 mg QD vs placebo	12	All-cause mortality	Significant mortality reduction (HR 0.66), reduced rate of sudden death and death from worsening HF
COPERNICUS [16]	NYHA class III–IV, LVEF ≤25%	2289	Carvedilol 25 mg BID vs placebo	10.4	All-cause mortality	Significant mortality benefit (HR 0.65), reduced risk of death/re-admission
CIBIS-II [17]	NYHA class III–IV, LVEF ≤35%	2647	Bisoprolol 10 mg QD vs placebo	15	All-cause mortality	Significant mortality reduction (HR 0.66), reduction in CV death and death/re-admission
BEST [18]	NYHA class III–IV, LVEF ≤35%	2708	Bucindolol 100 mg BID vs placebo	24	All-cause mortality	No significant mortality reduction
COMET [20]	NYHA class II–III, LVEF ≤35%	3029	Metoprolol 100 mg BID vs carvedilol 25 mg BID	58	All-cause mortality	Significant all-cause (HR 0.83) and CV (HR 0.80) mortality reduction with carvedilol, no difference in re-admission
SENIORS [21]	Age ≥70, EF ≤35%, or admit for HF within past year	2128	Nebivolol 10 mg QD vs placebo	21	Composite of all-cause mortality and CV re-admission	Reduction in composite endpoint (HR 0.86), no difference in mortality; benefits persist regardless of whether EF > or < 35%

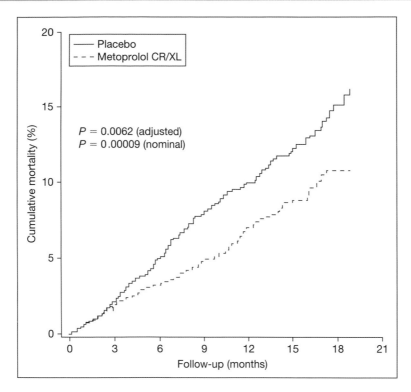

Figure 6.1 Kaplan-Meier mortality curves, metoprol CR/XL vs placebo, MERIT-HF trial. With permission [15].

MODERATE–SEVERE HF: COPERNICUS, CIBIS-II

The Carvedilol Prospective Randomized Cumulative Survival (COPERNICUS) study was a large, randomized, multicenter trial designed to explore the efficacy of β-blocker therapy in patients with severe chronic HF. A total of 2289 patients with severe chronic HF, defined by the occurrence of dyspnea or fatigue at rest or on minimal exertion for at least 2 months and a LVEF of <25% despite appropriate conventional therapy with ACE/ARB and diuretics, were enrolled. Patients with systolic blood pressure less than 85 mmHg, resting heart rate less than 68 bpm, creatinine higher than 2.8 mg/dl, or potassium greater than 5.2 mmol/l or less than 3.5 mmol/l were excluded. Patients received an initial dose of 3.125 mg of carvedilol or placebo twice daily for 2 weeks, which was then increased at 2-week intervals (if tolerated), first to 6.25 mg, then to 12.5 mg, and finally to a target dose of 25 mg twice daily. After 4 months, 65.1% of those in the carvedilol group were receiving the target dose of carvedilol, with mean dose 37 mg of carvedilol daily. This study was also terminated prematurely by its data and safety monitoring board due to a significant benefit of carvedilol on survival. There was a 35% reduction in all-cause mortality and a 24% reduction in the combined endpoint of death or hospitalization with carvedilol therapy compared to placebo (Figure 6.2) [16].

Because earlier studies had suggested that patients at the highest risk might respond poorly to β-blockade, further analyses were conducted to determine whether there were patients in COPERNICUS who had HF too advanced to benefit from treatment. These analyses consisted of assessments of the effects of carvedilol in a subgroup of patients at very high risk, defined as those with recent or recurrent cardiac decompensation or severely

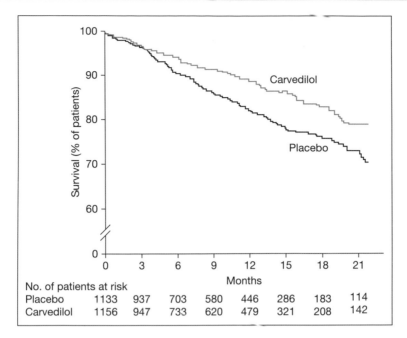

Figure 6.2 Kaplan-Meier survival curves, carvedilol vs placebo, COPERNICUS trial. With permission [16].

depressed cardiac function that was characterized by one or more of the following: the presence of pulmonary rales, ascites, or edema at randomization; three or more hospitalizations for HF within the previous year; hospitalization at the time of screening or randomization; the need for an intravenous positive inotropic agent or an intravenous vasodilator drug within 14 days before randomization; or a LVEF of 15% or lower. The baseline variables that defined this high-risk group were identified without knowledge of their influence on the effect of treatment. In this high-risk cohort, carvedilol reduced the risk of death by 39% and decreased the combined risk of death or hospitalization by 29% [16].

The Cardiac Insufficiency Bisoprolol Study II (CIBIS II) investigated the use of the β-blocker bisoprolol in reducing all-cause mortality in patients with NYHA class III or IV chronic HF and LVEF of 35% or less. Ninety-six percent and 99% of patients enrolled were on chronic therapy with ACE inhibitors and diuretics, respectively. This trial was stopped early due to a significant reduction in mortality in the bisoprolol group. At a mean follow-up of 15 months, chronic administration of bisoprolol resulted in a 34% reduction in all-cause mortality (Figure 6.3), 29% reduction in cardiovascular death, and 21% reduction in the combined endpoint of death or hospital admission [17]. Bisoprolol has an Food and Drug Administration (FDA) approved indication for the treatment of hypertension, but it is not FDA-approved for congestive HF.

'BEST': A FAILED CLINICAL TRIAL EXPERIENCE

The Beta blocker Evaluation of Survival Trial (BEST) evaluated the use of the β-blocker bucindolol in 2708 patients with NYHA class III (92% of patients) or IV (8% of patients) HF and LVEF ≤35%. At a mean follow-up of 2 years, therapy with bucindolol resulted in no significant difference in mortality vs placebo. The trial was terminated at this point by the

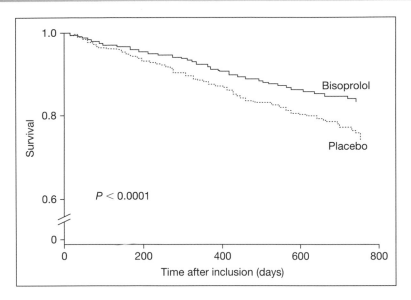

Figure 6.3 Kaplan-Meier survival curves, bisoprolol vs placebo, CIBIS-II trial. With permission [17].

data and safety monitoring board because other β-blockers, namely bisoprolol and carvedilol, had recently been found to have a survival advantage in a similar patient population and continued trial duration – i.e. further double–blind therapy with bucindolol – would therefore no longer have been ethical. Within this trial, there was no apparent benefit in the African-American cohort, and while benefit was seen in the Caucasian-American cohort, the magnitude of that benefit was approximately 50% less than that typically seen in prior β-blocker trials [18].

It has been subsequently demonstrated that bucindolol also displays partial intrinsic sympathomimetic (ISA) properties in human myocardium [19]. The β-agonist properties of bucindolol can be likened to therapy with inotropes, known to improve symptoms in the short term but also known to negatively impact survival. It is possible that ISA may result in cancellation of the benefit of this drug, namely β-adrenergic receptor antagonism. It is therefore recommended that β-blockers with ISA be avoided in patients with chronic HF.

THE COMET STUDY – CARVEDILOL OR METOPROLOL TARTRATE

The Carvedilol versus Metoprolol European Trial (COMET) randomized 3029 patients to receive either carvedilol (titrated to 25 mg BID) or immediate-release metoprolol (titrated to 50 mg BID), in addition to standard therapy including ACE inhibitors. The trial was designed to test the hypothesis that the differing properties of these compounds other than their antagonism of the β_1-adrenergic receptor may result in different treatment outcomes. Recruitment began in December 1996 and ended in January 1999. By the time the MERIT-HF study data became available, the study had nearly completed enrollment and it was therefore too late to modify the metoprolol preparation used in the study, thus COMET is a study that compares an evidence-based β-blocker with a non-evidence based β-blocker. Enrolled subjects were 80% male, 95% class II–III, 50% ischemic, and had an average EF of 26%. Follow-up for morbidity and mortality was concluded in 2002, with a mean duration of follow-up of 58 months. Relative to immediate-release metoprolol, therapy with carvedilol resulted in a 17% reduction in all-cause mortality and a 20% reduction in cardiovascular death. This mortality reduction persisted after multivariable analysis adjusting for known prognostic factors. There was no difference between the two therapies in terms of preventing hospital admission. No data were presented comparing the ability of the two drugs to induce favorable echocardiographic changes (i.e. 'reverse remodeling'). Nonetheless, based on this study, therapy with carvedilol should be considered superior to immediate-release metoprolol [20]. The results of COMET do not address whether carvedilol is superior to extended-release metoprolol. This question remains unanswered.

SENIORS: NEBIVOLOL; POTENTIAL USE OF β-BLOCKERS IN DIASTOLIC HF

The randomized trial to determine the effect of nebivolol on mortality and hospital admission in elderly patients with HF (SENIORS) randomized 2128 patients with age ≥70 with a history of HF (admitted for HF within past year or LVEF ≤35%) to placebo or therapy with nebivolol (starting dose 1.25 mg once daily, titrated to 10 mg once daily). The primary outcome was a composite of all-cause mortality or cardiovascular hospital admission. At a mean follow-up of 21 months, nebivolol therapy resulted in a 14% reduction in the composite endpoint, largely driven by a reduction in hospitalization. Nearly a third of patients in each group had LVEF >35%, ranging from 35% to 80%. This group had the same benefit from nebivolol therapy as those patients with LEVF <35%. The investigators reasoned that the vasodilator properties, which appear to be due to modulation of nitric oxide release that reduces peripheral vascular resistance, may contribute to the ability of nebivolol to improve HF outcomes in elderly patients, regardless of ejection fraction [21]. To date, this *post hoc* subgroup analysis of the SENIORS trial is the only randomized evaluation of the utility of β-blockers in the treatment of HF with preserved ejection fraction.

INITIATION OF β-BLOCKERS BEFORE ACE INHIBITORS OR ACE INHIBITORS BEFORE β-BLOCKERS: CIBIS III

As mentioned previously, sympathetic activation precedes RAAS activation in the pathogenesis of HF and also results in the further activation of RAAS, making antagonism of the SNS an equally if not more attractive therapeutic target than RAAS inhibition. However, at the time these discoveries were made, antagonism of the SNS was considered dangerous as it had the potential to interfere with the heart's attempt to maintain a compensated state. Investigation of ACE inhibitors in HF was more readily accepted given the absence of potential serious adverse effects and the general acceptance of vasodilator therapy in the management of HF. The CONSENSUS (Cooperative North Scandinavian Enalapril Survival Study) [22] trial and the SOLVD (Studies of Left Ventricular Dysfunction) prevention [23] and treatment [24] trials demonstrated a survival benefit over placebo in patients with HF treated with ACE inhibitors. This difference in survival was entirely due to a reduction in death from pump failure; sudden death was largely unaffected. The SOLVD Prevention study also demonstrated a reduction in the incidence of HF but not a reduction in mortality in patients with asymptomatic LV dysfunction. These trials made ACE inhibitor therapy standard of care in patients with left ventricular dysfunction. Upon the discovery that excess sympathetic stimulation was deleterious to the heart, carefully conducted trials examining the use of β-blockers in patients with chronic HF were undertaken as described in detail in the text above. These trials demonstrated a substantial clinical benefit with β-blocker therapy: an average of ~35% relative risk reduction in mortality, a reduction in both sudden death and pump failure death, and reduced left ventricular dimensions and improved left ventricular ejection. These data underscore the importance of β-blocker therapy in patients with chronic HF.

Given the relative benefits of β-blocker therapy, perhaps more than the benefits of ACE inhibitor therapy, and the knowledge that β-blocker penetration is significantly lower than

ACE inhibitor penetration in patients with chronic HF, a trial was undertaken to examine the effect of initiating therapy with a β-blocker prior to the initiation of an ACE inhibitor vs the conventional order. The Cardiac Insufficiency Bisoprolol Study III (CIBIS III) trial randomized approximately 1000 patients with class II and III HF over the age of 65 to therapy with bisoprolol, titrated to a target dose of 10 mg daily over 16 weeks, followed by the initiation of enalapril, titrated to a target dose of 10 mg twice daily, vs the reverse order (enalapril then bisoprolol). Patients had to be clinically stable for at least 7 days prior to randomization, with no prior therapy with ACE inhibitors or β-blockers for at least 3 months prior to randomization. Mean ejection fraction was 29%. After a mean follow-up of 1.22 years, there was no significant difference in the composite outcome of death and hospitalization, although criteria for non-inferiority were not met. Importantly, patients initiated on β-blocker therapy first achieved a higher mean dose of bisoprolol than those who were initiated on β-blockers after ACE inhibitors [25]. The data from this trial do not support a recommendation to initiate β-blocker therapy prior to ACE inhibitors in patients with symptomatic HF. However, in selected patients in whom there is concern about initiating an ACE inhibitor or ARB, these data indicate that initiation of a β-blocker without concomitant ACE inhibitor administration can be done safely.

GUIDELINES FOR THE USE OF β-BLOCKERS IN HF

The guidelines below regarding the use of β-blocker therapy in patients with left ventricular systolic dysfunction have been issued by the Heart Failure Society of America: [26]

1. β-blocker therapy should be routinely administered to clinically stable patients with left ventricular systolic dysfunction (LVEF ≤40%) and mild-to-moderate HF symptoms (i.e. NYHA class II–III) who are on standard therapy, which typically includes ACE inhibitors, diuretics as needed to control fluid retention, and digoxin (strength of evidence A).
2. β-blocker therapy should be considered for patients with left ventricular systolic dysfunction (LVEF ≤40%) who are asymptomatic (i.e. NYHA class I) and on standard therapy, including ACE inhibitors (strength of evidence C).
3. To maximize patient safety, a period of clinical stability on standard therapy should occur before β-blocker therapy is instituted. Initiation of β-blocker therapy in patients with HF requires a careful baseline evaluation of clinical status (strength of evidence B).
4. There is insufficient evidence to recommend the use of β-blocker therapy for inpatients or outpatients with symptoms of HF at rest (i.e. NYHA class IV) (strength of evidence C).
5. β-blocker therapy should be initiated at low doses and up-titrated slowly, generally no sooner than at 2-week intervals. Clinical re-evaluation should occur at each titration point and with worsening of patient symptoms. Patients who develop worsening HF or other side-effects after drug initiation or during titration require adjustment of concomitant medications. These patients may also require a reduction in β-blocker dose and, in some cases, temporary or permanent withdrawal of this therapy (strength of evidence B).
6. In general, patients who experience a deterioration in clinical status or symptomatic exacerbation of HF during chronic maintenance treatment should be continued on β-blocker therapy (strength of evidence C).
7. Patient education regarding early recognition of symptom exacerbation and side-effects is considered important. If clinical uncertainty exists, consultation with clinicians who have expertise in HF and/or specialized programs with experience in β-blocker use in patients with HF is recommended (strength of evidence B).

SUMMARY

How effective are β-blockers in the therapy of HF?

- Large, prospective, randomized clinical trials demonstrate an average mortality risk reduction of ~35% with the addition of β-blockers to ACE inhibitor therapy. These benefits extend to all patients with clinical HF and impaired systolic function.
- In contrast to therapy with ACE inhibitors only, addition of chronic β-blocker therapy results in a reduction in the incidence of sudden cardiac death.
- Also in contrast to therapy with ACE inhibitors only, addition of chronic β-blocker therapy results in dose-dependent reductions in left ventricular dimensions and significant improvements in ejection fraction.

Therapeutic strategies:

- Initiation of β-blockers is recommended in all patients with symptomatic HF and impaired systolic function, provided that they are in a compensated state.
- Initiation of β-blockers should be done slowly and carefully, allowing sufficient time (at least 2 weeks) for the patient to adjust to the new dose.
- Titration of β-blockers to the maximum tolerated dose is recommended, with a goal of achieving the evidence-based target for the selected agent.
- Should β-blocker titration be limited by hypotension or orthostatic symptoms, reduction of ACE inhibitor dose may allow escalation of β-blocker therapy. ACE inhibitors, unlike β-blockers, do not show dose-dependent associations with survival and ventricular remodeling.

REFERENCES

1. Packer M, Carver JR, Rodeheffer RJ *et al.* Effect of oral milrinone on mortality in severe chronic heart failure. The PROMISE Study Research Group. *N Engl J Med* 1991; 325:1468–1475.
2. Packer M. Evolution of the neurohormonal hypothesis to explain the progression of chronic heart failure. *Eur Heart J* 1995; 16(suppl F):4–6.
3. Francis GS. Pathophysiology of chronic heart failure. *Am J Med* 2001; 110(suppl 7A):37S–46S.
4. Schrier RW. Pathogenesis of sodium and water retention in high-output and low-output cardiac failure, nephrotic syndrome, cirrhosis, and pregnancy (2). *N Engl J Med* 1988; 319:1127–1134.
5. Chidsey CA, Braunwald E. Sympathetic activity and neurotransmitter depletion in congestive heart failure. *Pharmacol Rev* 1966; 18:685–700.
6. Thomas JA, Marks BH. Plasma norepinephrine in congestive heart failure. *Am J Cardiol* 1978; 41:233–243.
7. Levine TB, Francis GS, Goldsmith SR *et al.* Activity of the sympathetic nervous system and renin-angiotensin system assessed by plasma hormone levels and their relation to hemodynamic abnormalities in congestive heart failure. *Am J Cardiol* 1982; 49:1659–1666.
8. Colucci WS. The effects of norepinephrine on myocardial biology: implications for the therapy of heart failure. *Clin Cardiol* 1998; 21:I20–I24.
9. Rundqvist B, Elam M, Bergmann-Sverrisdottir Y *et al.* Increased cardiac adrenergic drive precedes generalized sympathetic activation in human heart failure. *Circulation* 1997; 95:169–175.
10. Bristow MR, Ginsburg R, Minobe W *et al.* Decreased catecholamine sensitivity and beta-adrenergic-receptor density in failing human hearts. *N Engl J Med* 1982; 307:205–211.
11. Mann DL, Cooper G. Neurohumoral activation in congestive heart failure: a double-edged sword? *Clin Cardiol* 1989; 12:485–490.
12. Swedberg K, Hjalmarson A, Waagstein F *et al.* Beneficial effects of long-term β-blockade in congestive cardiomyopathy. *Br Heart J* 1980; 44:117-133.

13. Engelmeier RS, O'Connell JB, Walsh R *et al.* Improvement in symptoms and exercise tolerance by metoprolol in patients with dilated cardiomyopathy: a double-blind, randomized, placebo-controlled trial. *Circulation* 1985; 72:536–546.
14. Packer M, Bristow MR, Cohn JN *et al.* The effect of carvedilol on morbidity and mortality in patients with chronic heart failure. U.S. Carvedilol Heart Failure Study Group. *N Engl J Med* 1996; 334:1349–1355.
15. Effect of metoprolol CR/XL in chronic heart failure: Metoprolol CR/XL Randomised Intervention Trial in Congestive Heart Failure (MERIT-HF). *Lancet* 1999; 353:2001–2007.
16. Packer M, Coats AJ, Fowler MB *et al.* Effect of carvedilol on survival in severe chronic heart failure. *N Engl J Med* 2001; 344:1651–1658.
17. The Cardiac Insufficiency Bisoprolol Study II (CIBIS-II): a randomised trial. *Lancet* 1999; 353:9–13.
18. A trial of the beta blocker bucindolol in patients with advanced chronic heart failure. *N Engl J Med* 2001; 344:1659–1667.
19. Andreka P, Aiyar N, Olson LC *et al.* Bucindolol displays intrinsic sympathomimetic activity in human myocardium. *Circulation* 2002; 105:2429–2434.
20. Poole-Wilson PA, Swedberg K, Cleland JG *et al.* Comparison of carvedilol and metoprolol on clinical outcomes in patients with chronic heart failure in the Carvedilol Or Metoprolol European Trial (COMET): randomised controlled trial. *Lancet* 2003; 362:7–13.
21. Flather MD, Shibata MC, Coats AJ *et al.* Randomized trial to determine the effect of nebivolol on mortality and cardiovascular hospital admission in elderly patients with heart failure (SENIORS). *Eur Heart J* 2005; 26:215–225.
22. Effects of enalapril on mortality in severe congestive heart failure. Results of the Cooperative North Scandinavian Enalapril Survival Study (CONSENSUS). The CONSENSUS Trial Study Group. *N Engl J Med* 1987; 316:1429–1435.
23. Effect of enalapril on mortality and the development of heart failure in asymptomatic patients with reduced left ventricular ejection fractions. The SOLVD Investigators. *N Engl J Med* 1992; 327:685–691.
24. Effect of enalapril on survival in patients with reduced left ventricular ejection fractions and congestive heart failure. The SOLVD Investigators. *N Engl J Med* 1991; 325:293–302.
25. Willenheimer R, van Veldhuisen DJ, Silke B et al. Effect on survival and hospitalization of initiating treatment for chronic heart failure with bisoprolol followed by enalapril, as compared with the opposite sequence: results of the randomized Cardiac Insufficiency Bisoprolol Study (CIBIS) III. *Circulation* 2005; 112:2426–2435.
26. Heart Failure Society of America (HFSA) practice guidelines. HFSA guidelines for management of patients with heart failure caused by left ventricular systolic dysfunction – pharmacologic approaches. *J Card Fail* 1999; 5:357–382.

7

Neurohormonal activation in heart failure: aldosterone antagonists

E. Hsich, R. C. Starling

INTRODUCTION

The use of neurohormonal antagonism to favorably influence the natural history of heart failure has been quite successful. The cornerstone of neurohormonal inhibition has been the use of angiotensin-converting enzyme (ACE) inhibitors and β-blockers. Additional antagonism of this cascade has been proven to be beneficial *via* the use of angiotensin receptor antagonists. Data are also consistent with favorable outcomes using aldosterone antagonists. Aldosterone levels are increased in heart failure and likely influence electrolyte homeostasis, ventricular remodeling and myocardial fibrosis. Major clinical trials have established a clear benefit from the use of aldosterone antagonists for advanced heart failure and for left ventricular dysfunction occurring subsequent to a myocardial infarction (MI). However, the risk of drug-related hyperkalemia is not trivial and appropriate caution must be exercised in patient selection, initiation of therapy and follow-up monitoring of renal function and potassium homeostasis. Given the multiple agents available to alter neurohormonal activation in heart failure, initiation of adjunctive neurohormonal antagonism should be guided by a patient's risk–benefit profile and guideline statements.

ROLE OF ALDOSTERONE

Patients with chronic heart failure (CHF) can have aldosterone levels 20 times as high as normal individuals. Aldosterone is a neurohormone secreted from the adrenal gland in response to elevated serum levels of angiotensin II, corticotropins, catecholamines, endothelins, and potassium. Aldosterone binds to mineralocorticoid receptors in the kidney, intestine, salivary glands and sweat glands to help achieve salt, potassium, and water homeostasis [1]. This neurohormone is also produced by endothelial cells and vascular smooth muscle cells in the heart and blood vessels [2–4]. Under normal conditions, aldosterone is beneficial. However, elevated levels or inappropriate secretion may cause myocardial and vascular fibrosis, baroreceptor dysfunction, inappropriate volume expansion, and inhibition of myocardial norepinephrine uptake [1, 5–8].

Eileen Hsich, MD, Heart Failure and Transplant Cardiologist, Department of Cardiology, Section of Heart Failure and Cardiac Transplant Medicine, Cleveland Clinic, Cleveland, Ohio, USA.

Randall C. Starling, MD, MPH, Medicak Director, Kaufman Center for Heart Failure, Section Head, Heart Failure and Cardiac Transplantation, Department of Cardiology, Section of Heart Failure and Cardiac Transplant Medicine, Cleveland Clinic, Cleveland, Ohio, USA.

ALDOSTERONE BLOCKADE

Drugs like ACE inhibitors can reduce the aldosterone levels initially but chronic usage is associated with a gradual rise in the aldosterone level [9, 10], i.e. 'aldosterone escape'. This rise may be due to non-angiotensin II stimulation of aldosterone (i.e. corticotropins, potassium) or angiotensin II production *via* an ACE independent pathway [9, 11]. Aldosterone antagonists block the effects of circulating aldosterone by binding to mineralocorticoid receptors. Currently, there are two aldosterone antagonists available: (1) spironolactone and (2) eplerenone. Spironolactone is a non-selective mineralocorticoid receptor antagonist which also up-regulates progesterone receptors and down-regulates androgen receptors. It is associated with hyperkalemia (related to the activation of the mineralocorticoid receptor), gynecomastia, impotence, irregular menses, and libido changes. Eplerenone is a selective mineralocorticoid receptor antagonist. Side-effects include hyperkalemia but it is not associated with gynecomastia, sexual dysfunction, or irregular menses. Both spironolactone and eplerenone are metabolized by the liver. The metabolites of spironolactone remain active whereas the metabolites of epleronone are inactive. The elimination half-life of spironolactone is 17–22 h and the elimination half-life of eplerenone is 4–6 h. Since both drugs are associated with hyperkalemia, they should not be used in patients with significant renal insufficiency. Potassium supplements and other potassium-sparing diuretics should be avoided if possible with the use of these drugs in order to prevent hyperkalemia. Non-steroidal anti-inflammatory drugs (NSAIDs) and high-dose salicylates should also be avoided in heart failure patients taking aldosterone antagonists due to concerns about causing renal failure which could lead to life-threatening or fatal hyperkalemia. It is also important to mention that spironolactone increases digoxin levels but eplerenone does not interact with digoxin [12, 13].

MAJOR CLINICAL TRIALS

There are two major clinical studies using aldosterone antagonists in heart failure patients: The Randomized Aldactone Evaluation Study (RALES) study [14] and the Eplerenone Post-Acute Myocardial Infarction Heart Failure Efficacy and Survival Study (EPHESUS) study [15]. Both trials noted a morbidity and mortality benefit with aldosterone antagonists but studied different patient populations using different aldosterone antagonists. These studies have impacted new heart failure practice guidelines as they were well designed, large, placebo-controlled, randomized, multicenter, double-blind clinical trials that had significant and meaningful endpoints.

The RALES trial studied the effects of spironolactone in CHF patients with moderate-to-severe symptoms (New York Heart Association [NYHA] functional class III–IV). Patients were eligible for enrollment if they had NYHA class IV heart failure within 6 months before enrollment and were in NYHA class III or IV at the time of enrollment, had been given a diagnosis of heart failure at least 6 weeks before enrollment, were being treated with an ACE inhibitor (if tolerated) and a loop diuretic, and had a left ventricular ejection fraction (LVEF) of no more than 35% within 6 months before enrollment (with no clinically significant intercurrent event). They included ischemic and non-ischemic patients but excluded those patients with potassium >5.0 mmol/l, creatinine >2.5 mg/dl, current usage of K^+ sparing diuretic, unstable angina, cancer, liver failure, operable valvular disease (except tricuspid regurgitation or mitral regurgitation), and those patients awaiting heart transplantation. There were a total of 1663 participants: 841 randomized to placebo and 822 randomized to spironolactone. Oral potassium supplementation was discouraged due to concern about the development of hyperkalemia with concomitant usage of an ACE inhibitor and an aldosterone antagonist. The spironolactone group was begun on 12.5 or 25 mg daily that could be increased to a maximum dose of 50 mg after 8 weeks of treatment and no evidence of hyperkalemia. Laboratory measurements of potassium were assessed on all patients at 4 weeks, 8 weeks, 12 weeks, then every 3 months for 1 year, and finally every 6 months. Patients on the higher dosage of spironolactone had additional laboratory testing and the study medication was stopped or reduced for all patients if they developed hyperkalemia. The primary endpoint was death from any cause and the secondary endpoints were cardiac death, cardiac hospitalizations, change in NYHA functional class, and combined cardiac death and cardiac hospital admissions. The study was prematurely stopped because a mortality benefit was noted early with the usage of spironolactone (mean dose 26 mg). There was a 30% reduction in the risk of death with usage of spironolactone and that was mostly due to a reduction in sudden death and death from heart failure. There was also a 30% reduction in the risk of cardiac hospitalizations and a greater improvement in NYHA functional class. It is noted that this was a fairly ill patient population given the requirement for recent documentation of class IV heart failure met by many of the patients enrolled in the study.

Spironolactone was overall well-tolerated with only 2% serious hyperkalemia and 10% gynecomastia compared to 1% hyperkalemia and 1% gynecomastia in the placebo group. The major limitation of the study was that it preceded the advent of evidence-based β-blocker usage for heart failure. Only 11% of the participants were using β-blockers which raised the concern whether aldosterone antagonism could provide additional benefits during concomitant usage of β-blockers [14].

The EPHESUS trial studied the effects of eplerenone in patients that developed heart failure with a LVEF <40% during an acute MI. They also included diabetic patients with an acute MI, left ventricular systolic dysfunction (LVEF <40%) and no heart failure, since this population has a similar prognosis to the non-diabetic who presented with heart failure during an acute MI. They excluded patients with potassium >5.0 mmol/l, creatinine >2.5 mg/dl, and current usage of potassium-sparing diuretics. There were a total of 6642 participants: 3313 randomized to placebo and 3319 randomized to eplerenone. All patients were randomized 3–14 days after a MI. Starting dose of eplerenone was 25 mg daily which could be increased to a maximum dose of 50 mg daily. Laboratory measurements of potassium were obtained 48 h after starting the study medication, 1 week, 4 weeks, 5 weeks, 3 months, and then every 3 months. Any changes in study doses required additional laboratory testing for potassium 1 week after the change. The primary endpoints were death from any cause and hospitalization or death from a cardiovascular event. Secondary endpoints included cardiovascular death, death from any cause, and any hospitalization. Patients were followed for a mean of 16 months and eplerenone was found to have both significant morbidity and mortality benefits. The reduction in cardiovascular death was mostly due to a reduction in sudden death and the reduction in hospitalization for a cardiovascular cause was mostly due to a reduction of heart failure. What was most impressive was the fact that the majority of patients were taking an ACE inhibitor (86%), a β-blocker (75%), and an aspirin (88%) and that the usage of eplerenone provided an additional benefit. Eplerenone was overall well-tolerated with only 5.5% serious hyperkalemia (defined as K^+ ≥6.0 mmol/l) compared to 3.9% hyperkalemia in the placebo group. Eplerenone was also not associated with gynecomastia, impotence, or breast pain in women [15] (Table 7.1).

SPECIAL SUBGROUPS

There are very few data regarding the benefits of any heart failure medication in women and/or the African-American population. Therefore, it is important to mention that aldosterone antagonists are one of the few medications deemed by subgroup analysis to have a total mortality benefit for women with systolic heart failure based on both the RALES [14] and EPHESUS trials [15]. Although potential mechanisms were not explored by these investigators, it is interesting to know that the Framingham Heart Study noted higher levels of

Table 7.1 Major clinical trials

Trial	Design	Inclusion	Exclusion	Endpoints	Results
RALES	Placebo/control Randomized Multicenter Double-blinded	NYHA III-IV, LVEF ≤35%	K^+ >5.0 mmol/l, Cr >2.5 mg/dl, K^+ sparing diuretic, unstable angina, cancer, liver failure, operable valvular disease (except TR/MR), awaiting heart transplantation	*Primary:* Death from any cause *Secondary:* Cardiac death, cardiac hospitalizations, change in NYHA class, combined cardiac death or cardiac admissions	Improved survival, improved NYHA class, and fewer cardiac admissions with spironolactone
EPHESUS	Placebo/control Randomized Multicenter Double-blinded	Acute MI, LVEF <40%, and evidence of CHF if non-diabetic	K^+ >5.0 mmol/l, Cr >2.5 mg/dl, K^+ sparing diuretic	*Primary:* (1) Time to death from any cause and (2) time to death from cardiovascular cause or first admission for cardiovascular event *Secondary:* Cardiac death, death from any cause, cardiovascular admissions	Improved survival and fewer cardiac admissions with eplerenone

LVEF = left ventricular ejection fraction; MR = mitral regurgitation; TR = tricuspid regurgitation

aldosterone in women compared to men prior to the development of heart failure. The Framingham Study also noted a significant correlation between increased aldosterone levels and increased ventricular wall thickness in women [16]. The association with increased ventricular wall thickness is important since left ventricular hypertrophy is considered a risk factor for the development of heart failure [17].

The RALES [14] and EPHESUS [15] trials did not provide subgroup analysis for the African-American participants and there are no large clinical studies comparing aldosterone levels in African-American to Caucasian heart failure participants. Only a small trial was performed noting racial differences in aldosterone levels and the development of ventricular hypertrophy. In that study 109 African-Americans with hypertension were compared to 73 French-Canadians with hypertension. Plasma aldosterone levels in the African-Americans were higher than the French-Canadians when hormone levels were obtained while patients were standing. Plasma renin levels were lower in the African-Americans in both the supine and standing positions. In the African-Americans, increased aldosterone levels were associated with increased left ventricular thickness. It is interesting to note that the majority of African-Americans studied in that trial were women (70%) which may have influenced the results although the investigators did not analyze the data by gender [18]. Genetic polymorphisms in the aldosterone synthase promoter may influence the outcomes of African-American heart failure patients. A recently published article analyzing a subgroup of heart failure patients in the African-American Heart Failure Trial (A-HeFT) noted that the aldosterone synthase promoter -344C allele was associated with higher mortality [19].

HYPERKALEMIA WITH ALDOSTERONE ANTAGONISTS

Hyperkalemia is a side-effect for both spironolactone and eplerenone. The risk of serious hyperkalemia in both the RALES and EPHESUS trials was low because of the following: careful selection criteria for participants, low dosages of aldosterone antagonists administered, and frequent laboratory monitoring for potassium levels. Both studies excluded patients with creatinine >2.5 mg/dl, potassium >5.0 mmol/l, and concomitant usage of other K^+ sparing agents. The maximum dose of aldosterone antagonists used in the RALES and EPHESUS trials was 50 mg daily but the mean doses were lower with mortality benefits still evident. For instance, the mean dose of spironolactone was 26 mg daily in the RALES trial and the mean dose of eplerenone was 43 mg daily in the EPHESUS trial [14, 15]. An earlier safety trial for a duration of 12 weeks comparing different dosages of spironolactone provided important background data. In that study serious hyperkalemia was defined as $K^+ \geq 5.5$ mmol/l and it occurred in 5% patients taking placebo, 5% patients taking spironolactone 12.5 mg daily, 13% patients taking 25 mg daily, 20% patients taking 50 mg daily, and 24% patients taking 75 mg daily. Since the risk of hyperkalemia increased with higher dosages of spironolactone, these investigators recommended that the maximum dose be 25 mg daily and higher doses should be very carefully monitored [20].

After the publication of the RALES and EPHESUS studies there was an increase in the usage of aldosterone antagonists for heart failure patients and this was associated with a higher rate of hyperkalemia than that observed in the RALES and EPHESUS trials. One of the most disturbing population-based studies was performed in Ontario, Canada which noted a five-fold increase in the usage of spironolactone after the publication of the RALES data. This higher usage of spironolactone was associated with 560 additional hospitalizations for hyperkalemia and 73 additional hospital deaths [21]. Although this study did not address the cause for the higher rate of hyperkalemia, a Medicare cross-sectional study performed in the US noted that 30% of patients with systolic heart failure ≥ 65 years of age who were prescribed spironolactone at hospital discharge did not meet the RALES criteria. Of those patients, 14.1%

had creatinine ≥2.5 mg/dl, 17.3% had severe renal failure with a estimated glomerular filtration rate (GFR) <30 ml/min × m², and 22.8% had potassium >5 mmol/l [22]. In another study, the higher than expected rate of hyperkalemia for heart failure patients prescribed an aldosterone antagonist was partially attributed to infrequent laboratory monitoring [23].

There are many factors that can contribute to the development of hyperkalemia during usage of an aldosterone antagonist in heart failure patients. As already mentioned, renal insufficiency, pre-existing hyperkalemia, and inadequate laboratory monitoring are common causes. In addition, using 50 mg or higher of an aldosterone antagonist increases the risk of hyperkalemia. Other possible reasons for hyperkalemia include diabetes mellitus which can cause type IV renal tubular acidosis, older age patients since the serum creatinine may not adequately reflect a reduced GFR, and concomitant usage of potassium supplementation, K^+ sparing diuretics, or drugs that directly/indirectly suppress renin (i.e. β-blocker antagonists and non-steroidal anti-inflammatory agents) or angiotensin II (i.e. ACE inhibitors or angiotensin receptor blockers [ARB]) [24].

POSSIBLE BENEFITS BASED ON SMALLER CLINICAL TRIALS

Aldosterone antagonists may reduce ventricular ectopy [8, 23] and arrhythmias [26] as demonstrated in small studies involving patients with systolic left ventricular dysfunction. This may be due to maintaining higher serum levels of potassium and magnesium than would be expected if the patients were on only a loop diuretic combined with an ACE inhibitor [26] or it may be due to the ability of aldosterone antagonists to reduce myocardial fibrosis [27, 28]. Aldosterone antagonists have also been shown to improve endothelial function in patients with systolic dysfunction by increasing nitric oxide bioactivity [29]. Prior investigations have attempted to assess whether the clinical benefits of aldosterone antagonists for patients with heart failure exist for those patients with preserved left ventricular systolic function (i.e. diastolic heart failure) [30, 31]. However, the design of the studies has been limited by the fact that diastolic heart failure remains a difficult diagnosis to establish non-invasively and echocardiographic endpoints for improvement in diastolic heart failure remain controversial. One study in patients with heart failure and preserved systolic function noted regression in the posterior wall thickness and increases in long-axis strain rate with usage of spironolactone [30].

CURRENT GUIDELINES

The current American College of Cardiology/American Heart Association (ACC/AHA) heart failure guidelines recommend an aldosterone antagonist for two groups of patients: (1) Those with systolic left ventricular dysfunction and moderate-to-severe symptoms (i.e. NYHA class III–IV) and (2) those patients with systolic left ventricular dysfunction early after a MI. An aldosterone antagonist is not indicated for patients with mild heart failure symptoms and systolic ventricular dysfunction or heart failure with preserved ventricular function (i.e. diastolic heart failure). Due to the potential risk of hyperkalemia the ACC/AHA Task Force discourages the use of aldosterone antagonists in women with creatinine >2.0 mg/dl, men with creatinine >2.5 mg/dl, any patient with creatinine clearance <30 ml, and patients already with hyperkalemia as defined as K^+ >5.0 mEq/l. They also discourage triple drug therapy with an aldosterone antagonist, an ACE inhibitor and an ARB, since the safety profile with all three drugs has not been studied. Potassium supplements should be discontinued or reduced and non-steroidal anti-inflammatory agents and cyclo-oxygenase-2 inhibitors should be avoided.

The initial dose of spironolactone should be 12.5 mg daily and eplerenone 25 mg daily if the estimated GFR is between 30 and 50 ml/min. If the estimated GFR is above 50 ml/min, the initial dose of both spironolactone and eplerenone should be 25 mg daily and can be titrated to a maximum dose of 50 mg daily. Laboratory monitoring of potassium should occur 3 days after initiating an aldosterone antagonist, then 1 week after initiating the drug, then every month for 3 months, and if it remains stable, the laboratory testing can be done every 3 months. Aldosterone antagonists should be stopped or reduced if K^+ >5.5 mEq/l unless the patient is taking potassium supplementation which could instead be discontinued. Aldosterone antagonists should also be transiently stopped if the patient develops diarrhea or has an interruption in loop diuretic therapy. Rigorous laboratory testing to monitor potassium should be performed upon reinitiating an aldosterone antagonist, increasing the dosage of an aldosterone antagonist, or increasing the dosage of either an ACE inhibitor or ARB while maintaining the same dosage of an aldosterone antagonist [17].

SUMMARY

Points of emphasis:

Risk:
- Hyperkalemia with eplerenone or spironolactone.
- Gynecomastia with spironolactone only.

ACC/AHA Guidelines:
- Indications: NYHA class III–IV with LVEF ≤35%
  Acute MI with LVEF <40% (and heart failure signs if non-diabetic)
- Exclusions: Cr >2.5 mg/dl men
  Cr >2.0 mg/dl women
  Cr clearance <30 ml
  K >5.0 mEq/l
  Concomitant usage of NSAIDs, cox-2 inhibitors, K+ sparing agents
  Concomitant usage of an ACE inhibitor with an ARB
- Dosages: If GFR = 30–50 ml/min, begin spironolactone 12.5 mg daily or eplerenone 25 mg daily
  If GFR >50 ml/min, begin spironolactone 25 mg daily or eplerenone 25 mg daily
  Up-titrate to spironolactone 50 mg daily or eplerenone 50 mg daily as maximum dose
- Laboratory monitoring:
  Laboratory tests: K+ and Cr
  Frequency: 3 days after initiation of drug, then 1 week after initiation then every month for 3 months, then every 3 months.
  Additional testing: Repeat above after increasing an aldosterone antagonist or increasing either an ACE inhibitor or angiotensin aldosterone antagonist
- Caveats: Potassium supplements should either be reduced or discontinued
  If K^+ >5.5 mEq/l, then either reduce or discontinue aldosterone antagonist
  Temporarily stop aldosterone antagonist if the patient has diarrhea or has stopped a loop diuretic

Definite benefits:
- Improved survival
- Fewer cardiac hospitalizations

Potential benefits:
- Reduced ventricular ectopy and arrhythmias
- Reduced myocardial fibrosis
- Improved endothelial function   } Retard or reverse ventricular remodeling
- Improved diastolic heart failure

REFERENCES

1. Weber KT. Aldosterone in congestive heart failure. *N Engl J Med*. 2001; 345:1689–1697.
2. Takeda Y, Miyamori I, Yoneda T *et al*. Production of aldosterone in isolated rat blood vessels. *Hypertension* 1995; 25:170–173.
3. Silvestre JS, Robert V, Heymes C *et al*. Myocardial production of aldosterone and corticosterone in the rat. Physiologic regulation. *J Biol Chem* 1998; 273:4883–4891.
4. Takeda Y, Miyamori I, Yoneda T *et al*. Regulation of aldosterone synthase in human vascular endothelial cells by angiotensin II and adrenocorticotropin. *J Clin Endocrinol Metab* 1996; 81:2797–2800.
5. Qin W, Rudolph AE, Bond BR *et al*. Transgenic model of aldosterone-driven cardiac hypertrophy and heart failure. *Circ Res* 2003; 93:69–76.
6. Sun Y, Ramires FJ, Weber KT. Fibrosis of atria and great vessels in response to angiotensin II or aldosterone infusion. *Cardiovasc Res* 1997; 35:138–147.
7. Wang W. Chronic administration of aldosterone depresses baroreceptor reflex function in the dog. *Hypertension* 1994; 24:571–575.
8. Barr CC, Lang CC, Hanson J, Arnott M, Kennedy N, Struthers AD. Effects of adding spironolactone to an angiotensin converting enzyme inhibitor in chronic congestive heart failure secondary to coronary artery disease. *Am J Cardiol* 1995; 76:1259–1265.
9. Borghi C, Boschi S, Ambrosioni E, Melandri G, Branzi A, Magnani B. Evidence of a partial escape of renin-angiotensin-aldosterone blockade in patients with acute myocardial infarction treated with ACE inhibitors. *J Clin Pharmacol* 1993; 33:40–45.
10. Staessen J, Lijnen P, Fagard R, Verschueren LJ, Amery A. Rise in plasma concentration of aldosterone during long-term angiotensin II suppression. *J Endocrinol* 1981; 91:457–465.
11. Urata H, Healy B, Stewart RW, Bumpus FM, Husain A. Angiotensin II-forming pathways in normal and failing human hearts. *Circ Res* 1990; 66:883–890.
12. Pitt B. The role of aldosterone blockade in patients with heart failure. *Heart Fail Rev* 2005; 10:79–83.
13. Brown NJ. Eplerenone: cardiovascular protection. *Circulation* 2003; 107:2512–2518.
14. Pitt B, Zannad F, Remme WJ *et al*. The effect of spironolactone on morbidity and mortality in patients with severe heart failure. Randomized Aldactone Evaluation Study Investigators. *N Engl J Med* 1999; 341:709–717.
15. Pitt B, Remme W, Zannad F *et al*. Eplerenone, a selective aldosterone blocker, in patients with left ventricular dysfunction after myocardial infarction. *N Engl J Med* 2003; 348:1309–1321.
16. Vasan RS, Evans JC, Benjamin EJ *et al*. Relations of serum aldosterone to cardiac structure: gender-related differences in the Framingham Heart Study. *Hypertension* 2004; 43:957–962.
17. Hunt SA, Abraham WT, Chin MH *et al*. ACC/AHA 2005 Guideline Update for the Diagnosis and Management of Chronic Heart Failure in the Adult: a report of the American College of Cardiology/American Heart Association Task Force on Practice Guidelines (Writing Committee to Update the 2001 Guidelines for the Evaluation and Management of Heart Failure): developed in collaboration with the American College of Chest Physicians and the International Society for Heart and Lung Transplantation: endorsed by the Heart Rhythm Society. *Circulation* 2005; 112:e154–e235.
18. El-Gharbawy AH, Nadig VS, Kotchen JM *et al*. Arterial pressure, left ventricular mass, and aldosterone in essential hypertension. *Hypertension* 2001; 37:845–850.
19. McNamara D, Tam W, Sabolinski ML *et al*. Aldosterone synthase promoter polymorphism predicts outcome in African-Americans with heart failure. *J Am Coll Cardiol* 2006; 48:1277–1282.
20. Effectiveness of spironolactone added to an angiotensin-converting enzyme inhibitor and a loop diuretic for severe chronic congestive heart failure (the Randomized Aldactone Evaluation Study [RALES]). *Am J Cardiol* 1996; 78:902–907.
21. Juurlink DN, Mamdani MM, Lee DS *et al*. Rates of hyperkalemia after publication of the Randomized Aldactone Evaluation Study. *N Engl J Med* 2004; 351:543–551.

22. Masoudi FA, Gross CP, Wang Y *et al.* Adoption of spironolactone therapy for older patients with heart failure and left ventricular systolic dysfunction in the United States, 1998–2001. *Circulation* 2005; 112:39–47.
23. Shah KB, Rao K, Sawyer R, Gottlieb SS. The adequacy of laboratory monitoring in patients treated with spironolactone for congestive heart failure. *J Am Coll Cardiol* 2005; 46:845–849.
24. McMurray JJ, O'Meara E. Treatment of heart failure with spironolactone – trial and tribulations. *N Engl J Med* 2004; 351:526–528.
25. Macdonald JE, Kennedy N, Struthers AD. Effects of spironolactone on endothelial function, vascular angiotensin converting enzyme activity, and other prognostic markers in patients with mild heart failure already taking optimal treatment. *Heart* 2004; 90:765–770.
26. Ramires FJ, Mansur A, Coelho O *et al.* Effect of spironolactone on ventricular arrhythmias in congestive heart failure secondary to idiopathic dilated or to ischemic cardiomyopathy. *Am J Cardiol* 2000; 85:1207–1211.
27. Zannad F, Alla F, Dousset B, Perez A, Pitt B. Limitation of excessive extracellular matrix turnover may contribute to survival benefit of spironolactone therapy in patients with congestive heart failure: insights from the Randomized Aldactone Evaluation Study (RALES). Rales Investigators. *Circulation* 2000; 102:2700–2706.
28. Fraccarollo D, Galuppo P, Hildemann S, Christ M, Ertl G, Bauersachs J. Additive improvement of left ventricular remodeling and neurohormonal activation by aldosterone receptor blockade with eplerenone and ACE inhibition in rats with myocardial infarction. *J Am Coll Cardiol* 2003; 42:1666–1673.
29. Farquharson CA, Struthers AD. Spironolactone increases nitric oxide bioactivity, improves endothelial vasodilator dysfunction, and suppresses vascular angiotensin I/angiotensin II conversion in patients with chronic heart failure. *Circulation* 2000; 101:594–597.
30. Mottram PM, Haluska B, Leano R, Cowley D, Stowasser M, Marwick TH. Effect of aldosterone antagonism on myocardial dysfunction in hypertensive patients with diastolic heart failure. *Circulation* 2004; 110:558–565.
31. Roongsritong C, Sutthiwan P, Bradley J, Simoni J, Power S, Meyerrose GE. Spironolactone improves diastolic function in the elderly. *Clin Cardiol* 2005; 28:484–487.

Section III

Emerging pharmacologic therapies for heart failure

8

Nitric oxide biology and oxidative stress in heart failure: heart failure in African-Americans

C. W. Yancy

INTRODUCTION

Over the last several decades, the US has realized a striking demographic shift. By the middle of the 21st century, there will no longer exist a majority population. As such, a number of significant special populations will constitute the US demographic and these individuals will share the burden of cardiovascular disease – a burden which may be distinct from traditional disease models. Evidence of important variances in the expression and treatment of cardiovascular disease is already visible in these emerging special populations. Heart failure as it occurs in African-Americans has become the prototypical model. Data are now available that attest to the differences that exist in the expression of heart failure in African-Americans, the variations in response to evidence-based therapies, new insights into the pathophysiology of heart failure and novel drug responses that appear to be uniquely beneficial in this cohort. At the core of these apparent nuances in disease expression and the natural history of heart failure in African-Americans is an emerging awareness of the role of nitric oxide (NO) deficiency and excessive oxidative stress in certain patients with cardiovascular disease.

HEART FAILURE: IS THIS A UNIQUE DISEASE IN AFRICAN-AMERICANS?

Recent discoveries have rendered chronic heart failure as something other than the fatalistic diagnosis it once was. Rather, it is a treatable disease entity with significant improvements in morbidity and mortality that, when best treated with evidence-based strategies, will result in annual mortality rates of less than 10%. However, although this is a remarkable improvement from historic expectations, the 3–5 year disease burden still carries nearly a 30–50% mortality risk [1]. Traditionally, the results of randomized controlled clinical trials have been extrapolated to the general patient population with expectations that all persons treated would experience similar outcomes. However, a critical review of clinical trials in heart failure questions the appropriateness of extrapolating these results to African-Americans with heart failure [2]. The data are not only inconsistent but are indeed worrisome. There are very real concerns that the same salutary benefits of neurohormonal antagonists seen in clinical trials cannot be fully realized in this patient cohort. These concerns may be based on variances in the pathophysiology of disease but the inconsistent representation of African-Americans in major heart failure clinical trials, the risk of undersized

Clyde W. Yancy, MD, FACC, FAHA, FACP, Medical Director and Chief, Cardiothoracic Transplantation, Baylor Heart and Vascular Institute, Baylor University Medical Center, Dallas, Texas, USA.

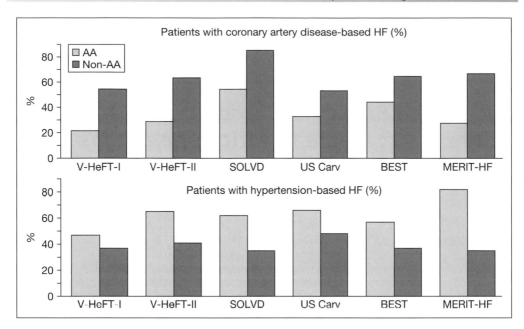

Figure 8.1 Etiology of congestive heart failure in African-Americans. Data from [9, 12, 14, 16, 17, 18, 20]. BEST = Beta-blocker Evaluation of Survival Trial; HF = heart failure; MERIT-HF = Metoprolol CR/XL Randomized Intervention Trial in Congestive Heart Failure; SOLVD = Studies of Left Ventricular Dysfunction; V-HeFI = Vasodilator Heart Failure Trial; US Carv = US Carvedilol Heart Failure Trial.

subgroups and the limitations of retrospective subgroup analyses all combine to confound the interpretation of those trials. Thus there is ambiguity concerning the expected responsiveness of African-Americans to evidence-based therapies. It is important to emphasize that, despite these concerns, there are no data to suggest harm and sufficient signals consistent with benefit that all persons with heart failure should be treated with guideline-based therapies irrespective of race, gender or age [3]. In this context, insights have been gleaned from the clinical trials that define heart failure in African-Americans.

Heart failure occurs more frequently in African-Americans. The prevalence of heart failure in African-Americans is 3% vs only 2% in whites [4]. In African-American women, the prevalence may be as high as 4% or nearly a 100% higher prevalence. When heart failure does occur in African-Americans, it has an enigmatic natural history. The disease occurs at an earlier age with a much higher incidence in the 30–64 age group in African-Americans than any other patient populations [4]. The degree of left ventricular dysfunction and severity of disease as measured by New York Heart Association (NYHA) class are worse at the time of diagnosis. Morbidity is a major issue as hospitalization rates are higher in African-Americans [2]. The rate of death due to heart failure is higher in younger cohorts of African-Americans (<65 years) but similar in the usual age range of heart failure (>65 years). Clinical trial data must be viewed very carefully as initial assessments would suggest a higher rate of death but when populations are matched for disease severity and disease etiology, the differences in mortality are much less and are no longer significant. The true cause of heart failure is often difficult to ascertain but concomitant other cardiac illnesses do suggest likely etiologies of left ventricular dysfunction. As such, the presumed etiology of left ventricular (LV) dysfunction in African-Americans is less likely to be due to coronary artery disease and more likely to be non-ischemic than that seen in whites. As seen in Figure 8.1, there is a lower likelihood of documented

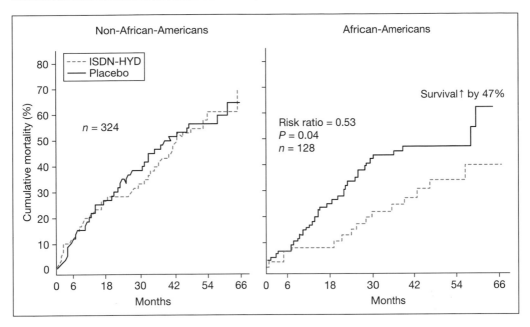

Figure 8.2 Mortality from congestive heart failure in African-American patients in V-HeFT. With permission [13]. ISDN-HYD = Isosorbide dinitrate and hydralazine; V-HeFT = Vasodilator Heart Failure Trial.

ischemic heart disease as the putative cause of left ventricular dysfunction and a greater likelihood of non-ischemic etiologies, principally hypertensive disease, as the sole potential explanation for left ventricular dysfunction. At best, only an association of hypertension and LV dysfunction can be implicated in this paradigm as there have to date not been cogent mechanisms to explain the progression from normal systolic function to left ventricular hypertrophy and eventually to impaired left ventricular systolic function.

Explanations for these nuances in disease and for this apparent heart failure enigma in African-Americans are frankly lacking. There is no accepted single proven causative theory. Candidate theories include issues related to the psychosocial burdens of race in North America, disparate healthcare [5], the excess burden of hypertension [5–7], genetic predispositions to hypertrophy and fibrosis, inherited variances in response to medical therapeutics and poor clinical trial design. Of these, the psychosocial burdens of the African- American culture cannot be minimized. Increasingly we must also acknowledge that disparate healthcare (i.e. differences in outcomes not based on physiology or patient choice but rather due to system or healthcare provider issues of access to care, language/cultural barriers and bias), is a real entity and is likely more prevalent than has been accepted [8] (Figure 8.2). The deleterious influence of malignant hypertension, obesity and diabetes must also be incorporated in any model of cardiovascular disease in African-Americans.

The most promising but also most troublesome explanation is in the field of genomic medicine. It is inappropriate to equate race and genetics but the likelihood of over-representation of certain at-risk genes in certain individuals that have a similar heritage, intermarry and share the same cultural environment cannot be discounted. Yet the African-American race is likely more heterogeneous than any other group and again caution must be exercised before generalizations are made. Finally, as a discipline, genomic medicine and pharmacogenomics remain quite incipient and at best are hypothesis generating but not yet capable of definitive statements in medicine.

CLINICAL TRIALS IN HEART FAILURE: WHAT HAVE WE LEARNED ABOUT HEART FAILURE IN AFRICAN-AMERICANS?

Several of the major published randomized controlled clinical trials in heart failure have reported data as a function of race. Perhaps the most descriptive data come from the Studies of Left Ventricular Dysfunction (SOLVD). Data derived from SOLVD were the first to suggest that mortality from heart failure was higher in African-Americans [9]. This *post hoc* analysis suggested a 1.8-fold increase in the risk of death for African-American men and a 2.4-fold increase for African-American women. This analysis was confounded by dissimilar patient populations. A subsequent re-analysis that adjusted for the degree of left ventricular dysfunction and for trial participation (i.e. SOLVD Prevention or SOLVD Treatment trial) yielded no differences in mortality [10]. However, even after matching the patient populations, a significantly higher risk (44%) for hospitalization due to heart failure was observed in the African-American patients compared with white patients. The conclusion from these findings was an apparent lesser responsiveness to angiotensin-converting enzyme (ACE) inhibitors in African-Americans [9, 10].

The data emanating from clinical trials testing β-blockers in heart failure are similarly confounded. A meta-analysis done by the RAND Corporation compiled data reported as a function of race from the major clinical trials using β-blocker trials in heart failure [11]. Whereas the aggregate benefit of β-blockers for white Americans was a 31% reduction in mortality, the apparent benefit of β-blockers in African-Americans was only 3%. These underwhelming data regarding the use of β-blockers in African-Americans with heart failure were heavily impacted by the negative outcomes seen in the African-American cohort from the Beta blocker Evaluation of Survival Trial (BEST) [12]. In this trial, non-blacks had a statistically significant survival advantage on bucindolol ($P = 0.014$) when compared to blacks. Subsequent further analyses of these data have provocatively suggested that the findings might be better explained by an over-representation of a loss-of-gain single nucleotide polymorphism affecting the functionality of the β_1 receptor in African-Americans [13]. However, the experience with carvedilol varies substantially from the experience with bucindolol. In both the US Carvedilol Heart Failure Trials program [14] and the Carvedilol Prospective Randomized Cumulative Survival Trial (COPERNICUS) [15], retrospective analyses by ethnicity were quite favorable and demonstrated consistency of response to an evidence-based β-blocker used for heart failure irrespective of race. A summary of major clinical trials in heart failure that reported data as a function of race can be found in Table 8.1.

Data gathered from the Vasodilator Heart Failure Trials (V-HeFT-I and II) have now become seminal in our understanding of this patient cohort. V-HeFT-I was the first clinical trial in heart failure to demonstrate that the natural history of heart failure could be modified by medical therapy [16]. The modest benefit on survival from the addition of isosorbide dinitrate and hydralazine (ISDN/HYD) was appropriately heralded as a landmark discovery. In the V-HeFT-I experience, 180 patients were African-American. A *post hoc* retrospective analysis of V-HeFT-I yielded the striking finding that the benefit of ISDN/HYD when added to diuretics and digoxin was seen almost exclusively in the African-American patients with heart failure. Thus the positive findings in this subgroup, specifically, a nearly incredible 47% mortality advantage, drove the results of the primary trial (Figure 8.3) [17]. A similar retrospective analysis of V-HeFT-II (ACE inhibitor therapy vs ISDN/HYD) confirmed the decided benefit of combined vasodilator therapy in African-Americans with heart failure. When V-HeFT-II was re-analyzed as a function of race, the white patients responded better to an ACE inhibitor than to ISDN/HYD while the African-American patients responded similarly on an ACE inhibitor or vasodilator regimen [17, 18]. These findings would suggest that, within the subgroup of African-Americans, a significant response to ISDN/HYD was once again realized. How might vasodilator therapy effect such significant improvement in heart failure? It is now apparent that the combination of

Table 8.1 Summary of major clinical trials in heart failure reporting data by race

Study	AA (%)	Design	Intervention	Results
V-HeFT-I (16)	29	Double-blind RCT; primary endpoint: mortality	Placebo vs hydralazine/isosorbide nitrate. Background: diuretics and digoxin	Annual mortality rate decreased from 17.9% to 9.7%; $P = 0.04$
V-HeFT-II (17, 18)	27	Double-blind RCT; primary endpoint: mortality	Hydralazine/isosorbide dinitrate vs enalapril. Background: diuretics and digoxin	Annual mortality rate: 12.9–12.8%; P = NS
SOLVD Treatment (10)	12	Double-blind RCT; primary endpoint: mortality	Placebo vs enalapril in NYHA class II/III HF	No mortality difference blacks vs non-blacks in a matched population, re: LVEF and clinical trial participation; RR 0.92 vs 0.95; higher hospitalization rate for blacks; RR 0.95 vs 0.54; $P = 0.005$
SOLVD Prevention (19)	9.8	Double-blind RCT; primary endpoint: mortality	Placebo vs enalapril in NYHA class I/II HF	No difference in the prevention of heart failure using enalapril; statistically significant difference in the incidence of heart failure; RR 1.81; $P < 0.001$
BEST (12)	23	Double-blind RCT; primary endpoint: all-cause mortality	Placebo vs bucindolol in NYHA class III and IV; randomization stratified for women and blacks. Background: diuretics, ACE inhibitors; digoxin at investigator's discretion	Non-significant 17% increase in risk of death on bucindolol; $P = 0.27$
MERIT-HF (20)	<5	Double-blind RCT; primary endpoint: mortality	Placebo vs metoprolol succinate in NYHA class II/IV; mostly II/III	Insufficient numbers to ascertain efficacy

Table 8.1 (continued)

Study	AA (%)	Design	Intervention	Results
US Carvedilol Trials Program (14)	20	Four concurrent trials; double-blind RCT design; mortality was not a predetermined endpoint	Placebo vs carvedilol in NYHA class II–IV; mostly II/III with protocol participation determined by 6-minute walk time; Background: diuretics, ACE inhibitors and digoxin at investigator's discretion	Similar efficacy between black and non-black groups; reduction in death for any cause or hospitalization for any cause – 48%; reduction in worsening of heart failure – 54%
COPERNICUS (15)	5	Double-blind RCT design; primary endpoint: all-cause mortality	Placebo vs carvedilol in NHYA class III/IV; LVEF <0.25 (mean 0.19)	Similar efficacy between black and non-black groups despite small number of blacks

LVEF = left ventricular ejection fraction; RCT = randomized controlled trial; RR = relative risk

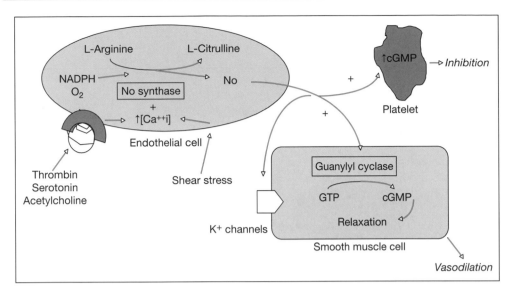

Figure 8.3 NO synthesis and actions. NO = Nitric oxide; NADPH = reduced nicotinamide adenine dinucleotide phosphate; cGMP = cyclic guanosine monophosphate; GTP = guanosine triphosphate.

ISDN/HYD represents more than a balanced vasodilating regimen. Isosorbide dinitrate is a NO donor, and hydralazine has important antioxidant properties. NO plays an important role in the stabilization of vascular endothelium and a deficient state of NO, theorized to occur more frequently in African-Americans, may lead to cardiovascular disease.

NITRIC OXIDE BIOLOGY

NO, originally named 'endothelium-derived relaxation factor' is fairly ubiquitous with functions that include vasodilation, neurotransmission and elimination of pathogens. It is produced by endothelial cells from a family of oxidoreductases that bear close homology to the cytochrome P_{450} system of enzymes [21, 22].

Three 'synthases' have been identified: NOS I (neuronal NOS or nNOS), NOS 2 (inducible NOS or iNOS) and NOS 3 (endothelial NOS or eNOS). NOS 3 is activated by agonists acting on G protein coupled receptors and by shear forces and changes in O_2 delivery. L-arginine and oxygen serve as substrates for NOS while nicotinamide adenine dinucleotide phosphate (NADPH), serves as one of several cofactors. The byproduct of NO synthesis is L-citrulline plus $NADP^+$. NO produces vasodilation by activating soluble guanylate cyclase (sGC) with subsequent production of cyclic guanosine monophosphate (cGMP) (Figure 8.4). NO influences organ function by its post-translational effects on effector molecules. This occurs most often at cysteine residues and is termed S-nitrosylation. S-nitrosylation of ion channels within the heart maintains normal calcium flux important in systolic and diastolic function.

Superoxide $[O_2^-]$ facilitates S-nitrosylation at physiologic levels but disrupts S-nitrosylation at pathologic levels. It does so by targeting the same cysteine residues as NO and prevents S-nitrosylation from occurring. Pathologic levels of superoxide will also react with NO and lead to the production of peroxynitrite. This process of excess superoxide production and disruption of S-nitrosylation is characteristic of oxidative stress. The balance between the effects of NO and superoxide has been termed the 'nitroso-redox' balance (Figure 8.4). If this balance is inclined towards low NO and excess superoxide, cell injury may ensue [21, 22].

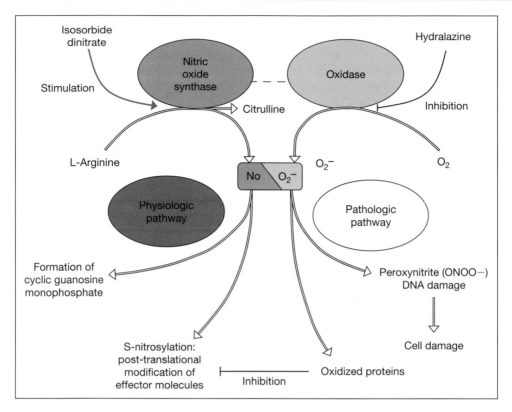

Figure 8.4 Consequences of NO and superoxide balance disruption in heart failure patients. With permission [21].

African-Americans have demonstrable evidence of diminished NO bioavailability and enhanced production of peroxynitrite. It is plausible (but not yet proven) that the progression of cardiovascular disease, especially, heart failure, in African-Americans might be a result not only of an activated neurohormonal system but also a deficient endogenous vasodilator/growth-inhibiting system. If this is a valid hypothesis, then an adjunctive approach in the management of heart failure in African-Americans might be an increase in NO bioavailability along with a decrease in oxidant stress in a background consisting of traditional neurohormonal blockade (Figure 8.5). These issues may have direct bearing on the results of the African-American Heart Failure Trial (A-HeFT).

THE AFRICAN-AMERICAN HEART FAILURE TRIAL

The A-HeFT represents yet another landmark study [23]. In a population exclusively represented by African-Americans with heart failure, the adjunctive benefit of a fixed dose combination of ISDN/HYD was tested in a randomized double-blind placebo-controlled manner. One thousand and fifty African-Americans with predominantly NYHA class III heart failure were randomized to a fixed dose combination of ISDN/HYD vs placebo in the setting of contemporary medical therapy for heart failure. The primary endpoint was a composite of all-cause mortality, time to first hospitalization for heart failure and quality of life.

Inclusion criteria for this trial were left ventricular dysfunction with a measured ejection fraction of 35% or less, or 45% or less with a left ventricular internal dimension in diastole of 6.5 cm or greater; clinical stability on an evidence-based medical regimen; and heart failure disease severity of either NYHA class III or IV. The usual exclusionary criteria applied,

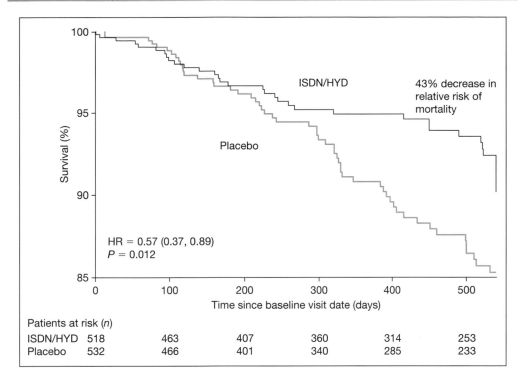

Figure 8.5 African-American Heart Failure Trial: mortality results.

e.g. pregnancy, recent acute coronary syndromes, atypical causes of heart failure and presence of other life-threatening illnesses.

Patients were treated with a fixed dose combination tablet of isosorbide dinitrate 20 mg/hydralazine 37.5 mg given as one or two tabs three times daily. The target dose was isosorbide dinitrate 120 mg and hydralazine 225 mg daily. Follow-up was for up to 18 months with periodic assessment of left ventricular size and function, B-type natriuretic peptide and quality of life along with assessment for the primary events. The study was terminated early (1050 of 1100 patients had been enrolled), due to a survival benefit of active therapy on the recommendation of an independent data safety and monitoring board. The patient characteristics are noted in Table 8.2. Background therapy in this trial was exceptional and consistent with contemporary evidence-based therapy for heart failure: renin–angiotensin system blockade was present in 87%. β-blockers were present in 77% of all patients. Aldosterone antagonism was utilized in nearly 40% of all patients.

The target dose of ISDN/HYD was achieved in 68% of subjects. The mean dose of isosorbide dinitrate was 88 mg daily and the mean dose of hydralazine was slightly less than 200 mg qd. Adverse effects of therapy included headaches (47%) and dizziness (29.3%) but headaches of the severity to require discontinuation of study drug occurred in only 7% of cases. There was only one adjudicated case of lupus but the incidence of joint pain was higher in those on study drug compared to placebo.

The results demonstrated a statistically significant reduction in the primary composite score consistent with a favorable effect of therapy. The individual components of the composite were positive as well. All-cause mortality was reduced by 43%, time to first hospitalization was reduced by 39% and the quality of life scores reflected an improvement in quality of life [23]. The implications of these findings are remarkable. Given the excellent utilization

Table 8.2 A-HeFT baseline characteristics

	ISDN/HYD (n = 518)	Placebo (n = 532)
Age	57	57
Male gender (%)	56	64
Weight (kg)	93	94
NYHA class III/IV (%)	97/3	95/5
Etiology of LV dysfunction (%)	–	–
Ischemic heart disease	23	23
Hypertension	40	37
Idiopathic dilated cardiomyopathy	25	28
Systolic BP (mmHg)	127	125
Diastolic BP (mmHg)	78	76
Ejection fraction (%)	24	24
Diabetes (%)	45	37
Renal insufficiency (%)	16	18
Implantable cardiac defibrillator (%)	17	17
Cardiac resynchronization therapy (%)	2	2

of evidence-based medical therapy for heart failure, the 'placebo' group provided an opportunity to evaluate the benefit of standard medical therapy for heart failure in African-Americans. The 1-year survival of ~90% in this group on standard medical therapy is consistent with that which would be anticipated for patients with stable, chronic ambulatory class III heart failure. Thus, to achieve a further 43% reduction in the risk of death with the adjunctive administration of isosorbide dinitrate/hydralazine is quite remarkable. No other adjunctive treatment regimens for heart failure, including angiotensin receptor antagonists, aldosterone antagonists and even implantable defibrillators, have achieved a similar magnitude of benefit when added to ACE inhibitors and β-blockers as background therapy for heart failure. When interpreted in the context of the 47% mortality advantage seen in V-HeFT-I, the similarity of benefit irrespective of background therapy (i.e. 47% when background therapy is digoxin and diuretics vs 43% when background therapy is diuretics, ACE inhibitors and β-blockers), would implicate a novel mechanism of action that is not otherwise modulated by standard therapies. Neither V-HeFT-I or A-HeFT were designed to test the benefit of NO enhancement so caution is exercised in implicating certainty regarding the mechanisms of the salutary benefit of isosorbide dinitrate/hydralazine. Nevertheless it is at least hypothesis-generating to consider enhanced NO availability and a reduction in oxidative stress as imputed mechanisms of action. The most recent data outputs from A-HeFT have now suggested the potential of genetic biomarkers to predict responsiveness to this therapy. Further research is required to better understand the potential advantages of NO enhancement and, importantly, to identify the more precise markers of responsiveness to this regimen other than race.

ADDITIONAL THERAPEUTIC COMMENTS

None of the trials investigating angiotensin receptor antagonists had a sufficiently sized sub-group of African-Americans to derive any meaningful data on responsiveness. Similarly, the two major trials using aldosterone antagonists were almost devoid of African-American participation – even though signals from genomic investigations might suggest the potential for unique responsiveness of aldosterone antagonism in African-Americans [24, 25]. Early retrospective analyses of the implantable cardioverter defibrillator (ICD) trials in heart failure have suggested a similar responsiveness to ICD therapy in African-Americans yet ICDs may be underutilized in African-Americans with left ventricular dysfunction.

DISPARATE HEALTHCARE

No discussion of the impact of race on clinical outcomes in cardiovascular disease can be complete without consideration of the non-physiologic factors that are operative and that do indeed affect the health status of certain 'special populations' affected by heart failure. Access to healthcare remains a challenge for at-risk racial/ethnic populations and a lack of cultural awareness within healthcare systems and healthcare providers exerts a negative impact as well. The A-HeFT data derived from a clinical trial with an intensive patient support infrastructure demonstrate the expected survival benefit from standard therapies for heart failure yet epidemiologic data suggest a higher risk of observed mortality in this same cohort. Almost assuredly these observations are not due to physiologic differences but more global quality of care concerns and indeed represent perhaps the largest challenge in appropriately managing heart failure in special populations.

CONCLUSIONS

Symptomatic left ventricular dysfunction may not be the same illness in all patient types. Heart failure in African-Americans is likely to be a unique disease entity. Its natural history, epidemiology, and disease outcomes vary from heart failure in white patients. The influence of hypertension is inescapable and carries with it important public health concerns for more proactive disease prevention through effective treatment. Even though tantalizing genetic data are emerging, it is still too early in the process to supplant race for genetics – much more work needs to be done to better understand the context in which genetic data should be best interpreted. The data regarding responsiveness to contemporary evidence-based medical therapy are inconsistent but there are no data to support avoidance of evidence-based standard therapy, specifically, ACE inhibitors and β-blockers.

Ongoing efforts to explain the excess cardiovascular disease burden in African-Americans have targeted mechanisms that lead to more malignant expressions of hypertension and physiologic/genetic profiles that might predispose patients to more advanced left ventricular dysfunction and/or lesser responsiveness to medical therapy. The newest theory focuses on endothelial homeostasis with diminished NO bioavailability as the primary variable. The vasodilating regimen of ISDN/HYD has been identified as one that potentially increases NO bioavailability. A-HeFT tested the benefit of a fixed dose combination of the vasodilators ISDN/HYD in a group of patients self-identified as African-American with class III heart failure already on appropriate medical therapy. The striking findings of an additional 43% improvement in mortality, 39% decrement in time to first hospitalization and improved quality of life represent landmark data. At present, major guidelines now strongly suggest that African-Americans with class III heart failure should be treated with ACE inhibitors and β-blockers as cornerstone therapy with strong consideration given to the addition of ISDN/HYD.

REFERENCES

1. Hunt SA, Abraham WT, Chin MH et al. ACC/AHA 2005 guideline update for the diagnosis and management of chronic heart failure in the adult: a report of the American College of Cardiology/American Heart Association Task Force on Practice Guidelines (Writing Committee to Update the 2001 Guidelines for the Evaluation and Management of Heart Failure): developed in collaboration with the American College of Chest Physicians and the International Society for Heart and Lung Transplantation: endorsed by the Heart Rhythm Society. *Circulation* 2005; 112:e154–e235.
2. Yancy CW. Heart failure in African Americans: a cardiovascular enigma [editorial]. *J Card Fail* 2000; 6:183–186.
3. Adams KF, Lindenfeld J, Arnold MJ, Baker DW, Barnard DH et al. Heart Failure Society of America 2006 Comprehensive Heart Failure Practice Guideline. Available at www.hfsa.org
4. American Heart Association. Heart Disease and Stroke Statistics–2006 Update. Dallas, TX: American Heart Association; 2006.

5. Williams DR, Rucker TD. Understanding and addressing racial disparities in health care. *Health Care Financ Rev* 2000; 21:75–90.

6. Chobanian AV, Bakris GL, Black HR *et al.* Seventh report of the Joint National Committee on Prevention, Detection, Evaluation, and Treatment of High Blood Pressure. *Hypertension* 2003; 42:1206–1252.

7. Douglas JG, Bakris GL, Epstein M *et al.* Management of high blood pressure in African Americans: consensus statement of the Hypertension in African Americans Working Group of the International Society on Hypertension in Blacks. *Arch Intern Med* 2003; 163:525–541.

8. Smedley BD, Stith AY, Nelson AR (eds). Unequal Treatment: Confronting Racial and Ethnic Disparities in Health Care. Washington, DC: The National Academies Press, 2003.

9. Dries DL, Exner DV, Gersh BJ, Cooper HA, Carson PE, Domanski MJ. Racial differences in the outcome of left ventricular dysfunction. *N Engl J Med* 1999; 340:609–616.

10. Exner DV, Dries DL, Domanski MJ, Cohn JN. Lesser response to angiotensin-converting-enzyme inhibitor therapy in black as compared with white patients with left ventricular dysfunction. *N Engl J Med* 2001; 344:1351–1357.

11. Shekelle PG, Rich MW, Morton SC, Atkinson SW, Tu W, Maglione M, Rhodes S, Barrett M, Fonarow GC, Greenberg B, Heidenreich PA, Knabel T, Konstam MA, Steimle A, Stevenson LW. Efficacy of angiotensin-converting enzyme inhibitors and beta-blockers in the management of left ventricular systolic dysfunction according to race, gender, and diabetic status: a meta-analysis of major clinical trials. *J Am Coll Cardiol* 2003; 41:1529–1538.

12. The Beta-Blocker Evaluation of Survival Trial Investigators. A trial of the beta-blocker bucindolol in patients with advanced chronic heart failure. *N Engl J Med* 2001; 344:1659–1667.

13. Unpublished data; personal communication. L. Waggoner.

14. Yancy CW, Fowler MB, Colucci WS, Gilbert EM, Bristow MR, Cohn JN, Lukas MA, Young ST, Packer M, for the US Carvedilol Heart Failure Study Group. Race and the response to adrenergic blockade with carvedilol in patients with chronic heart failure. *N Engl J Med* 2001; 344:1358–1365.

15. Packer M, Coats AJS, Fowler MB, Katus HA, Krum H, Mohacsi P, Rouleau JL, Tendera M, Castaigne A, Roecker EB, Schultz MK, DeMets DL, for the Carvedilol Prospective Randomized Cumulative Survival Study Group. Effect of carvedilol on survival in severe chronic heart failure. *N Engl J Med* 2001; 344:1651–1658.

16. Cohn JN, Archibald DG, Ziesche S, Franciosa JA, Harston WE, Tristani FE, Dunkman WB, Jacobs W, Francis GS, Flohr KH, Goldman S, Cobb FR, Shah PM, Saunders R, Fletcher RD, Loeb HS, Hughes VC, Baker B. Effect of vasodilator therapy on mortality in chronic congestive heart failure: results of a Veterans Administration Cooperative Study. *N Engl J Med* 1986; 314:1547–1552.

17. Carson P, Ziesche S, Johnson G, Cohn JN, for the Vasodilator-Heart Failure Trial Study Group. Racial differences in response to therapy for heart failure: analysis of the Vasodilator-Heart Failure Trials. *J Card Fail* 1999; 5:178–187.

18. Cohn JN, Johnson G, Ziesche S *et al.* A comparison of enalapril with hydralazine-isosorbide dinitrate in the treatment of chronic congestive heart failure. *N Engl J Med* 1991; 325:303–310.

19. Dries DL, Strong MH, Cooper S, Drazner MH. Efficacy of angiotensin-converting enzyme inhibition in reducing progression from asymptomatic left ventricular dysfunction to symptomatic heart failure in black and white patients. *J Am Coll Cardiol* 2002; 40:311–317.

20. MERIT-HF Study Group. Effect of metoprolol CR/XL in chronic heart failure: Metoprolol CR/XL Randomised Intervention Trial in Congestive Heart Failure (MERIT-HF). *Lancet* 1999; 353:2001–2007.

21. Hare JM. Nitroso-redox balance in the cardiovascular system. *N Engl J Med* 2004; 351:2112–2114.

22. Prabhu SD. Nitric oxide protects against pathologic ventricular remodeling: reconsideration of the role of NO in the failing heart. *Circ Res* 2004; 94:115–157.

23. Taylor AL, Ziesche S, Yancy C, Carson P, D'Agostino R Jr, Ferdinand K, Taylor M, Adams K, Sabolinski M, Worcel M, Cohn JN, for the African-American Heart Failure Trial Investigators. Combination of isosorbide dinitrate and hydralazine in blacks with heart failure. *N Engl J Med* 2004; 351:2049–2057.

24. McNamara DM, Holubkov R, Postava L, Ramani R, Janosko K, Mathier M, MacGowan GA, Murali S, Feldman AM, London B. Effect of the Asp298 variant of endothelial nitric oxide synthase on survival for patients with congestive heart failure. *Circulation* 2003; 107:1598–1602.

25. McNamara DM, Tam SW, Sabolinski ML, Tobelmann P, Janosko K, Taylor AL, Cohn JN, Feldman A, Worcel M. Aldosterone synthase promoter polymorphism predicts outcome in African Americans with heart failure: results from the A-HeFT Trial. *J Am Coll Cardiol* 2006; 48:1277–1282.

9

B-type natriuretic peptides in heart failure

J. Patel, J. Thomas Heywood

INTRODUCTION

The development of the therapeutic use of B-type natriuretic peptides (BNP) began in 1956 with the publication by Kirsch [1] of electron micrographs of dense granules seen in guinea pig atria which resembled secretory granules seen in the pancreas. The concentration of these granules was later shown to change with alterations of water and electrolyte balances in experimental animals [2]. Jamieson and Palade [3] reported similar granules in human atria in 1964. Baines *et al.* [4] injected an extract of rodent atrial wall intravenously into a second animal with a marked diuretic effect. A similar preparation *in vitro* caused relaxation of aortic rings, therefore demonstrating a vascular effect in addition to their natriuretic properties [5]. Sudoh *et al.* [6] in 1988 described a natriuretic-like peptide found in porcine brains and named this substance 'brain natriuretic peptide'. Several years later 'brain' natriuretic peptide (BNP) was found in human ventricular tissue [7]. The levels of BNP have been shown to be nearly twice as high in the cardiac tissue of New York Heart Association Class I (NYHA I) and II patients as compared to controls, and nearly 7-fold higher in NYHA III and IV patients as compared to controls [8]. In the early 1990s human BNP was synthesized (nesiritide, Scios, Sunnyvale, California) and the neurohormonal, hemodynamic, and renal effects were reported [9–14]. Clinical trials demonstrated symptomatic and hemodynamic benefits, and the drug was approved for use in the US in 2001 [15–17].

PHYSIOLOGIC EFFECTS OF BNP INFUSIONS

Since its discovery in 1988 and its isolation and sequencing in 1990 [18], the physiologic effects of the infusion of human BNP produced by recombinant DNA technology has been elucidated in a series of elegant studies [9–11, 18]. BNP is a potent vasodilator; studies have shown a consistent fall in right atrial, pulmonary artery and pulmonary artery wedge pressure [9, 11, 12]. In addition, mean arterial pressure and systemic vascular resistance fall while the cardiac index increases [9, 12]. At low doses of the agent (≤ 0.01 µg/kg/min), the heart rate declines, while at higher doses it may increase [9]. Elkayam *et al.* [19] demonstrated renal artery dilation with intravenous BNP infusion.

In addition to these hemodynamic effects, there are important neurohormonal responses that have been described. Based on animal studies, BNP is thought to act as a neurotransmitter causing changes in salt appetite, vasopressin secretion from the hypothalamus, and

---

Jigar D. Patel, MD, Fellow, Heart Failure Program, Scripps Clinic, Department of Cardiology, La Jolla, California, USA.

J. Thomas Heywood, MD, FACC, Director, Heart Failure Recovery and Research Center, Scripps Clinic, Department of Cardiology, La Jolla, California, USA.

angiotensin A-II induced water intake [20]. In patients with congestive heart failure, aldosterone levels consistently fall with short-term BNP infusions [10, 11, 15]. The effects of BNP on serum norepinephrine levels have been more variable, with some investigators reporting reductions and others reporting no effect [10, 12, 15]. BNP infusion also reduced local norepinephrine spillover from the heart and kidneys in CHF patients, more so than in normal subjects [21].

RENAL EFFECTS

The renal effects of BNP are more difficult to study and hence there are much fewer data concerning them. Moreover, the effects may be complicated by the interplay of the drug's hemodynamic effects versus its intrarenal actions on the glomerular vascular bed and renal tubular handling of sodium and water. As its name implies, BNP produces a natriuresis when infused into subjects without heart failure [11]. In addition, urine volume and glomerular filtration rate (GFR) increase significantly [22]. On the other hand, in subjects with congestive heart failure, no study has demonstrated an improvement in GFR [9, 11, 12, 14]. Sodium excretion and urine volume have increased with BNP infusions in two studies [9, 11] and have not increased in two others [12, 14]. The two studies that did demonstrate increased urine output and sodium excretion used higher doses of BNP than are currently used. However, Abraham et al. [12] presented data that the diuretic response to BNP was variable with some subjects showing a brisk diuresis. Urinary sodium excretion in this study correlated extremely well with increased lithium clearance, suggesting that BNP may have increased distal tubular sodium delivery in some patients but not in others. Resistance to natriuretic peptides, especially atrial natriuretic peptide, has been described in animals with experimentally induced heart failure [23]. Thus, despite favorable hemodynamic and neurohormonal effects, BNP infusion has been shown to have less of an effect on urinary output and sodium excretion in subjects with heart failure than those with normal cardiac function, and no statistically significant improvement in GFR in those with heart failure. However, the effect on sodium excretion and urinary volume appears to be heterogeneous in heart failure patients [12].

Whereas the above studies of renal function were done while diuretics and other medication were held, Wang et al. [24] studied 15 patients with worsening renal function and decompensated heart failure in a randomized, double-blind, placebo-controlled, crossover trial of a 24-hour infusion of nesiritide vs placebo combined with diuretics. GFR was measured using iothalamate clearance and renal plasma flow via para-amino hippurate clearance. Furosemide dose was constant for each patient on both days and administered at 6 h into the infusion; it varied widely from 40 mg orally to 240 mg intravenously based on the patient history. There was no significant difference between nesiritide and placebo in terms of urine output, net sodium excretion, GFR or effective renal plasma flow. This study has several limitations: nesiritide was given to some of the patients after several days of diuretic administration, so that the renal effects of nesiritide may have been blunted; the total diuretic dose was high which may have impaired renal function; and the cohort studied was quite small [25]. Nonetheless this is one of the best designed trials evaluating the renal effects of nesiritide in a real world setting and no benefit was seen in terms of renal function.

MAJOR CLINICAL TRIALS

EFFICACY TRIAL

Several randomized clinical trials have been conducted with synthetic human BNP (Nesiritide, Scios – Sunnyvale, California). The first of these was the Efficacy/Comparative Trial [15]. The Efficacy arm was a randomized, double-blind trial, conducted in 23 US medical centers, that allocated patients in 1:1:1 fashion to either (1) placebo of 5% dextrose in water, (2) nesiritide 0.3 μg/kg bolus followed by 0.015 μg/kg/min infusion, or (3) nesiritide 0.6 μg/kg bolus followed by 0.03 μg/kg/min infusion. The use of dopamine, dobutamine, milrinone, and intravenous vasodilators was discontinued prior to the study. The allocation was blinded for the 6 h of the infusion, following which the allocation was revealed to the investigator clinicians. During the 6-h infusion and in the 4 h prior, all oral and intravenous vasoactive medications and all intravenous diuretics were withheld.

The main inclusion criteria for the Efficacy arm were symptomatic heart failure sufficient to warrant hospital admission for treatment with one or more intravenous vasoactive agents in addition to diuretics. They were also required to have hemodynamic monitoring *via* a pulmonary artery catheter. The hemodynamic inclusion criteria were pulmonary capillary wedge pressure at least 18 mmHg, cardiac index no greater than 2.7 l/min, and systolic blood pressure at least 90 mmHg.

The exclusion criteria for the Efficacy arm were recent myocardial infarction or unstable angina (within prior 48 h), constrictive pericarditis, and active myocarditis. Also, patients with history of clinically important valvular stenosis, hypertrophic cardiomyopathy, restrictive cardiomyopathy, or primary pulmonary hypertension were excluded.

The primary endpoint measured in the Efficacy trial was change in pulmonary capillary wedge pressure after 6 h of blinded infusion. The secondary endpoints included global clinical status, clinical symptoms, cardiac index, mean arterial pressure, mean pulmonary artery pressure, systolic blood pressure, serum aldosterone levels, and serum norepinephrine levels.

Results from the Efficacy trial, which randomized 127 patients, showed that pulmonary capillary wedge pressure was lowered 26–32% in the nesiritide groups, which was significantly better than placebo, $P < 0.001$. Also significantly better than placebo were reductions in right atrial pressure ($P < 0.001$), systemic vascular resistance ($P < 0.001$), systolic blood pressure ($P = 0.001$), mean pulmonary artery pressure ($P < 0.001$), and systolic pulmonary artery pressure ($P < 0.001$). Heart rate was unchanged by nesiritide ($P = 0.22$). Symptoms were also significantly improved, such as dyspnea, which was improved in 50–56% of the nesiritide group, vs 12% of placebo group ($P < 0.001$). Fatigue was improved in 32–38% of nesiritide-treated patients, vs 5% of placebo-treated patients ($P < 0.001$). Global clinical status was better in 60–67% of the nesiritide-treated group, vs only 14% of placebo-treated patients ($P < 0.001$). All of the improvements in symptom measurements were statistically significant. The Efficacy trial also showed significant reductions in plasma aldosterone levels ($P = 0.03$), and increase in urine output ($P = 0.004$), with the two nesiritide groups compared to placebo.

The Comparative arm was essentially another randomized trial conducted concurrently with the Efficacy trial. The Comparative trial was meant to compare nesiritide with standard intravenous agents used in the treatment of decompensated heart failure. This was a randomized open-label trial, at 46 US medical centers. Subjects were randomized in 1:1:1 fashion to receive either (1) standard therapy – a single intravenous vasoactive agent (57% dobutamine, 19% milrinone, 18% nitroglycerin, 6% dopamine, or 1% amrinone), routinely used in the management of decompensated heart failure, according to physician judgment, (2) nesiritide 0.3 μg/kg bolus followed by 0.015 μg/kg/min infusion, or (3) nesiritide 0.6 μg/kg bolus followed by 0.03 μg/kg/min infusion. The dose of nesiritide was blinded to the treating investigator/physicians. Intravenous diuretics could be added, as could a second intravenous vasoactive agent. The duration of therapy was 1–5 days.

Similar to the Efficacy trial, patients were included in the Comparative arm if they had symptomatic heart failure requiring admission to the hospital for treatment with an intravenous vasoactive agent, in addition to intravenous diuretics. However, a pulmonary artery catheter was not required. The exclusion criteria included all the exclusion criteria from the Efficacy trial described above. Additionally, patients were also ineligible for the Comparative trial if they had been given intravenous vasoactive agent for more than 4 h.

The endpoints of the Comparative trial were global clinical status and clinical symptoms. The results showed that global clinical status was significantly improved in all three groups. Dyspnea and fatigue were similarly improved in all groups but not at a statistically significant threshold. The use of intravenous diuretics was 84% in the nesiritide 0.015 μg/kg/min group, 74% in the nesiritide 0.03 μg/kg/min group, and 96% in the standard therapy group; $P < 0.001$ for both nesiritide groups (Table 9.1).

PRECEDENT

The Prospective Randomized Evaluation of Cardiac Ectopy with Dobutamine or Natrecor Therapy (PRECEDENT) trial was intended to compare the effect of nesiritide vs dobutamine on healthcare utilization and long-term mortality and morbidity outcomes [16]. Patients were recruited if they had symptomatic decompensated heart failure requiring hospital admission for treatment with intravenous vasoactive agents. They were excluded if they had been treated with intravenous vasoactive agents in the 4 h prior to randomization, if they were in shock, or if they had systolic blood pressure <90. Valvular stenosis, hypertrophic cardiomyopathy, constrictive pericarditis, acute myocarditis, and complex congenital heart disease were also reasons for exclusion from the study.

Patients were randomized in 1:1:1 allocation to either (1) standard vasoactive therapy (dobutamine), (2) nesiritide 0.3 μg/kg bolus followed by 0.015 μg/kg/min infusion, or (3) nesiritide 0.6 μg/kg bolus followed by 0.03 μg/kg/min infusion. The randomization was open-label, but the participating centers were blinded to dose of nesiritide.

The endpoints of the PRECEDENT study included duration of treatment with intravenous vasoactive medication and need for additional vasoactive agents. Healthcare utilization was also analyzed by the endpoints of hospital length-of-stay, and hospital re-admissions through day 21 following randomization. Finally, 6-month mortality was also examined.

The PRECEDENT trial recruited 305 patients. The standard therapy group consisted of 102 patients, but the study analyzed only 58 who were treated with dobutamine. The results of the PRECEDENT study showed that duration of intravenous vasoactive treatment was significantly shorter in the nesiritide groups – 42 h with nesiritide 0.015 μg/kg/min, 41 h with nesiritide 0.03 μg/kg/min, and 65 h with dobutamine; $P = 0.016$. Intravenous diuretic use was significantly lower in the nesiritide groups – 100% with dobutamine, 82% with nesiritide 0.01 μg/kg/min, 74% with nesiritide 0.03 μg/kg/min; $P < 0.001$. Endpoints that did not reach statistical significance included initial hospital length-of-stay ($P = 0.411$), and all-cause re-admission ($P = 0.085$). Mortality at 6 months was 18% with nesiritide 0.015 μg/kg/min group compared to 31% with dobutamine, statistically significant at $P = 0.04$.

VMAC

The Vasodilatation in the Management of Acute CHF (VMAC) trial was devised to examine the hemodynamic and clinical effects of a natriuretic peptide added to standard care, compared with intravenous nitroglycerin and standard care for patients with decompensated heart failure [17]. Patients were included if they had dyspnea at rest requiring hospitalization for intravenous vasoactive therapy. In those patients that had pulmonary artery catheters, the pulmonary capillary wedge pressure was required to be at least 20 mmHg. Patients also had to satisfy two of the following criteria: (1) jugular venous distention, (2) paroxysmal nocturnal dyspnea or 2-pillow orthopnea within 72 h of study entry, (3) abdominal discomfort due to mesenteric congestion, or (4) chest X-ray findings consistent with decompensated congestive heart failure. Patients were excluded if they had systolic blood pressure <90 mmHg, shock, volume depletion, or unstable clinical status that precluded

Table 9.1 Summary of major clinical trials

Trial	Design	Inclusion/exclusion	Endpoints	Results
Efficacy	Randomized, double-blind, 1:1:1 (1) Placebo (2) Nesiritide 0.3 μg/kg bolus, then 0.015 μg/kg/min (3) Nesiritide 0.6 μg/kg bolus, then 0.03 μg/kg/min duration infusion for 6 h Dopamine, dobutamine, milrinone, and vasodilators stopped before study IV diuretics not permitted	HF warranting admission Swan–Ganz catheter PCWP ≥18 mmHg CI ≤2.7 l/min SBP ≥90 mmHg Exclusion: MI or unstable angina within 48 h Constrictive pericarditis Active myocarditis Valvular stenosis HCM or RCM Primary pulmonary hypertension	Primary: change in PCWP Secondary: global clinical status Clinical symptoms Change in CI Change in MAP, RAP, mPAP, SBP Serum aldosterone and norepinephrine levels	§ PCWP lowered – 6.0–9.6 mmHg nesiritide, raised by 2.0 mmHg placebo § Nesiritide lowered RAP, SVR, SBP, mPAP § Dyspnea improved – 50–56% nesiritide, 12% placebo § Fatigue improved – 32–38% nesiritide, 5% placebo § Global clinical status improved – 60–67% nesiritide, 14% placebo * Nesiritide reduced aldosterone and increased urine output
Comparative	Randomized, open-label, dose of nesiritide was blinded (1) Standard care – single IV vasoactive agent (2) Nesiritide 0.3 μg/kg bolus, then 0.015 μg/kg/min (3) Nesiritide 0.6 μg/kg bolus, then 0.03 μg/kg/min Duration 1–5 days IV diuretics permitted	HF warranting admission Exclusion: MI or unstable angina within 48 h Constrictive pericarditis Active myocarditis Valvular stenosis HCM or RCM Primary pulmonary hypertension Received IV vasoactive agents for more than 4 h	Primary: global clinical status Clinical symptoms Secondary: Use of IV diuretics	(NS) Global clinical status equally improved in all three groups (NS) Dyspnea and fatigue equally improved in all three groups Use of IV diuretics: 96% in standard therapy vs §84% in nesiritide 0.015 μg/kg/min §74% in nesiritide 0.03 μg/kg/min

Table 9.1 (continued)

Trial	Design	Inclusion/exclusion	Endpoints	Results
PRECEDENT	Randomized, open-label, blinded to dose of nesiritide (1) Standard therapy (dobutamine) (2) Nesiritide 0.3 µg/kg bolus, then 0.015 µg/kg/min (3) Nesiritide 0.6 µg/kg bolus, then 0.03 µg/kg/min	Decompensated HF requiring hospital admission Exclusion: treatment with IV vasoactive agents in prior 4 h Shock or SBP <90 mmHg Valvular stenosis HCM Constrictive pericarditis Acute myocarditis Complex congential heart disease	Prospective: duration of treatment with IV vasoactive agents Need for additional vasoactive agents Hospital LOS All-cause hospital re-admissions through day 21 Retrospective: 6-month mortality	Duration of IV vasoactive therapy: 65 h with dobutamine vs **42 h with nesiritide 0.015 **41 h with nesiritide 0.03 IV diuretic use 100% for dobutamine vs §82% with nesiritide 0.015 §74% with nesiritide 0.03 Hospital LOS – median 4.5 days for dobutamine vs (NS) 5 days for nesiritide 0.015 (NS) 5 days for nesiritide 0.03 Re-admissions through day 21 – 20% with dobutamine vs *8% nesiritide 0.015 (NS) 11% nesiritide 0.03 6-month mortality: 31% with dobutamine *18% nesiritide 0.015 (NS) 24% nesiritide 0.03
VMAC	Randomized, double-blind, double-dummy Non-PA catheter group: (1) Placebo (2) Nitroglycerin dose-titrated (3) Nesiritide 2 µg/kg bolus, then 0.01 µg/kg/min fixed dose PA catheter group: (1) Placebo	Dyspnea due to decompensated HF requiring hospital admission Two of following: (1) Jugular venous distention (2) Nocturnal dyspnea or orthopnea (3) Abdominal discomfort (4) CXR – decompensated HF	Primary: At 3 h, change in PCWP Change in self-assessment dyspnea Secondary: time to onset change in PCWP At 24 h, change in PCWP 24 h self-assessment dyspnea Self-assess global clinical status	3-h PCWP reduction (−3.8 mmHg) nitroglycerin vs *(−5.8 mmHg) nesiritide 3-h self-assess dyspnea (NS) nesiritide vs nitroglycerin 24-h PCWP reduction (−6.3 mmHg) nitroglycerin

		Overall safety profile	
	(2) Nitroglycerin dose-titrated (3) Nesiritide 2 μg/kg bolus, then 0.01 μg/kg/min fixed dose (4) Same as (3) except nesiritide could be increased every 3 h to max 0.03 μg/kg/min	Catheter group: PCWP ≥20 mmHg Exclusion: SBP <90 mmHg or shock Volume depletion Too unstable for 3-h placebo Mechanical ventilation Contraindication to IV vasodilators Estimated survival <35 days	*(−8.2 mmHg) nesiritide 24-h self-assess dyspnea and global clinical status (NS) nitroglycerin vs nesiritide Any adverse event: 14% placebo 27% nitroglycerin *18% nesiritide
FUSION I	Randomized, open-label groups: (1) Nesiritide 1.0 μg/kg bolus, then 0.005 μg/kg/min (2) Nesiritide 2.0 μg/kg bolus, then 0.01 μg/kg/min (3) Usual care each infusion 4–6 h once-weekly infusion for 12 weeks Patients classified as high risk if: (1) Diabetes mellitus (2) NYHA class IV (3) Renal insufficiency (4) Ischemic left ventricular dysfunction (5) Documented ventricular arrhythmias (6) Serum creatinine >2.0 mg/dl	NYHA III or IV HF for ≥60 days prior to study Appropriate background therapy 6-minute walk <400 m Two hospitalizations in past year, 1 of which in past 30 days Instead of hospitalization, could also use unscheduled outpatient visit for IV vasoactive drugs Exclusion: past or imminent organ transplant hemodialysis or anticipated MI in past 30 days Biventricular pacemaker in past 60 days ICD in past 30 days	Primary: Adverse events (investigator-report) Serious adverse events Premature stopping of infusion Laboratory results Vital signs Increased creatinine Retrospective: (*post hoc* analysis) Combined endpoint death and hospitalization All-cause death All-cause hospitalization	210 patients, 1645 infusions 1% of infusions stopped prematurely Usual care vs either dose nesiritide: (NS) worsening HF (NS) hypotension (NS) renal adverse effects (NS) increased creatinine All-cause death/hospitalization: 58% usual care vs: (NS) 46% nesiritide 0.005 (NS) 49% nesiritide 0.01 For high-risk group, all-cause death/hospitalization: 78% usual care vs *42% nesiritide 0.005 (NS) 65% nesiritide 0.01 For high-risk group, median days alive out of hospital:

Table 9.1 (continued)

Trial	Design	Inclusion/exclusion	Endpoints	Results
	(7) Recent outpatient parenteral agents			67 days usual care vs *76 days nesiritide 0.005 (NS) 77 days nesiritide 0.01
PROACTION	Randomized, double-blind (1) Placebo (2) Nesiritide 2 µg/kg bolus, then 0.01 µg/kg/min infusion 12 h (12 h more by choice) At least 1 dose IV diuretics Must receive oral ACE inhibitor 3 h after study	Presented to ED with history of HF, fluid overload by exam, evidence of increased filling pressures by exam, dyspnea at rest or minimal exertion (walking 20 ft) Judged to require 12 h treatment in observation unit or hospital Classified as HF if two of the following: (1) Nocturnal dyspnea or orthopnea within 72 h (2) Jugular venous distention (3) Abdominal symptoms (4) 5 pound weight gain in past month (5) CXR consistent with heart failure (6) Pulmonary rales Exclusion: SBP <90 mmHg Contraindication to vasodilator Elevated cardiac enzymes IV vasodilators or oral ACE inhibitor in 24 h before enrollment Chronic dialysis Estimated survival <30 days	Primary: Adverse events Serious adverse events Vital signs Hospital admission Re-admission in 30 days LOS on initial visit LOS on subsequent visits within 30 days Self-assessed dyspnea scores (seven-point scale) at 12 h	250 patients Any adverse events 12 h: 25% placebo vs (NS) 31% nesiritide Any adverse events 24 h: 37% placebo (NS) 45% nesiritide Asymptomatic hypotension 24 h: 3% placebo vs *10% nesiritide Symptomatic hypotension 24 h: 1% placebo vs (NS) 4% nesiritide LOS median on initial visit: 5.5 days placebo vs (NS) 5.1 days nesiritide LOS on subsequent admissions: 7.1 days placebo vs *3.1 days nesiritide Re-admission rate: 23% placebo vs *10% nesiritide Dyspnea score improvement: 2 points better placebo vs (NS) 2 points better nesiritide

Trial	Design / Treatment	Inclusion / Exclusion	Endpoints	Results
FUSION II	Randomized, double-blind Once or twice weekly infusions: (1) nesiritide bolus 2 mcg/kg, then 0.01 mcg/kg/min infusion (2) placebo	NYHA class IV NYHA class III only if CrCl <60 ml/min LVEF <40% ≥2 hospitalizations in last 12 months, with last within 60 days but no closer than 5 days Optimal treatment with chronic oral medications unless documented intolerance Exclusion: SBP <90 mmHg, >2 outpatient infusions of vasoactive therapy within last 30 days without hospitalization, biventricular pacemaker within 45 days or ICD within 15 days, dialysis, acute MI within 30 days	Primary: time to all-cause death or first hospitalization for CV or renal causes Secondary: # of CV or renal hospitalizations Days alive and out of hospital Time to CV death	Patients:: 300 placebo, 600 nesiritide (NS) Primary endpoint: 36.7% nesiritide, 36.8% placebo (NS) Mortality: 9.5% nesiritide, 9.6% placebo # hospitalizations: 1.0 nesiritide, 0.8 placebo
NAPA	double-blind, exploratory study, randomized to minimum of 24 hour infusion of: (1) nesiritide, no bolus, infusion 0.01 mcg/kg/min (2) placebo	Undergoing CABG with or without mitral replacement or repair NYHA II – IV LVEF ≤40% Exclusion: aortic valve repair or replacement, dialysis, restrictive or obstructive cardiomyopathy; pericarditis, pericardial tamponade, PCWP <15, CVP <6, SBP <90, congenital heart	Primary: Max rise in SCr in 14d Max decline GFR Use of IV inotrope, vasopressor, or vasodilator Max decline PCWP up to 24 hours Urine output up to 24 hours Secondary: Duration of intubation, ICU LOS, hospital LOS, 30 day mortality, 180 day mortality	272 patients § Max rise SCr nesiritide 0.15 mg/dl placebo 0.34 mg/dl § Max decline GFR nesiritide 10.2 ml/min placebo 17.8 ml/min (NS) Inotrope or vasoactive use nesiritide 96% placebo 95% (NS) Max decline PCWP nesiritide 2.8 placebo 1.9 § Urine output nesiritide 2926 placebo 2350

CABG = coronary artery bypass graft; CI = cardiac index; CVP = central venous pressure; Crcl = creatinine clearance; CXR = chest X-ray; ED = Emergency Department; GFR = glomerular filtration rate; HCM = hypertrophic cardiomyopathy; HF = heart failure; ICD = implantable cardioverter-defibrillator; ICU = intensive care unit; LOS = length of stay; LVEF = left ventricular ejection fraction; MAP = mean arterial pressure; MI = myocardial infarction; mPAP = mean pulmonary artery pressure; NS = not significant; PA = pulmonary artery; PCWP = pulmonary capillary wedge pressure; RAP = right atrial pressure; RCM = restrictive cardiomyopathy; SBP = systolic blood pressure; SCr = serum creatinine; SVR = systemic vascular resistance; § = significant of the $P \leq 0.001$ level; * = significant at the $P \leq 0.005$ level

waiting 3 h through a potential placebo period. Other exclusion criteria included mechanical ventilation, and any contraindications to intravenous vasodilators. Also, patients were excluded if their estimated survival was <35 days.

The VMAC trial was a randomized, double-blind, double-dummy trial. The investigator-clinician decided if the subjects warranted placement of pulmonary artery catheter to aid in the management of the decompensated heart failure episode. The presence of pulmonary artery catheter determined stratification into two groups. The non-catheter group was randomly assigned to placebo, nitroglycerin that could be dose-titrated, or fixed-dose nesiritide at 2 μg/kg bolus followed by 0.01 μg/kg/min infusion. The catheter group was randomly assigned to these same three groups or to adjustable-dose nesiritide – 2 μg/kg bolus, 0.01 μg/kg/min infusion for 3 h, then infusion of nesiritide that could be increased every 3 h (if the pulmonary capillary wedge pressure was 20 mmHg or higher, and systolic blood pressure was at least 100 mmHg), to a maximum dose of nesiritide of 0.03 μg/kg/min.

Primary endpoints for the VMAC trial were changes by 3 h in pulmonary capillary wedge pressure (for the group with pulmonary artery catheter), and patient self-assessment of dyspnea. Other endpoints included time to onset of effect on pulmonary capillary wedge pressure, effect on pulmonary capillary wedge pressure 24 h after the start of the study drug, self-assessed dyspnea and global clinical status, and overall safety profile.

The VMAC trial was conducted at 55 US medical centers, and recruited 248 patients in the non-catheterized group, and 246 patients in the catheterized group. At 3 h, the pulmonary capillary wedge pressure was reduced by 5.8 mmHg with nesiritide and 2 mmHg with placebo ($P < 0.05$); the reduction with nesiritide was also significant when compared to nitroglycerin ($P < 0.05$). The right atrial pressure was also reduced more by nesiritide than nitroglycerin or placebo at 3 h (−3.1 mmHg and −2.6 mmHg respectively; $P < 0.05$. At 24 h, nesiritide still showed significantly greater reduction in pulmonary capillary wedge pressure than nitroglycerin; $P = 0.04$. At 24 h, the reduction in systolic blood pressure was not significantly different between the groups, −8.7 mmHg with nesiritide, and −8.1 mmHg with nitroglycerin; $P = 0.54$. The patient's self-assessment of dyspnea at 3 h was significantly better in nesiritide vs placebo groups ($P = 0.03$), but no different between nesiritide and nitroglycerin ($P = 0.56$). The 24-hour self-assessment of dyspnea ($P = 0.13$) and global clinical status ($P = 0.08$) were also not significantly different in the nesiritide and nitroglycerin groups.

The VMAC trial also examined safety data. The rate of any adverse event after 3 h of infusion was significantly lower in nesiritide vs nitroglycerin (51% and 68% respectively; $P < 0.001$). The rate of headache was also significantly lower (8% with nesiritide, 20% with nitroglycerin; $P < 0.001$). There was no difference between the two drugs in the rate of serious adverse events or change in serum creatinine at 30 days. Six-month mortality was also not different between the two (25% with nesiritide, 20% with nitroglycerin; $P = 0.32$).

FUSION

The Follow-Up Serial Infusion of Nesiritide (FUSION) trial was designed to examine the safety and feasibility of outpatient administration of nesiritide [26]. Patients were included if they had NYHA III or IV heart failure for at least 60 days prior to the study enrollment, and they were on appropriate background medical therapy. They also had to have 6-minute walk time of <400 m. They had to have two hospitalizations (or unscheduled outpatient visits for intravenous vasoactive therapy) for heart failure in the previous year, with one in the previous 30 days. Patients were excluded if they had past or imminent organ transplant, if they were on current hemodialysis, if they were anticipated to have hemodialysis, or if they had myocardial infarction in the previous 30 days. Other criteria for exclusion were biventricular pacemaker placement in the prior 60 days, or implantable cardioverter-defibrillator in the prior 30 days.

The FUSION trial was a randomized, open-label trial of usual care vs once-weekly nesiritide. Nesiritide was given as 1.0 µg/kg bolus followed by 0.005 µg/kg/min infusion for 4–6 h, or 2.0 µg/kg bolus followed by 0.01 µg/kg/min infusion for 4–6 h. The trial continued for 12 weeks, and then patients were followed for 4 weeks. No outpatient inotropes were permitted in the nesiritide groups. Patients were classified into a high risk group for a further analysis if they had at least four risk factors of the following: (1) diabetes mellitus, (2) NYHA class IV, (3) renal insufficiency, (4) ischemic left ventricular dysfunction, (5) documented ventricular arrhythmias, (6) serum creatinine >2.0 mg/dl, or (7) recent outpatient parenteral agents.

Since the FUSION trial was designed primarily to assess the safety and tolerability of nesiritide in the outpatient setting, the primary measures that were examined were investigator reports of adverse events, serious adverse events, stopping of the infusion, laboratory results, vital signs, and incidence of increased creatinine. Other parameters that were subsequently examined in *post hoc* analysis were combined endpoint of death and hospitalization, all-cause death, and all-cause hospitalizations.

During this study, 210 patients were recruited from 48 medical centers. There were 1645 total infusions given, of which 99% were completed. Of the 1% that were discontinued, two were stopped due to symptomatic hypotension, four due to asymptomatic hypotension, one due to angina, one due to myocardial infarction, one due to dehydration, and six due to administrative reasons. Of the completed infusions, there was no difference in the rate of worsening heart failure, symptomatic hypotension, asymptomatic hypotension, or renal adverse effects (such as increased serum urea nitrogen, increased serum creatinine, acute kidney failure, or oliguria). For the secondary endpoint of combined death and hospitalization, there was no significant difference between the nesiritide and usual care groups (58% with usual care; 46% with nesiritide 0.005 µg/kg/min, $P = 0.175$; 49% with nesiritide 0.01 µg/kg/min, $P = 0.385$). In the high-risk group (with four or more risk factors), the combined secondary endpoint of death or hospitalization was significantly lower in the nesiritide 0.005 µg/kg/min infusion group than the usual care group (42% and 78% respectively; $P = 0.017$), while there was no difference between nesiritide 0.01 µg/kg/min and usual care (65% and 78% respectively; $P = 0.323$). For this higher risk group, number of days alive and out of hospital was also significantly lower in the nesiritide 0.005 µg/kg/min infusion group than the usual care (76 and 67 days respectively; $P = 0.028$).

PROACTION

The Prospective Randomized Outcomes study of Acutely decompensated CHF Treated Initially as Outpatients with Nesiritide (PROACTION) trial was intended to examine the efficacy of early initiation of nesiritide by Emergency Departments, along with examination of the safety of such practice in the observation unit, where intensive monitoring is not routinely provided [27]. Patients were included if they presented to the Emergency Department with a medical history consistent with heart failure, fluid overload or evidence of increased filling pressures by clinical exam, and dyspnea at rest or with minimal exertion (walking 20 feet) judged to require at least 12 h of treatment in the observation unit or hospital setting. Heart failure was the etiology of dyspnea if at least two of the following criteria were met: (1) nocturnal dyspnea or two-pillow orthopnea within 72 h of presentation, (2) jugular venous distention, (3) abdominal symptoms such as discomfort, loss of appetite, or nausea, felt to be sequelae of congestion of intra-abdominal organs, (4) 5 pound weight gain in past month, (5) chest X-ray findings consistent with heart failure, or (6) pulmonary rales. Patients were excluded if systolic blood pressure was <90 mmHg, if they had medical contraindications to intravenous vasodilators, or if they had received intravenous vasodilators or oral ACE inhibitors in the 24 h before enrollment. Other contraindications included cardiac markers of myocardial necrosis, admission for rule out of acute coronary syndrome, chronic dialysis, or presence of medical condition that made survival past 30 days unlikely.

The PROACTION study was a randomized, double-blind study. Patients were randomized 1:1 to either placebo or nesiritide for 12 h in the observation unit, after which the investigator could continue the study drug infusion for another 12 h. After 24 h in the observation unit, the clinician decided on hospital admission or discharge. Nesiritide was given as 2 μg/kg bolus followed by 0.01 μg/kg/min infusion. The infusion could be increased every 3 h to a maximum rate of 0.03 μg/kg/min if systolic blood pressure was >100 mmHg. Patients were required to receive at least one dose of intravenous diuretics for their symptoms. They were also required to receive an oral ACE inhibitor 3 h after initiation of the study drug, unless contraindicated. Subjects were followed for 30 days after receiving the study drug in the observation unit.

The endpoints in PROACTION were safety endpoints of adverse effects, serious adverse effects (life-threatening, and including hospitalization for worsening heart failure), and vital signs. Efficacy endpoints included admission to the hospital after the index visit, re-admission within 30 days for any reason, length-of-stay on the index visit and assessments of dyspnea by the investigator.

The PROACTION trial enrolled 250 patients, 237 of whom received the study drug. Adverse events were no different in placebo vs nesiritide. At 24 h, asymptomatic hypotension was significantly higher in the nesiritide group than the placebo group (10% vs 3%; $P = 0.03$). Symptomatic hypotension was not significantly different ($P = 0.23$). Total length of stay for re-admissions through day 30, excluding index hospitalization was significantly lower with nesiritide vs placebo (3.1 days and 7.1 days respectively; $P = 0.032$), even though length of stay on index visit was not different (5.1 days with nesiritide, 5.5 days with placebo; $P = 0.618$). Hospitalization rates on the index visit, as well as readmission rates after the index visit, were not different between the two groups. Dyspnea scores were not significantly different between the two groups ($P = 0.95$).

FUSION II

Following up on the positive results of FUSION I, the FUSION II was designed to evaluate the efficacy of serial outpatient infusions of nesiritide [28]. Patients were included if they had chronic decompensated heart failure, at least 2 hospitalizations in the prior year, or LVEF <40%. Patients were required to be NYHA class IV, but NYHA class III patients were included if their creatinine clearance was <60ml/min. Exclusion criteria included continuous or intermittent use of intravenous vasoactive drugs, or systolic blood pressure <90 mmHg.

The study protocol called for randomization in a 2:1 fashion to nesiritide or placebo. The drug group received nesiritide once or twice weekly, at a dose of 2 μg/kg bolus followed by 0.01 μg/kg/min infusion for 4–6 hours. The groups were treated for 12 weeks, followed by a 4-week taper and 8-week follow-up. Standard heart failure therapies were continued during the study, under the direction of the treating physician.

Patients in FUSION II were noted to have better adherence to heart failure guidelines, with respect to use of implantable cardiac defibrillators and biventricular pacemakers, as well as use of beta-blockers such as carvedilol. Also, no patients in FUSION II were given inotropes.

The results of FUSION II are as yet unpublished, but the results were presented at the 2007 annual scientific sessions of the American College of Cardiology. According to that presentation, the study enrolled 920 patients, and had a mean follow-up of 24 weeks. 47% of the patients had NYHA class IV, 53% had NYHA class III, 64% had ischemic heart disease, and 51% of the patients had diabetes. The primary endpoint was a composite of all-cause death, cardiovascular hospitalization, or renal hospitalization; and 36.7% of the nesiritide group vs 36.8% of the placebo group reached this endpoint ($P = 0.79$). The secondary endpoint of mortality was reached by 9.5% of the nesiritide group and 9.6% of the placebo group ($P = 0.98$). The other secondary endpoints of hospitalization and quality of life (QOL) measurements were also not significantly different between the groups.

Adverse event rate was 42.0% in the nesiritide group and 27.5% in the placebo group ($P < 0.01$), primarily due to more incidence of hypotension in the nesiritide group. Increase in serum creatinine more than 0.5mg/dL was observed in 32% in the nesiritide group vs 39% in the placebo group ($P < 0.05$ in favor of nesiritide).

NAPA

The Nesiritide Administered Peri-Anesthesia in patients undergoing cardiac surgery (NAPA) trial was a exploratory study into the usefulness of nesiritide in the perioperative period for patients with left ventricular dysfunction undergoing coronary artery bypass grafting surgery [29]. This was a prospective, randomized, double-blind trial, which enrolled patients with NYHA class II to IV heart failure and LVEF ≤40%. Exclusion criteria were dialysis, restrictive or obstructive cardiomyopathy, pericarditis, pericardial tamponade, systolic blood pressure <90mmHg, congenital heart disease, evidence of ongoing infection, or pulmonary disease requiring hospitalization within 60 days. Patients were also excluded if Swan-Ganz catheter readings revealed pulmonary capillary wedge pressure <15mmHg, central venous pressure <6 mmHg.

Patients were, on average, 64 years old, 78% male, 86% white, 86 kg, and 50% had diabetes. Patients were randomized to nesiritide 0.01 µg/kg/min without bolus or placebo, both started after induction of anesthesia but before chest incision. The study drugs were required to be continued for a minimum of 24 hours and up to 96 hours, at the discretion of the treating physician. The mean duration observed during the study was 39 hours for nesiritide and 40 hours for placebo. During the study, reductions in study drug occurred in 9.2% for nesiritide and 8.0% for placebo ($P = 0.83$). Follow up data was available at 30 days for 93% of the nesiritide group and 92% of the placebo group. Follow up was obtained at 180 days for 66% of the nesiritide group and 68% of the placebo group.

Although 279 patients received the study drug, 7 of these had surgery with 'off-pump' techniques, so they were subsequently excluded from the efficacy analysis, but still included in the safety analysis. The five primary endpoints were:

1. Change in serum creatinine during the hospitalization up to 14 days.
2. Decline in glomerular filtration rate by the MDRD equation during the hospitalization up to 14 days.
3. Intravenous inotrope, vasopressor, and vasodilator use
4. Reduction in pulmonary artery pressure until removal of the Swan-Ganz catheter up to 24 hours
5. Urine output during the initial stay in the intensive care unit up to 24 hours.

During the hospital stay of up to 14 days, the nesiritide group had a maximum increase in serum creatinine of 0.15 mg/dl, whereas the placebo group had a maximum increase of 0.34 mg/dl ($P < 0.001$ in favour of nesiritide). Also during this timeframe, the maximum decline in glomerular filtration rate, which was calculated by the Modification of Diet in Renal Disease equation, was 10.2 ml/min/1.73 m^3 for the nesiritide group, and 17.8 ml/min/1.73 m^3 for the placebo group ($P = 0.001$ in favour of nesiritide). The investigators observed that, among patients with baseline creatinine >1.2 mg/dl (29 in the nesiritide group and 33 in the placebo group), this effect was even more pronounced, with the nesiritide group experiencing rise in serum creatinine of 0.02 mg/dl, and the placebo group experiencing rise in serum creatinine of 0.48 mg/dl ($P = 0.001$).

Use of inotropes or vasopressors was observed in 96% of the nesiritide group and 95% of the placebo group (P = ns). Inodilators, primarily milrinone, were used in 44% of the nesiritide group and 47% of the placebo group. For the endpoint regarding mean pulmonary capillary wedge pressure, there was reduction of 2.8 ± 7.9 mmHg in the nesiritide group and 1.9 ± 7.8 mmHg in the placebo group (P = 0.297).

For the endpoint of urine output during the initial 24 hours in the Intensive Care Unit, there was 2926 ± 1179 ml in the nesiritide group, and 2350 ± 1066 ml in the placebo group ($P < 0.001$).

There were several secondary endpoints, including hospital length of stay, which was 9.1 ± 6 days in the nesiritide group, and 11.5 ± 9.8 days in the placebo group (P = 0.043). Intensive care unit length-of-stay was not significantly different between groups. Thirty-day mortality was also not significantly different, at 2.8% in the nesiritide group and 5.9% in the placebo group. 180-day mortality was 6.6% in the nesiritide group and 14.7% in the placebo group (P = 0.046), but was limited by the low rate of follow-up at 180 days (66% of the nesiritide group and 68% of the placebo group).

THE NESIRITIDE CONTROVERSY – RENAL DYSFUNCTION AND BNP INFUSIONS

In 2005, Sackner-Bernstein *et al.* published a meta-analysis of five nesiritide trials with data on renal function [30]. Using a definition of renal dysfunction of serum creatinine increase of >0.5 mg/dl at any time during the inpatient portion of the trial, the relative risk of worsening renal function was 1.54 for nesiritide versus placebo (P = 0.001). The risk of worsening renal function was also seen with lower doses of nesiritide (<0.015 μg/kg/min). The concomitant administration of inotropes did not change the results. As a consequence of renal dysfunction, 32 of 288 nesiritide patients versus 6 of 144 of the control patients (P = 0.03) required medical intervention. However, the need for dialysis was not increased. Understandably, this report, along with other studies, led to widespread concern over the use of nesiritide in these patients already prone to renal dysfunction [31]. Worsening renal function is a significant risk factor for both mortality and prolonged length of stay in patients with heart failure [32–34].

Since these reports, FUSION II, a well-powered trial, and NAPA, an exploratory trial, found no increase in the risk of renal dysfunction with the use of nesiritide. There are several possible explanations for the discrepant findings by Sackner-Bernstein meta-analysis. Most of the early trials reported were dose-ranging trials, in which doses of nesiritide were frequently higher than the 0.01 μg/kg/min dose currently recommended. In the VMAC trial, the initial dose was 0.01 μg/kg/min in all patients, although the dose could be up-titrated if the pulmonary capillary wedge pressure was >20 mmHg. It is important to make this distinction of nesiritide dose, because there is a dose-dependent risk of worsening renal function as nesiritide infusion concentrations increase [35]. However, at 0.01 μg/kg/min of nesiritide, there is no significant increase in worsening renal function [35].

Another explanation for the renal dysfunction observed by Sackner-Bernstein *et al.* was less control of concomitant therapy in the trials included, which is an inherent limitation of meta-analyses. In a *post hoc* evaluation of the VMAC trial, renal dysfunction did not occur during the infusion or several days later, but did occur at 30 days, suggesting that concomitant therapy may have been important [36]. Patients in the VMAC trial who received lower doses of diuretics during the nesiritide infusion (defined as ≤160 mg per day of furosemide or its equivalent, and only one type of diuretic) had a similar frequency of renal insufficiency as those receiving nitroglycerin [37]. Many investigators have observed an association between diuretics and worsening renal function [25, 38, 39]. It is very likely that nesiritide has a heterogeneous effect on renal function in patients with heart failure; including neutral, deleterious and beneficial effects in various patient groups, as shown by Abraham *et al.* [12].

NESIRITIDE INFUSION AND MORTALITY

Unfortunately, of the nine nesiritide clinical trials, only FUSION II was clinically powered to assess effect on mortality. This is a curious omission, insofar as the mortality endpoint in heart failure has been the major driver as to whether a drug or therapy is approved or not. However, there are some exceptions, such as diuretics and digoxin, which are so entrenched (digoxin) or viewed as so necessary (diuretics) that they still maintain a role in the therapeutic armamentarium. Still others, such as inotropes, despite their clearly recognized drawbacks, are seen as life saving for very select patient groups and hence still are used, perhaps too frequently [40].

In an effort to address the issue of mortality, Sackner-Bernstein *et al.* conducted a meta-analysis that found an increase in the 30-day mortality for those given nesiritide [41]. Three trials (Efficacy, VMAC, and FUSION I) were included in the meta-analysis, and six were excluded (two because of lack of 30-day follow-up, one because patients did not have acute decompensated heart failure, two were open label, and one because nesiritide was given serially in an outpatient setting). The risk ratio for mortality using the Mantel-Haenszel Test using a fixed effect model was 1.74 for nesiritide (CI 0.97–3.12; $P = 0.059$). The Kaplan-Meier curves showed a HR of 1.86 (CI 1.02–3.41; $P = 0.04$). As with all meta-analyses, these findings are tenuous because of significant differences in the patient groups, such as increased inotrope use in the nesiritide group.

Two separate meta-analyses were conducted to address the same issue. The first, by Abraham, analyzed the then-current seven trials with 30-day mortality and the six trials with 6-month mortality, and adjusted the risk ratio to avoid inequalities in the patient groups [42]. The unadjusted harms ratio for the seven trials at 30 days was 1.27 ($P = 0.30$) and at six months was 1.05 ($P = 0.73$). The adjusted harms ratio at 30 days was 1.12 ($P = 0.63$) and at six months was 0.98 ($P = 0.085$).

Because of these concerns, a panel chaired by Eugene Braunwald was convened to examine the renal and mortality risks with the use of nesiritide [43]. They concluded:

"The panel noted that completed trials show that the use of nesiritide was associated with a trend toward an increase in mortality rate at 30 days, with a hazard ratio of approximately 1.3, a 30% increase. However, the confidence intervals around this ratio are wide and the number of deaths in a pooled analysis of all six of the controlled clinical trials (84) is insufficient to identify or exclude, with confidence, a moderate excess of risk to survival. Also, there are potentially important imbalances in baseline characteristics and in other treatments received concomitantly, and the trials differ with respect to the treatments with which nesiritide was compared. No increased hazard is observed at 180 days. Because of the small numbers of events in the current database and the inconclusive nature of these findings, the panel recommends that additional studies be conducted to assess the effect of nesiritide on survival."

The panel made several recommendations:

1. Continued enrollment in ongoing nesiritide trials.
2. The conduct of a large, placebo controlled outcomes trial of several thousand patients, adequately powered to detect a 15% difference in mortality between nesiritide and standard therapy. Endpoints of such a trial should be mortality in a 30–90 day window, 180-day mortality and renal dysfunction. Important mortality variables such as inotrope use and renal function should be stratified to ensure equal distribution between groups.
3. Other mechanistic trials to explore lower doses of nesiritide and subgroup analysis of completed trials to detect differences in the response to nesiritide infusions.
4. Nesiritide infusions should be limited to those patients who are hospitalized and present with dyspnea, and where the benefit of the infusion outweighs the potential risks discussed above.
5. Nesiritide infusions should not replace diuretics, and outpatient scheduled use of the drug should be not be done.

FUTURE DIRECTIONS

The recommendations of the Braunwald panel guided the design of the FUSION II trial. Based on the findings from FUSION I, the investigators designed a randomized trial for NYHA class III and IV heart failure patients, and powered it to find a 20% reduction in mortality with serial outpatient nesiritide infusions, compared with placebo [44]. However, the trial found no significant difference in mortality between the groups. The reason for the neutral findings could be that the estimated effect size was overly generous, because a smaller effect size would necessitate a larger sample size to achieve statistically significant results. Perhaps this shortcoming will be addressed by the ongoing ASCEND-HF (Acute Study of Clinical Effectiveness of Nesiritide in Decompensated Heart Failure) study, which plans to ultimately recruit 7,000 patients in a multicenter, international effort.

A significant limitation with nesiritide administration currently is the need for continuous intravenous dosing. This limitation is being addressed in several ways. Synthetic BNP has been given in repeated subcutaneous doses with positive effects on hemodynamics and cyclic GMP [45]. A study utilizing this delivery mode is currently underway. Amino acid sequences have been added to BNP to protect it from enzymatic degradation in the stomach but still allow intestinal absorption and receptor stimulation [46]. This modified form of BNP has been demonstrated to increase cyclic GMP and produce hemodynamic effects. If chronic oral administration of BNP were to be proven useful, this would clearly be a preferred method of administration. Finally, other modifications of the molecule have been made to increase its efficacy. Such 'designer molecules' could improve the renal effects of BNP while limiting untoward vascular effects such as excessive arteriolar vasodilation [47].

What are the benefits and concerns regarding the therapeutic use of BNP infusions?

1. Human recombinant BNP reduces right atrial, pulmonary artery and pulmonary artery wedge pressure with reduction in systemic vascular resistance. Plasma aldosterone levels fall and with a variable effect on norephinephrine in patients with heart failure.
2. In the VMAC trial nesiritide plus standard therapy improved pulmonary capillary wedge pressures more rapidly than nitroglycerine with standard therapy or standard therapy alone. In addition, patients' symptoms improved with nesiritide compared to placebo. However there was not a significant difference between nesiritide and nitroglycerine with regard to symptomatic improvement at 3h. Ventricular arrhythmias are reduced with nesiritide compared to dobutamine.

In patients with congestive heart failure early physiologic trials showed no change in GFR in patients with heart failure given BNP although GFR improved in those without heart failure. Studies do not consistently show increased urine output with nesiritide in patients with heart failure although a diuretic effect is seen in some patients. When clinical studies are combined, the risk of an increase in serum creatinine of 0.5 mg/dl or greater is 28% with nesiritide.

No trial of nesiritide has been sufficiently powered to determine its effect on short-term mortality. The resolution of this question awaits prospectively acquired randomized placebo-controlled data.

SUMMARY

Therapeutic strategies

- Nesiritide is a useful adjunct to standard therapy for acute decompensated heart failure. Because it reduces symptoms and improves hemodynamics it would be most useful in symptomatic patients who are not hypotensive.
- The hemodynamic effects of nesiritide are dose-dependent as are the significant adverse effects such as hypotension and renal dysfunction. Thus use of the 0.01mg/kg/min dose is recommended.

The use of high-dose diuretics (more than 160 mg per day of furosemide or its equivalent) when combined with nesiritide is associated with an increased risk of renal dysfunction. Therefore diuretic doses should probably be reduced when nesiritide is added to standard therapy.

As with all therapy for congestive heart failure the patient's volume status and renal function should be carefully monitored. This is especially important during nesiritide infusions.

REFERENCES

1. Kirsch B. Electron microscopic investigation of the heart of cattle. *Exp Med Surg* 1959; 17:247.
2. Okamoto H. An electron microscopic study of the specific granules in the atrial muscle cell upon the administration of agents affecting autonomic nerves. *Arch Histol* 1969; 30:467–478.
3. Jamieson JD, Palade GE. Specific granules in atrial muscle cells. *J Cell Biol* 1964; 23:151–172.
4. Baines AD, DeBold AJ, Sonnenberg H. Natriuretic effect of atrial extract on isolated perfused rat kidney. *Can J Physiol Pharmacol* 1983; 61:1462–1466.
5. Zhou HL, Fiscus RR. Brain natriuretic peptide (BNP) causes endothelium-independent relaxation and elevation of cyclic GMP in rat thoracic aorta. *Neuropeptides* 1989; 14:161–169.
6. Sudoh T, Kangawa K, Minamino N, Matsuo H. A new natriuretic peptide in porcine brain. *Nature* 1988; 332:78–81.
7. Hosoda K, Nakao K, Mukoyama M *et al.* Expression of brain natriuretic peptide gene in human heart. Production in the ventricle. *Hypertension* 1991; 17:1152–1155.
8. Wei CM, Heublein DM, Perrella MA *et al.* Natriuretic peptide system in human heart failure. *Circulation* 1993; 88:1004–1009.
9. Marcus LS, Hart D, Packer M *et al.* Hemodynamic and renal excretory effects of human brain natriuretic peptide infusion in patients with congestive heart failure. A double-blind, placebo-controlled, randomized crossover trial. *Circulation* 1996; 94:3184–3189.
10. Holmes SJ, Espiner EA, Richards AM, Yandle TG, Frampton C. Renal, endocrine, and hemodynamic effects of human brain natriuretic peptide in normal man. *J Clin Endocrinol Metab* 1993; 76:91–96.
11. Yoshimura M, Yasue H, Morita E *et al.* Hemodynamic, renal, and hormonal responses to brain natriuretic peptide infusion in patients with congestive heart failure. *Circulation* 1991; 84:1581–1588.
12. Abraham WT, Lowes BD, Ferguson DA *et al.* Systemic hemodynamic, neurohormonal, and renal effects of a steady-state infusion of human brain natriuretic peptide in patients with hemodynamically decompensated heart failure. *J Card Fail* 1998; 4:37–44.
13. Mills RM, LeJemtel TH, Horton DP *et al.* Sustained hemodynamic effects of an infusion of nesiritide (human b-type natriuretic peptide) in heart failure: a randomized, double-blind, placebo-controlled clinical trial. Natrecor Study Group. *J Am Coll Cardiol* 1999; 34:155–162.
14. Jensen KT, Eiskjaer H, Carstens J, Pedersen EB. Renal effects of brain natriuretic peptide in patients with congestive heart failure. *Clin Sci (Lond)* 1999; 96:5–15.
15. Colucci WS, Elkayam U, Horton DP *et al.* Intravenous nesiritide, a natriuretic peptide, in the treatment of decompensated congestive heart failure. Nesiritide Study Group. *N Engl J Med* 2000; 343:246–253.
16. Silver MA, Horton DP, Ghali JK, Elkayam U. Effect of nesiritide versus dobutamine on short-term outcomes in the treatment of patients with acutely decompensated heart failure. *J Am Coll Cardiol* 2002; 39:798–803.
17. Publication Committee for the VMAC Investigators (Vasodilatation in the Management of Acute CHF). Intravenous nesiritide vs nitroglycerin for treatment of decompensated congestive heart failure: a randomized controlled trial. *JAMA* 2002; 287:1531–1540.
18. Kambayashi Y, Nakao K, Mukoyama M *et al.* Isolation and sequence determination of human brain natriuretic peptide in human atrium. *FEBS Lett* 1990; 258:341–345.
19. Elkayam U, Singh H, Akhter MW *et al.* Effects of intravenous nesiritide on renal hemodynamics in patients with congestive heart failure [abstract #256]. *J Card Fail* 2004; 10(suppl):S88.
20. Koller KJ, Goeddel DV. Molecular biology of the natriuretic peptides and their receptors. *Circulation* 1992; 86:1081–1088.
21. Brunner-La Rocca HP, Kaye DM, Woods RL, Hastings J, Esler MD. Effects of intravenous brain natriuretic peptide on regional sympathetic activity in patients with chronic heart failure as compared with healthy control subjects. *J Am Coll Cardiol* 2001; 37:1221–1227.

22. La Villa G, Fronzaroli C, Lazzeri C *et al*. Cardiovascular and renal effects of low dose brain natriuretic peptide infusion in man. *J Endocrinol Metab* 1994; 78:1166–1171.

23. Koepke JP, DiBona GF. Blunted natriuresis to atrial natriuretic peptide in chronic sodium-retaining disorders. *Am J Physiol* 1987; 252:F865–F871.

24. Wang DJ, Dowling TC, Meadows D *et al*. Nesiritide does not improve renal function in patients with chronic heart failure and worsening serum creatinine. *Circulation* 2004; 110:1620–1625.

25. Gottlieb SS, Skettino SL, Wolff A *et al*. Effects of BG9719 (CVT-124), an A1-adenosine receptor antagonist, and furosemide on glomerular filtration rate and natriuresis in patients with congestive heart failure. *J Am Coll Cardiol* 2000; 35:56–59.

26. Yancy CW, Saltzberg MT, Berkowitz RL *et al*. Safety and feasibility of using serial infusions of nesiritide for heart failure in an outpatient setting (from the FUSION I trial). *Am J Cardiol* 2004; 94:595–601.

27. Peacock WF 4th, Holland R, Gyarmathy R *et al*. Observation unit treatment of heart failure with nesiritide: results from the proaction trial. *J Emerg Med* 2005; 29:243–252.

28. Unpublished results, presented at the Annual Scientific Sessions of the American College of Cardiology, March 2007.

29. Mentzer RM, Oz MC, Sladen RN, Graeve AH, Hebeler RF, Luber JM, Smedira NG, on behalf of the NAPA investigators. Effects of perioperative nesiritide in patients with left ventricular dysfunction. *J Am Coll Cardiol* 2007; 49:716–726.

30. Sackner-Bernstein JD, Skopicki HA, Aaronson KD. Risk of worsening renal function with nesiritide in patients with acutely decompensated heart failure. *Circulation* 2005; 111:1487–1491.

31. Hauptman PJ, Schnitzler MA, Swindle J, Burroughs TE. Use of nesiritide before and after publications suggesting drug-related risks in patients with acute decompensated heart failure. *JAMA* 2006; 296:1877–1884.

32. Smith GL, Vaccarino V, Kosiborod M *et al*. Worsening renal function: what is a clinically meaningful change in creatinine during hospitalization with heart failure? *J Card Fail* 2003; 9:13–25.

33. Gottlieb SS, Abraham W, Butler J *et al*. The prognostic importance of different definitions of worsening renal function in congestive heart failure. *J Card Fail* 2002; 8:136–141.

34. Forman DE, Butler J, Wang Y *et al*. Incidence, predictors at admission, and impact of worsening renal function among patients hospitalized with heart failure. *J Am Coll Cardiol* 2004; 43:61–67.

35. Heywood JT. Clinical predictors of worsening renal function in patients hospitalized for heart failure. *Circulation* 2005; 112(supp II):II-589.

36. Heywood JT. Combining nesiritide with high-dose diuretics may increase the risk of increased serum creatinine. *Circulation* 2005; 112(supp II):II-451.

37. Abraham WT. Serum creatinine elevations in patients receiving nesiritide are related to starting dose. *J Card Fail* 2005; 11(suppl):S156.

38. Weinfeld MS, Chertow GM, Stevenson LW. Aggravated renal dysfunction during intensive therapy for advanced chronic heart failure. *Am Heart J* 1999; 138:285–290.

39. Domanski M, Norman J, Pitt B, Haigney M, Hanlon S, Peyster E. Diuretic use, progressive heart failure, and death in patients in the studies of left ventricular dysfunction (SOLVD). *J Am Coll Cardiol* 2003; 42:705–708.

40. Stevenson LW. Clinical use of inotropic therapy for heart failure: looking bacward or forward? Part I: Inotropic infusions during hospitalization. *Circulation* 2003; 108:367–372.

41. Sackner-Bernstein JD, Kowalski M, Fox M, Aaronson K. Short-term risk of death after treatment with nesiritide for decompensated heart failure: a pooled analysis of randomized controlled trials. *JAMA* 2005; 293:1900–1905.

42. Abraham WT. Nesiritide does not increase 30-day or 6-month mortality risk. *Circulation* 2005; 112(suppl II): II-676.

43. Press Release – Scios, Inc. Web address as of 11/29/05: http://www.sciosinc.com/scios/pr_1118721302.

44. Yancy CW, Krum H, Massie BM, Silver MA, Stevenson LW, Cheng M, Kim SS, Evans R; FUSION II Investigators. *Am Heart J* 2007; 153:478–484.

45. Chen HH, Grantham JA, Schirger JA, Jougasaki M, Redfield MM, Burnett JC Jr. Subcutaneous administration of brain natriuretic peptide in experimental heart failure. *J Am Coll Cardiol* 2000; 36:1706–1712.

46. Cataliotti A, Schirger JA, Martin FL *et al*. Oral human brain natriuretic peptide activates cyclic guanosine 3′,5′-monophosphate and decreases mean arterial pressure. *Circulation* 2005; 112:836–840.

47. Lisy O, Kurlansky P, Burnett JC. Cardiac and renal actions of a new designer peptide BD-NP are superior to human BNP. *Circulation* 2005; 112:II-253.

Section IV

Future pharmacologic therapies for
heart failure

10

Arginine vasopressin antagonism in heart failure

J. Finley, O. Hedrich, M. A. Konstam, J. E. Udelson

INTRODUCTION

Arginine vasopressin (AVP) has recently attracted attention as a potentially important neurohormonal mediator of the heart failure (HF) syndrome in humans [1]. A neurohypophysial hormone, vasopressin (also called antidiuretic hormone or ADH) helps regulate free water reabsorption, body fluid osmolality, blood volume, blood vessel vasoconstriction, and myocardial contractile function [2, 3]. These biological functions are subtended by two distinct receptors (V_{1a} and V_2), which in turn activate intracellular second messenger pathways with diverse effects [4]. Effects are seen with changes in hemodynamics (vasoconstriction and water retention resulting in increased systemic vascular resistance [SVR], increased pulmonary wedge pressure, decreased cardiac output [CO], and decreased stroke volume [SV]) and in terms of cardiac remodeling and cardiomyocyte hypertrophy [4]. Accordingly, this system represents a potentially novel target for the treatment of HF. In an effort to mediate the potential detrimental effects of vasopressin in this syndrome, selective and potent vasopressin receptor antagonists have been developed in recent years, several of which have reached the late regulatory stage of human clinical trials.

Two specific and selective non-peptide V_2 receptor antagonists without intrinsic agonist properties, tolvaptan (OPC-41061) and lixivaptan (VPA-985), have shown efficacy in clinical trials (Table 10.1). In the multicenter, randomized, double-blind, placebo-controlled ACTIV in CHF trial [5], tolvaptan, in acutely decompensated HF patients, caused significant volume loss, decreased body weight by increasing urine output, normalized serum sodium concentration in hyponatremic patients, and possibly prevented a concomitant decline in renal function or significant electrolyte derangement commonly encountered with traditional diuretic regimens. No significant differences were observed in rates of rehospitalization or outpatient visits for HF. However, there was a trend toward improved event-free survival in the tolvaptan groups compared to placebo. This finding is now being explored further in a larger, pivotal phase 3 trial – the Efficacy of Vasopressin Antagonism in Heart Failure Study with Tolvaptan (EVEREST) trial [6] – examining long-term impact in regards to all-cause mortality and time to cardiovascular mortality or HF mortality.

John J. Finley IV, MD, Chief Medical Resident, Department of Medicine, Tufts-New England Medical Center, Boston, Massachusetts, USA.

Olaf Hedrich, MD, Cardiology Fellow, Department of Cardiology, Tufts-New England Medical Center, Boston, Massachusetts, USA.

Marvin A. Konstam, MD, Chief, Division of Cardiology, Professor of Medicine, Division of Cardiology, Tufts-New England Medical Center, Tufts University School of Medicine, Boston, Massachusetts, USA.

James E. Udelson, MD, Associate Chief, Division of Cardiology, Tufts-New England Medical Center, Tufts University School of Medicine, Boston, Massachusetts, USA.

Table 10.1 Arginine vasopressin receptor antagonists for chronic heart failure – major findings of clinical trials

Clinical trial [reference]	Design	Drug	Inclusion/ exclusion criteria	Endpoints	Results
ACTIV in CHF [5]	Multicenter; placebo-controlled; double-blinded (30, 60, or 90 mg orally daily up to 60 days) $n = 319$	Tolvaptan	Class III/IV HF patients with LVEF ≤40% and two clinical signs of HF	Body weight Urine volume (day 1)	Decrease in body weight Increase in urine volume No impact on rehospitalization at 60 days Trend to decrease mortality at 60 days No change in BUN, Cr, K^+
Gheorghiade et al. [37, 38]	Placebo-controlled, double-blinded, multidose (30, 45, or 60 mg orally daily for 25 days) $n = 254$	Tolvaptan	HF patients irrespective of LVEF	Body weight Urine volume (day 1) Edema Serum sodium	Decrease in body weight and edema in modestly volume-overloaded CHF patients Increased urinary volume, and normalization of hyponatremia
EVEREST [6]	Multicenter, placebo-controlled, double-blinded, single dose (30 mg orally daily for up to 60 days), short- and long-term outcomes, $n = \sim 4000$/until 1065 deaths	Tolvaptan	Acute decompensated HF patients with LVEF ≤40%	Long-term: all-cause mortality/first occurrence of cardiovascular mortality or heart failure hospitalization Short-term: symptom improvement in hospital	Ongoing
Abraham et al. [7]	Placebo-controlled, double-blinded, multidose (10, 30, 75, 150, 250, or 400 mg single oral dose) $n = 42$	Lixivaptan	Class II/III HF patients with LVEF ≤35%	Urine volume; urine osmolality; solute-free water excretion; serum osmolality; serum sodium; serum electrolytes	Increase significant and dose-dependent effect on urine volume at 4 h (for doses >10 mg) and 24 h Increase in solute-free water excretion Increase in serum sodium with higher doses

Study	Design	Drug	Patient population	Outcome measure	Results
Wong et al. [8]	Multicenter, placebo-controlled, double-blinded, multidose (25, 125, or 250 mg orally twice daily for 7 days) n = 44	Lixivaptan	Hyponatremic patients (HF, cirrhosis, SIADH)	Free water clearance (P < 0.05) and serum sodium (P < 0.05)	Overall increased aquaretic response without significant changes in orthostatic blood pressure or serum creatinine levels. Higher dose (250 mg) led to dehydration
Udelson et al. [9]	Multicenter, placebo-controlled, double-blinded, multidose (10, 20, or 40 mg single intravenous dose) n = 142	Conivaptan	Class III/IV HF patients with LVEF 21–26%	Changes in hemodynamic parameters (PCWP, RAP, CI, SVR, PVR, SAP, HR) and urine output and urine osmolality	Reduction in PCWP and RAP with 20 and 40 mg doses without changes in other hemodynamic parameters. Decrease in urine output and in urine osmolality without changes in serum osmolality, sodium, or potassium
Russell et al. [10]	Multicenter, placebo-controlled, double-blinded, multidose (10, 20, or 40 mg orally twice daily) n = 343	Conivaptan	Class III HF patients	Exercise tolerance and functional capacity	No improvement in overall functional capacity, exercise tolerance or quality of life
Goldsmith et al. [45]	Multicenter, placebo-controlled, double-blinded, multidose (20 mg bolus and cont. IV 40, 80, 120 mg/day) n = 160	Conivaptan	Acute decompensated HF patients	Subjective patient and clinician global assessments; Objective lab measurements	Pending

Table 10.1 (continued)

Clinical trial [reference]	Design	Drug	Inclusion/ exclusion criteria	Endpoints	Results
Verbalis et al. [46]	Multicenter, placebo-controlled, double-blinded, multidose (20 mg bolus and cont. IV 40 or 80 mg/day × 4 days) n = 84	Conivaptan	Hyponatremic patients	Change in serum sodium over treatment duration	Increases serum sodium concentration and effective water clearance

ACTIV in CHF = Acute and Chronic Therapeutic Impact of a Vasopressin Antagonist in Congestive Heart Failure; BUN = blood urea nitrogen; CI = cardiac index; Cr = creatinine; EVEREST = Efficacy of Vasopressin Antagonism in Heart Failure Study with Tolvaptan; HF = heart failure; HR = heart rate; IV = intravenous; K = potassium; LVEF = left ventricular ejection fraction; METEOR = Multicenter Evaluation of Tolvaptan Effect On Remodeling; PCWP = pulmonary capillary wedge pressure; PVR = peripheral vascular resistance; RAP = right atrial pressure; SAP = systemic arterial pressure; SIADH = syndrome of inappropriate antidiuretic hormone; SVR = systemic vascular resistance.

Using lixivaptan, an agent more highly V_2 receptor specific, dose-dependent increases in solute-free aquaresis and serum sodium concentration have been demonstrated in studies of New York Heart Association (NYHA) class II and III HF patients [7]. In conditions associated with water retention (congestive heart failure [CHF], cirrhosis, syndrome of inappropriate antidiuretic hormone [SIADH]) lixivaptan may hold promise in correcting abnormal renal water handling and hyponatremia [8]. Both of these agents, tolvaptan and lixivaptan, may have the added benefit of sparing any decline in renal function, unlike loop diuretics.

Conivaptan (YM-087), an intravenously or orally administered, non-peptide vasopressin antagonist with high affinity for both V_{1a} and V_2 receptors, also results in significant aquaretic and hemodynamic effects (decreased pulmonary capillary wedge pressure [PCWP] and right atrial pressure [RAP]) in patients with advanced (NYHA class III/IV) HF [9], when administered as a single intravenous dose. The US Food and Drug Administration (FDA) has recently approved the intravenous form of conivaptan for use as an infusion for treatment of hyponatremia.

However, not all of the clinical trials looking at vasopressin antagonists have yielded consistently favorable results. A preliminary, clinical study of oral conivaptan did not demonstrate efficacy in terms of improving exercise tolerance or quality of life over several months of therapy [10].

In conclusion, these novel vasopressin inhibitors reduce body fluid volume by promotion of aquaresis with maintenance of electrolyte homeostasis (with potential consequent symptomatic and hemodynamic improvements) and correction of hyponatremia all while appearing to preserve renal function. Whether these changes translate to long-term outcome benefit is still in question. Nevertheless, these agents may offer an alternative in HF management to current diuretic regimens, which can be detrimental to renal function and electrolyte maintenance.

More comprehensive neurohormonal antagonism beyond ACE inhibition, β-adrenergic receptor-blockade and aldosterone antagonism holds potential promise in modulating the long-term adverse effects of neurohormonal activation in patients with HF and left ventricular (LV) dysfunction. AVP has recently attracted attention as a potentially important neurohormonal mediator of the HF syndrome in humans [1]. A neurohypophysial hormone, vasopressin (also called antidiuretic hormone or ADH) helps regulate free water reabsorption, body fluid osmolality, blood volume, blood vessel vasoconstriction, and myocardial contractile function [2, 3]. These biological functions are subtended by two distinct receptors (V_{1a} and V_2), which in turn activate intracellular second messenger pathways with diverse effects [4]. Accordingly, this system represents a novel target for the treatment of HF, and several vasopressin antagonists are currently under development [11].

PATHOPHYSIOLOGY OF VASOPRESSIN AND VASOPRESSIN RECEPTORS

There are three distinct vasopressin receptors through which vasopressin exerts its biological effects (Table 10.2) [4]. V_{1a} ('vascular') receptors are located on several diverse cell types including vascular smooth muscle cells and cardiomyocytes, and it is through this receptor that vasopressin assists in maintaining and regulating vascular tone and myocardial function [3]. V_2 ('renal') receptors are expressed on the basolateral membrane of the renal collecting ducts, and mediate the antidiuretic effects of vasopressin. Intracellular events triggered by binding of vasopressin to the V_2 receptor include 'shuttling' of aquaporin 2 (AQP-2) water channels from cytoplasmic vesicles to the luminal surface of the renal collecting duct cells where they are inserted into the cell membrane and facilitate water transport across the collecting duct cells (Figure 10.1) [12, 13]. V_2 receptor agonism appears also to promote increased *de novo* synthesis of AQP-2 channels. V_{1b} ('pituitary') receptors are

Table 10.2 Vasopressin levels measured by radio-immunosorbent assay (RIA) in HF and other populations

Reference	Patients	Mean AVP levels (pg/ml)	Comments
Creager et al. [29]	CHF, $n = 10$	2.4 ± 0.6	Vasodilators held
	Normals	1.1 ± 0.2	$\times$ 48 h
Nicod et al. [48]	CHF, $n = 10$	2.3 ± 0.8	
Pruszczynski et al. [49]	CHF, $n = 14$	4.6 ± 0.3	On diuretics
	HTN, $n = 8$	2.9 ± 0.1	On diuretics
	CAD, $n = 11$	3.4 ± 0.2	Not on diuretics
Goldsmith et al. [14]	CHF, $n = 31$	9.5 ± 0.9	Vasodilators/diuretics
	Normals, $n = 51$	4.7 ± 0.7	held $\times$ 48 h, low-Na diet
Goldsmith et al. [50]	CHF, $n = 15$	11.6 ± 5.5	Elevated baseline
	Normals, $n = 9$	5.3 ± 2.3	levels in HF patients did not increase in response to orthostatic stress
Szatalowicz et al. [15]	CHF, $n = 9$	4.6 ± 2.1	At serum [Na] 137 mEq/l
Riegger and coworkers [17]	CHF, $n = 20$		
	'High AVP' for Posm	14.5 ± 8.8	
	'Low AVP' for Posm	3.9 ± 1.0	
Rouleau et al. [51]	Asx LVD, $n = 534$	1.8 ± 6.7	SAVE trial population, 27% 'activated', i.e. >1.96 SD above age-matched controls
Gavras et al. [52]	Normals, $n = 12$	1.1 ± 0.2	
Francis et al. [16]	CHF, $n = 80$	3.5	Range 2.3–4.4
	Asx LVD, $n = 147$	2.6	Range 1.7–3.0
		2.9	Range 1.4–2.3
	Normals, $n = 54$		(SOLVD population)
Uretsky et al. [20]	CHF, $n = 42$	3.0 ± 2.5	
	Normals, $n = 10$	1.0 ± 0.4	
Udelson et al. [40]	CHF, n = 142	Median levels 2.1–2.9	

AVP = arginine vasopressin; CHF = congestive heart failure; HTN = hypertension; CAD = coronary artery disease; Asx LVD = asymptomatic left ventricular dysfunction; Posm = plasma osmolality; SOLVD = Studies of Left Ventricular Dysfunction.

expressed on the surfaces of corticotrophic cells in the anterior pituitary, where they potentiate the release of adrenocorticotropic hormone (ACTH).

VASOPRESSIN IN HEART FAILURE

GENERAL CONCEPTS

Several studies have shown a significant elevation in plasma vasopressin concentration in the setting of HF [11, 14–16]. In the neuroendocrine substudy of the Studies of Left Ventricular Dysfunction (SOLVD), patients with LV dysfunction were shown to have higher

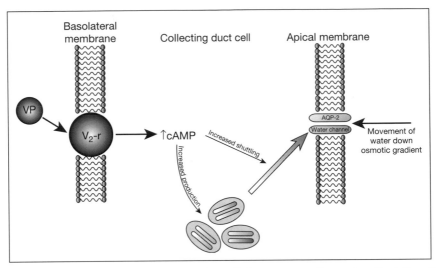

Figure 10.1 Intracellular events in renal collecting duct cells in response to V_2 receptor stimulation. Upon binding with vasopressin, the V_2 receptor (on the basolateral membrane of the renal collecting duct cells) causes activation of adenylyl cyclase and subsequent synthesis of intracellular cAMP. AQP-2 water channels are 'shuttled' from their cytoplasmic vesicles to the apical membrane, where they facilitate movement of free water across the apical membrane down an osmotic gradient. AQP-2 synthesis is also increased (with permission from [7]).

levels of vasopressin compared to an age-matched reference group [16]. Patients with asymptomatic LV dysfunction (LV ejection fraction [LVEF] $\leq$ 35%) had higher mean vasopressin levels (AVP = 2.2 pg/ml) than controls (AVP = 1.8 pg/ml). Individuals with mild-to-moderate symptoms of HF had even higher mean levels (AVP = 3.0 pg/ml) than their asymptomatic counterparts. Not all studies, nor all patients in these studies demonstrate consistently elevated vasopressin levels compared to normals. However, these levels may be 'inappropriately' elevated in HF relative to the state of plasma volume or osmolality, although studies are not often analyzed as such [17]. Studies reporting vasopressin levels in patients with HF and/or LV dysfunction are summarized in Table 10.2.

Whereas in the normal physiologic state, there is a close relationship between plasma vasopressin levels and osmolality, this relationship appears to be disrupted in HF [18, 19]. In a population of patients with HF who received an osmotic load by means of mannitol infusion, vasopressin levels were demonstrated to increase to a greater degree than in non-HF subjects, and baseline levels of vasopressin relative to plasma osmolality were found to be higher in the HF patients than in their normal counterparts [20]. Although dysregulated, the overall sensitivity of the system appears to remain intact, but with an 'upward shift' in plasma vasopressin levels.

PATHOPHYSIOLOGIC EFFECTS OF VASOPRESSIN IN HEART FAILURE

To assess whether vasopressin is truly a neuroendocrine pathogen in the development and progression of HF, consideration must be given to its potential pathophysiologic role, and its association with long-term outcomes [21, 22]. In multivariate analysis, vasopressin levels obtained 1 month after myocardial infarction in patients enrolled in the Survival and Ventricular Enlargement (SAVE) study correlated independently with severe HF (RR = 1.6), recurrent myocardial infarction (RR = 2.3) and a combined endpoint measure of cardiovascular mortality or HF or myocardial infarction (RR = 1.6) [23]. This tends to suggest that vasopressin levels in this setting do have prognostic significance.

EFFECTS ON WATER BALANCE

Elevated plasma vasopressin concentrations appear to be associated with impaired free water excretion in patients with HF [15, 18]. Rats with an elevated LV end-diastolic pressure (LVEDP) and reduced plasma sodium were found to have a significantly increased expression of AQP-2 mRNA when compared to rats with mild compensated HF without elevated LVEDP or reduced plasma sodium concentration [24]. While these observations are helpful in explaining the clinical observations of volume expansion and hyponatremia in HF, the role for implicating vasopressin in these processes is strengthened by further experimental observations regarding selective inhibition of V_2 receptors in animals with HF.

Lixivaptan (VPA-985), a specific and selective non-peptide V_2 receptor antagonist, has been shown to be a potent aquaretic compound in dogs and rats [25]. Furthermore, in humans, a randomized, placebo-controlled dose-ranging study administering lixivaptan resulted in a significant, dose-related increase in solute-free water excretion and resulting elevation of serum sodium concentration and serum osmolality in patients with mild-to-moderate HF [7]. In this study, an observed reduction in urinary AQP-2 protein levels suggested that the observed aquaresis may have been secondary to a reduction in AQP-2 expression at the level of the renal collecting duct.

EFFECTS ON HEMODYNAMICS

Under normal physiologic conditions, the vasoconstrictive effects of vasopressin are usually not associated with appreciable changes in arterial blood pressure at plasma levels within physiologic range [26]. However, in patients with HF, intravenous infusion of vasopressin results in a variety of hemodynamic effects [27]. SVR and PCWP increase, while SV and CO decrease with dose-dependent increments of vasopressin infusion (Figure 10.2).

These hemodynamic effects are thought to be primarily mediated *via* activation of V_{1a} receptors on vascular smooth muscle cells, which promotes an increase in afterload by means of arteriolar vasoconstriction [28, 29]. However, indirect effects mediated by V_2 receptor agonism may result in increased water retention, which increases circulating blood volume and hence preload, with concomitant increases in PCWP and LV filling pressure. At the myocyte level, vasopressin may be positively inotropic, yet when factoring in the effects of vasoconstriction on the coronary arteries resulting in decreased coronary flow, elevated levels of vasopressin may on balance have a negatively inotropic effect on the failing heart, with an attending decline in SV and CO [21].

Supportive evidence for these hypotheses once again comes from observational data employing selective V_{1a} receptor antagonists *in vivo* [29], where significant improvements in SVR and CO were recorded when vasopressin levels were elevated (Figure 10.2). In a dog model of CHF induced by rapid ventricular pacing, administration of the non-peptide vasopressin antagonist OPC-21268 resulted in significantly increased CO and reduced total peripheral resistance [30]. A porcine model of CHF revealed improved ventricular loading conditions when the non-peptide V_1 receptor antagonist SR49059 was administered, with reduced LV end-diastolic dimension and peak wall stress [31].

EFFECTS ON THE MYOCARDIUM

Vasopressin has been implicated in cardiac remodeling, and structural changes in myocardium exposed to high levels have been demonstrated in both neonatal and adult myocytes [32–34]. In cultured neonatal rat myocardial cells, cellular hypertrophy by means of enhanced protein synthesis has been observed [32, 33]. By means of exposure to V_{1a} receptor antagonists, the observed hypertrophy was significantly inhibited [32, 33]. Myocardial V_{1a} receptor agonism results in an increase in intracellular calcium concentration

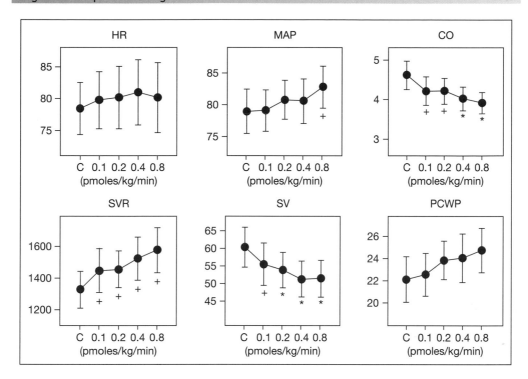

Figure 10.2 Hemodynamic effects of vasopressin in HF. Overall hemodynamic responses to infused arginine vasopressin. Data are shown as mean ± SD for each infusion rate. The mean basal plasma arginine vasopressin level was 6.4 ± 2.7 pg/ml, and increased to 63 ± 39 pg/ml at peak infusion rate. During the infusion, heart rate (HR, beats/min) and mean arterial pressure (MAP, mmHg) did not change, except for a small increase in blood pressure at the highest infusion rate. A statistically significant decline in cardiac output (CO, l/min) and stroke volume (SV, ml) was recorded, as was a statistically significant increase in systemic vascular resistance (SVR, dynes · s · cm^{-5}). There was significant overall variation ($P < 0.01$) in the pulmonary capillary wedge pressure (PCWP, mmHg), but no individual pairs attained statistical significance. RAP and pulmonary artery pressure (not shown) did not change. $^{+}P < 0.05$; $^{*}P < 0.01$; C denotes control group (no vasopressin). With permission [27].

as well as protein kinase C activity [32, 33], which is thought to be central in mediating the observed hypertrophic myocardial cell growth, not unlike effects ascribed to angiotensin II. Whether these structural changes translate into clinically significant outcomes in HF, or contribute to progression of the disease, is currently unknown.

CLINICAL TRIALS OF VASOPRESSIN ANTAGONISTS

V_2 RECEPTOR ANTAGONISTS

V_2 receptor antagonism has been demonstrated to result in stimulation of aquaresis in humans, with net loss of free water. Unlike with the administration of loop diuretics, antagonism of V_2 receptors appears not to increase activation of the renin–angiotensin–aldosterone system (RAAS) [35].

Tolvaptan

Tolvaptan (OPC-41061) is a specific and selective non-peptide V_2 receptor antagonist without intrinsic agonist properties, shown to have potent aquaretic properties in an animal

Table 10.3 Properties of vasopressin receptor blockers (adapted from [48])

	Tolvaptan (OPC-41061)	Lixivaptan (VPA-985)	SR-121463	Conivaptan (YM-087)
Receptor	V_2	V_2	V_2	V_{1a}/V_2
Selectivity $(K_iV_{1a}:K_iV_2)$	29:1	100:1	100:1	10:1
Administration route	Oral	Oral	Oral	Intravenous/oral
Urine volume	↑	↑	↑	↑
Urine osmolality	↓	↓	↓	↓
Sodium excretion/24 h	↔	↔Low dose ↑High dose	↔	↔

↑Increases; ↓decreases; ↔remains overall unchanged.

model [36]. In cloned human receptors, the $V_2:V_{1a}$ receptor selectivity was 29:1 (Table 10.3) [36]. Tolvaptan's half-life is between 6 and 8 h. Dose-dependent responses demonstrated in rats include markedly increased free water clearance, significantly less urinary loss of sodium than furosemide, and no significant effect on serum creatinine or blood urea nitrogen (BUN) [35]. In comparison with furosemide, serum sodium increased in a dose-dependent fashion in those animals given tolvaptan [30], highlighting the drug's potential benefit in hyponatremia.

Prospective randomized trials assessing the clinical utility of tolvaptan published to date have focused on its use in chronic HF [37], and more recently in patients admitted with acutely decompensated HF, to evaluate its short- and intermediate-term effects [5].

In a double-blinded study conducted in a group of 254 HF patients, three oral doses of tolvaptan (30, 45 or 60 mg) given daily for 25 days were evaluated [37]. The study enrolled patients irrespective of LVEF. Interestingly, abnormally elevated plasma concentrations of vasopressin (>8.0 pg/ml) were observed at baseline in only 6.3% of the patient population. Hyponatremia at baseline (defined as serum sodium ≤136 mEg/l) was encountered in approximately 30% of the population [38]. This study demonstrated a significant decrease in body weight and edema in modestly volume-overloaded CHF patients, increased urinary volume, and normalization of hyponatremia [37]. These effects were all sustained over the full course of therapy.

In the multicenter, randomized, double-blind, placebo-controlled, ACTIV in CHF trial, three oral, once-daily doses of tolvaptan (30, 60 or 90 mg) were compared with placebo in patients hospitalized with acute decompensated HF [5]. Body weight decreased significantly from baseline in all tolvaptan-treated groups on day 1 after admission (a primary endpoint) when compared with placebo, and decreased further during the course of hospitalization, remaining stable after discharge. This effect did not appear to be dose-dependent. Similarly, urine volume on day 1 was significantly higher in all groups treated with tolvaptan than placebo, and this effect was also maintained throughout the period of hospitalization. Diuretic use (defined by furosemide equivalents) decreased in all groups after discharge, but the mean dosage reduction was not significant. Hyponatremia (defined as serum sodium concentration <136 mEq/l) was observed in 16% of patients randomized to tolvaptan. Serum sodium concentrations were observed to rise and often normalize, in this cohort [5]. In the ACTIV in CHF trial, tolvaptan did not cause a decline in renal function, and no changes in serum potassium were noted. The absence of adverse effects on renal function seen in this trial [5] and other single-dose investigations [39] is potentially advantageous, as worsening renal function during hospitalization for decompensated HF is common [23], and associated with an unfavorable hospital course and outcome.

While no significant differences were observed in rates of rehospitalization or outpatient visits for HF, there was a trend toward longer event-free survival in the tolvaptan groups compared to placebo. In *post hoc* subgroup analysis, patients with elevated BUN levels and severe systemic congestion who were treated with tolvaptan experienced lower total mortality rates, although it should be noted that the study was not sufficiently powered or prospectively designed to assess mortality, and these results should be viewed in this light.

An important point to be noted from the ACTIV in CHF trial is that acutely decompensated HF patients with elevated BUN or severe congestion were at very high risk for short-term (60 days) mortality (22.5% and 17.8%, respectively). Whether the possible mortality benefit observed with tolvaptan in these groups is significant requires confirmation in appropriately powered studies.

Another randomized, placebo-controlled investigation of 83 NYHA functional class II and III patients with CHF and congestion who were taken off background diuretic therapy, salt restricted, and given either tolvaptan monotherapy (30 mg/day), furosemide monotherapy (80 mg/day) or a combination for 7 days, aimed at comparing tolvaptan with furosemide for volume reduction [40]. Tolvaptan-treated patients demonstrated a significant decline in body weight and increase in urine output when compared with furosemide, while serum sodium increased within normal range without a change in serum potassium. These preliminary data suggest that vasopressin receptor antagonism in stable HF patients may allow reduction or even discontinuation of loop diuretics in some cases.

In a small open-label, randomized, placebo-controlled, crossover study in patients with mild-to-moderate CHF designed to assess the effects of tolvaptan and furosemide on renal function and renal hemodynamics [39], tolvaptan was found to increase urine output, glomerular filtration rate (GFR), and renal blood flow (RBF) to statistical significance. By comparison, furosemide increased urine output to a comparable degree, but at the expense of a decreasing GFR and RBF. These results support the possibility that V_2 receptor antagonism may help preserve renal function in HF patients while promoting aquaresis.

In another recent study, Multicenter Evaluation of Tolvaptan Effect On Remodeling (METEOR), tolvaptan was evaluated on its potential effects on ventricular remodeling [41]. The primary endpoint of the study, change from baseline in LV end-diastolic volume index over 1 year of treatment, was not statistically significant in the tolvaptan group, although tolvaptan was equally as safe as placebo with equal number of adverse effects and no adverse effects in regards to ventricular remodeling or blood pressure (thought to theoretically occur with vasopressin 1_a receptor stimulation) [41]. There were favorable though not pre-specified effects on 1-year morbidity and mortality outcomes.

Currently, phase 3 studies are underway to further assess the potential for benefit of tolvaptan in acute decompensated HF (particularly from a standpoint of mortality and outcome), as well as for the specific treatment of hyponatremia associated with a variety of conditions including HF. The EVEREST trial is evaluating mortality, morbidity, and patient-assessed global clinical status in patients treated with tolvaptan compared with standard care (including diuretics) [6]. Patients are eligible for inclusion if they have a reduced LVEF (≤40%) and are hospitalized for worsening HF (class III/IV) with evidence of systemic congestion. This double-blind, multicenter trial randomizes patients to either tolvaptan 30 mg/day or matching placebo for a minimum of 60 days. Time to all-cause mortality and time to cardiovascular mortality or HF hospitalization are the co-primary endpoints. Patient-assessed global clinical status and quality of life are also being evaluated. EVEREST will be continued until 1065 deaths occur [6].

In summary, the trial data suggest that tolvaptan possesses several properties of significant potential benefit in the treatment of chronic HF, including: decreasing body weight and therefore congestion by increasing urine output; normalizing serum sodium concentration in hyponatremic patients, and possibly preventing a concomitant decline in renal function or significant electrolyte derangement commonly encountered with traditional diuretic regimens. The results of EVEREST will determine whether these effects translate into improved clinical outcomes (reduced cardiovascular mortality and/or reduced HF hospitalizations). Patient-assessed global clinical status and quality of life are also being evaluated, as well as symptom parameters.

Lixivaptan

Lixivaptan (VPA-985) is a non-peptide, orally active, specific antagonist of the V_2 receptor currently undergoing clinical evaluation. Its binding affinity for V_2 receptors is approximately 100 times greater than for V_1 receptors. Dose-dependent increases in urine output, solute-free water clearance, and serum sodium concentration have been demonstrated in preliminary human studies of single doses of lixivaptan administered to patients with NYHA class II and III HF [7]. In this double-blind trial, 42 patients were randomized to receive a single dose of either placebo or lixivaptan at a dose of 10, 30, 75, 150, 250, or 400 mg. Endpoints were measured after 4 h of fluid restriction followed by another 20 h of liberal fluid intake. Dose-related increases in urinary flow were observed after 4 h for all doses >10 mg of lixivaptan when compared to placebo. After 24 h, an absolute increase of 2.1 l urine volume was seen between those receiving a maximum 400 mg dose of the study drug compared to placebo. These effects were complemented by increases in solute-free water excretion and serum sodium levels (at higher levels). AVP antagonism was well-tolerated, with no serious events reported [7].

Lixivaptan has also been evaluated in a multiple dose study of 44 patients with hyponatremia (etiologies of which included cirrhosis, CHF, and SIADH) receiving doses of 25, 125, or 250 mg orally twice daily for 7 days [8]. The observed effects included a significant overall aquaretic response compared with placebo, with significant dose-related increases in free water clearance ($P < 0.05$) and serum sodium ($P < 0.05$), without significant changes in orthostatic blood pressure or serum creatinine levels. This agent may therefore hold promise in correcting abnormal renal water handling and hyponatremia in conditions associated with water retention. Of note is that, although safe and effective at lower doses, the higher dose (250 mg) resulted in significant dehydration requiring withholding of doses in 50% of the patients receiving this dose. Further studies are required to determine the optimal dose and indication for this new vasopressin antagonist.

V_{1a}/V_2 RECEPTOR ANTAGONISTS

Due to the hemodynamic effects attributed to activation of the V_{1a} receptor in HF, there lies a theoretical advantage in antagonizing both the V_{1a} and V_2 receptor simultaneously. The result is conceivably a synergistic effect on systemic hemodynamic and renal parameters. The most extensively studied dual receptor vasopressin antagonist is conivaptan.

Conivaptan

Conivaptan (YM-087) is a non-peptide vasopressin antagonist with high affinity for both V_{1a} and V_2 receptors. Its binding affinities suggest somewhat more potent V_2 inhibition than V_{1a} inhibition [42]. Conivaptan may be administered by oral and intravenous routes [43]. The effects of conivaptan on urinary parameters in the rat model, either with or without captopril, have been demonstrated to lead to an increase in both urine volume and sodium concentration when compared with placebo [44]. These results were sustained after a 25-day period of administration of conivaptan. Additionally, decreased intracellular free calcium and mitogen-activated protein kinase activity were observed to occur in a dose-dependent manner [21], suggesting a reduction of intracellular protein synthesis and, by extrapolation, perhaps of cardiomyocyte hypertrophy. These observations are bolstered by the results of a rat infarct study of ventricular mass after 4 weeks of treatment with conivaptan, captopril, or combination [44], demonstrating a decrease in right ventricular mass when compared to placebo, while the combination of captopril and conivaptan yielded a greater decrease in both left and right ventricular mass, suggesting that vasopressin inhibition may play a role in remodeling after myocyte injury.

Single-dose studies with conivaptan in humans with advanced HF demonstrate that dual V_{1a}/V_2 antagonism results in significant, positive aquaretic and hemodynamic effects. In a multicenter study of 142 patients with advanced HF (NYHA class III or IV, LVEF 21–26%), conivaptan was administered as a single intravenous dose (10, 20 or 40 mg) and compared with placebo [9]. Both PCWP and RAP were significantly reduced after drug administration in the 20 mg ($P < 0.01$) and 40 mg ($P < 0.05$) conivaptan groups when compared with placebo, without significant change in cardiac index, pulmonary artery pressures, systemic or pulmonary vascular resistance, systemic arterial pressure, or heart rate. The peak effect on PCWP was sustained for approximately 8 hours after administration.

Urine output in the conivaptan-treated group was significantly greater than in the placebo group ($P < 0.001$), and demonstrated a dose-dependent response that peaked at 2–3 h after the dose was administered. Similarly, urine osmolality was significantly reduced by all doses of conivaptan ($P < 0.05$), without a significant change in serum osmolality, serum sodium, or serum potassium levels. Both AVP and serum sodium concentrations were within a relatively normal range on average, and there was no significant correlation between conivaptan effects and baseline levels of either. This suggests that the effects of conivaptan are apparent in a patient population beyond merely those with hyponatremia or elevated vasopressin levels.

A preliminary study of *oral conivaptan* in relation to potential effects on functional capacity yielded less promising results, as conivaptan did not demonstrate efficacy in terms of improving exercise tolerance or quality of life [10].

The intravenous form of conivaptan, for use as a several day infusion, has undergone investigations in trials for potential use in hyponatremic states and acute decompensated HF [45]. Recent data suggest that intravenous administration of conivaptan causes a significant and dose-dependent improvement in serum sodium in hyponatremic subjects [46]. This intravenous form of conivaptan has been approved by the US FDA.

In summary, conivaptan has been demonstrated to have promising properties for the treatment of HF, particularly with regard to increasing urine output and consequently improving hemodynamic parameters of congestion, as well as normalization of serum sodium concentrations in hyponatremic subjects.

FUTURE DIRECTIONS

Non-peptide vasopressin antagonists have been developed that have several beneficial effects on the clinical syndrome of HF. These include a reduction in body fluid volume by promotion of aquaresis with maintenance of electrolyte homeostasis and correction of hyponatremia in HF as well as other hyponatremic states. Of potentially major importance is that vasopressin antagonism has been shown largely to maintain renal function in acute decompensated HF while producing these favorable effects on volume retention and congestion. Since volume reduction with standard diuretics, particularly in advanced disease states requiring high doses, is often accompanied by hyponatremia and renal function impairment (both of which have been associated with poor outcomes), this property may prove to be highly valuable in managing HF in the future. In addition to the established methods of neurohormonal blockade, vasopressin antagonism may become an important tool in the pharmacologic armamentarium against the syndrome of HF.

SUMMARY

Does antagonism of AVP improve management of HF?

▪ Vasopressin (also called antidiuretic hormone or ADH), a neurohypophysial hormone, helps regulate free water reabsorption, body fluid osmolality, blood volume, blood vessel vasoconstriction, and myocardial contractile function

▪ Novel vasopressin inhibitors, such as tolvaptan, lixivaptan, and conivaptan reduce body fluid volume by promotion of aquaresis with maintenance of renal function.

▪ The long-term effects of vasopressin antagonists on mortality and HF hospitalizations are still unclear at the present time but the ongoing EVEREST trial should help answer these questions.

Therapeutic strategies:

▪ Further phase 3 trials need to be completed before vasopressin antagonists can be adopted as a new therapy for the treatment of acute and chronic HF in clinical practice.

REFERENCES

1. Schrier RW, Abraham W. Hormones and hemodynamics in heart failure. *N Engl J Med* 1999; 341:577–585.
2. Thibonnier M. Vasopressin receptor antagonists in heart failure. *Curr Opin Pharmacol* 2003; 3:683–687.
3. Penit J, Faure M, Jard S. Vasopressin and angiotensin II receptors in rat aortic arch smooth muscle cells in culture. *Am J Physiol* 1983; 244:E72–E82.
4. Carmichael MC, Kumar R. Molecular biology of vasopressin receptors. *Semin Nephrol* 1994; 14:341–348.
5. Gheorghiade M, Gattis WA, O'Connor CM *et al*. Effects of tolvaptan, a vasopressin antagonist, in patients hospitalized with worsening heart failure: a randomized controlled trial. *JAMA* 2004; 291:1963–1971.
6. Gheorghiade M, Orlandi C, Burnett JC *et al*. Double-blind, placebo-controlled study to evaluate the efficacy of vasopressin antagonism in heart failure: Outcome study with tolvaptan (EVEREST). *J Card Fail* 2005; 11:260–269.
7. Abraham WT, Shamshirsaz AA, McFann K *et al*. Aquaretic effect of lixivaptan, an oral, non-peptide, selective V2 receptor vasopressin antagonist, in New York Heart Association Functional Class II and III Chronic Heart Failure Patients. *J Am Coll Cardiol* 2006; 47:1615–1621.
8. Wong F, Blei AT, Blendis LM, Thuluvath PJ. A vasopressin receptor antagonist (VPA-985) improves serum sodium concentration in patients with hyponatremia: a multicenter, randomized, placebo-controlled trial. *Hepatology* 2003; 37:182–191.
9. Udelson JE, Smith WB, Hendrix GH *et al*. Acute hemodynamic effects of conivaptan, a dual V_{1a} and V_2 vasopressin receptor antagonist, in patients with advanced heart failure. *Circulation* 2001; 104:2417–2423.
10. Russell SD, Adams KF, Shaw JP, Gattis WA, O'Connor CM. Results of a twelve week double-blind, placebo controlled, multicenter study of oral conivaptan to assess functional capacity in patients with class III chronic heart failure. *J Card Fail* 2003; 9(suppl):S60.
11. Lee CR, Watkins MI, Patterson JH *et al*. Vasopressin: a new target for the treatment of heart failure. *Am Heart J* 2003; 146:9–18.
12. Nielsen S, Chou CL, Marples D, Christensen EI, Kishore BK, Knepper MA. Vasopressin increases water permeability of kidney collecting duct by inducing translocation of aquaporin-CD water channels to plasma membrane. *Proc Natl Acad Sci USA* 1995; 92:1013–1017.
13. Kalra PR, Anker SD, Coats AJS. Water and sodium regulation in chronic heart failure: the role of natriuretic peptides and vasopressin. *Cardiovasc Res* 2001; 51:495–509.
14. Goldsmith SR, Francis GS, Cowley AW, Levine TB, Cohn JN. Increased plasma arginine vasopressin levels in patients with congestive heart failure. *J Am Coll Cardiol* 1983; 1:1385–1390.

15. Szatalowicz VL, Arnold PE, Chaimovitz C, Bichet D, Schrier RW. Radioimmunoassay of plasma arginine vasopressin in hyponatremic patients with congestive heart failure. *N Engl J Med* 1981; 305:263–266.

16. Francis GS, Benedict C, Johnstone DE *et al.* Comparison of neuroendocrine activation in patients with left ventricular dysfunction with and without congestive heart failure. A substudy of the Studies of Left Ventricular Dysfunction (SOLVD). *Circulation* 1990; 82:1724–1729.

17. Kramer BK, Schweda F, Riegger GAJ. Diuretic treatment and diuretic resistance in heart failure. *Am J Med* 1999; 106:90–96.

18. Goldsmith SR, Cowley AW, Francis GS, Cohn JN. Arginine vasopressin and the renal response to water loading in congestive heart failure. *Am J Cardiol* 1986; 58:295–299.

19. Bichet DG, Kortas C, Mettauer B *et al.* Modulation of plasma and platelet vasopressin by cardiac function in patients with heart failure. *Kidney Int* 1986; 29:1188–1196.

20. Uretsky BF, Verbalis JG, Generalovich T, Valdes A, Reddy PS. Plasma vasopressin response to osmotic and hemodynamic stimuli in heart failure. *Am J Physiol* 1985; 248:H396–H402.

21. Goldsmith SR. Vasopressin: a therapeutic target in congestive heart failure? *J Card Fail* 1999; 5:347–356.

22. Francis GS, Tang WHW. Vasopressin receptor antagonists. Will the 'vaptans' fulfill their promise? *JAMA* 2004; 291:2017–2018.

23. Forman DE, Butler J, Wang Y *et al.* Incidence, predictors at admission, and impact of worsening renal function among patients hospitalized with heart failure. *J Am Coll Cardiol* 2004; 43:61–67.

24. Xu DL, Martin PY, Ohara M *et al.* Upregulation of aquaporin-2 water channel expression in chronic heart failure rat. *J Clin Invest* 1997; 97:1500–1505.

25. Chan PS, Coupet J, Park HC *et al.* VPA-985, a nonpeptide orally active and selective vasopressin V_2 receptor antagonist. In: Zingg HH, Bourque CW, Bichet D (eds). *Vasopressin and Oxytocin. Molecular, Cellular, and Clinical Advances.* Plenum Press, New York, NY, 1998, vol 449, pp 439–443.

26. Goldsmith SR. Vasopressin as vasopressor. *Am J Med* 1987; 82:1213–1219.

27. Goldsmith SR, Francis SG, Cowley AW, Goldenberg I, Cohn JN. Hemodynamic effects of infused arginine vasopressin in congestive heart failure. *J Am Coll Cardiol* 1986; 8:779–783.

28. Monos E, Cox RH, Peterson CH. Direct effects of physiologic doses of arginine vasopressin on the arterial wall in vivo. *Am J Physiol* 1978; 243:H167–H173.

29. Creager MA, Faxon DP, Cutler SS, Kohlman O, Ryan TJ, Gavras H. Contribution of vasopressin to vasoconstriction in patients with congestive heart failure: comparison with the renin-angiotensin system and the sympathetic nervous system. *J Am Coll Cardiol* 1986; 7:758–765.

30. Naitoh M, Suzuki H, Murakami M *et al.* Effects of oral AVP receptor antagonists OPC-21268 and OPC-31260 on congestive heart failure in conscious dogs. *Am J Physiol* 1994; 267:H2245–H2254.

31. Clair MJ, King MK, Goldberg AT *et al.* Selective vasopressin, angiotensin II, or dual receptor blockade with developing congestive heart failure. *J Pharmacol Exp Ther* 2000; 293:852–860.

32. Nakamura Y, Haneda T, Osaki J *et al.* Hypertrophic growth of cultured neonatal rat heart cells mediated by vasopressin V_{1a} receptor. *Eur J Pharmacol* 2000; 391:39–48.

33. Tahara A, Tomura Y, Wada K *et al.* Effect of YM087, a potent nonpeptide vasopressin antagonist, on vasopressin-induced protein synthesis in neonatal rat cardiomyocyte. *Cardiovasc Res* 1998; 38:198–205.

34. Fuzukawa J, Haneda T, Kikuchi K. Arginine vasopressin increases the rate of protein synthesis in isolated perfused adult rat heart via the V_1 receptor. *Mol Cell Biochem* 1999; 195:93–98.

35. Hirano T, Yamamura Y, Nakamura S, Onogawa T, Mori T. Effects of the V_2-receptor antagonist OPC-41061 and the lop diuretic furosemide alone and in combination in rats. *J Pharmacol Exp Ther* 2000; 292:288–294.

36. Yamamura Y, Nakamura S, Ito S *et al.* OPC-41061, a highly potent human vasopressin V2-receptor antagonist: pharmacologic profile and aquaretic effect by single and multiple oral dosing in rats. *J Pharmacol Exp Ther* 1998; 287:860–867.

37. Gheorghiade M, Niazi I, Ouyang J *et al.*, for the Tolvaptan Investigators. Vasopressin V_2-receptor blockade with tolvaptan in patients with chronic heart failure: results from a double-blind, randomized trial. *Circulation* 2003; 107:2690–2696.

38. Gheorghiade M, Konstam MA, Udelson JE *et al.* Vasopressin receptor blockade with tolvaptan in chronic heart failure: differential effects in normonatremic and hyponatremic patients (Abstract). *J Am Coll Cardiol* 2002; 39(suppl A):171A.

39. Costello-Boerrigter LC, Smith WB, Boerrigter G *et al.* Vasopressin-2-receptor antagonism augments water excretion without changes in renal hemodynamics or sodium and potassium excretion in human heart failure. *Am J Physiol Renal Physiol* 2006; 290:F273–F278.

40. Udelson JE, Orlandi C, O'Brien T, Sequiera R, Ouyang J, Konstam MA. Vasopressin receptor blockade in patients with congestive heart failure: results from a placebo-controlled, randomized study comparing the effects of tolvaptan, furosemide and their combination. *J Am Coll Cardiol* 2002; 39:156A.

41. Udelson JE, the METEOR Trial Investigators. Multicenter, randomized double-blind, placebo-controlled, efficacy study on the effects of oral tolvaptan on LV dilatation and function in patients with HF and LV systolic dysfunction. Program and abstracts from the 9th Annual Scientific Meeting of the Heart Failure Society of America, September 18–21, 2005, Boca Raton, Florida.

42. Thibonnier M, Coles P, Thibonnier A, Shoham M. The basic and clinical pharmacology of nonpeptide vasopressin receptor antagonists. *Annu Rev Pharmacol Toxicol* 2001; 41:175–202.

43. Burnier M, Fricker AF, Hayoz D *et al*. Pharmacokinetic and pharmacodynamic effects of YM087, a combined V_1/V_2 vasopressin receptor antagonist in normal subjects. *Eur J Clin Pharmacol* 1999; 55:633–637.

44. Naitoh M, Risvanis J, Balding LC *et al*. Neurohormonal antagonism in heart failure; beneficial effects of vasopressin V_{1a} and V_2 receptor blockade and ACE inhibition. *Cardiovasc Res* 2002; 54:51–57.

45. Goldsmith SR, Bisaha JG, Smith N. Evaluating the efficacy and safety of the novel vasopressin V_{1a} and V_2 receptor antagonist conivaptan for the treatment of acute decompensated chronic heart failure: Study Protocol. *J Card Fail* 2004; 10(suppl):S85.

46. Verbalis JG, Bisaha JG, Smith N. Novel vasopressin V_{1a} and V_2 antagonist (conivaptan) increases serum sodium concentration and effective water clearance in patients with hyponatremia. *J Card Fail* 2004; 10(suppl):S27.

47. Lee CR, Watkins ML, Patterson JH *et al*. Vasopressin: a new target for the treatment of heart failure. *Am Heart J* 2003; 146:9–18.

48. Nicod P, Waeber B, Bussien JP *et al*. Acute hemodynamic effect of a vascular antagonist of vasopressin in patients with congestive heart failure. *Am J Cardiol* 1985; 55:1043–1047.

49. Pruszczynski W, Vahanian A, Ardaillou R, Acar J. Role of antidiuretic hormone in impaired water excretion of patients with congestive heart failure. *J Clin Endocrinosl Metab* 1984; 58:599–605.

50. Goldsmith SR, Francis GS, Levine TB, Cowley AW Jr, Cohn JN. Impaired response of plasma vasopressin to orthostatic stress in patients with congestive heart failure. *J Am Coll Cardiol* 1983; 2:1080–1083.

51. Rouleau JL, de Champlain J, Klein M *et al*. Activation of neurohormonal systems in postinfarction left ventricular dysfunction. *J Am Coll Cardiol* 1993; 22:390–398.

52. Gavras H, Ribeiro AB, Kohlmann O *et al*. Effects of a specific inhibitor of the vascular action of vasopressin in humans. *Hypertension* 1984; 6:I156–I160.

11

Extracellular remodeling in heart failure – potential use of MMP inhibitors

D. S. Feldman, F. G. Spinale

INTRODUCTION

Matrix metalloproteinase (MMP) inhibitors (MMPIs) are an emerging class of therapeutic agents that may be utilized to attenuate the progression of pathologic remodeling of diseased hearts. In many types of heart failure (HF), there is an up-regulation in matrix metallo-proteinases that degrade the extracellular matrix (ECM). This phenomenon is, in part, due to an imbalance of discrete MMPIs and their specific tissue inhibitors (TIMPs). With the use of animal models, a causal relationship has been developed between MMPI expression and ventricular remodeling. Over the last decade, several MMPIs have been developed and studied extensively in cancer, arthritis and heart disease. Specifically, recent studies of select-ive MMPI pharmacologic inhibitors have been shown to decrease ventricular dilatation and decrease myocardial infarct size. In this chapter, the basic concepts of extracellular matrix degradation, pharmacotherapy of MMPIs, and the future application of MMPIs and other signaling targets involving the extracellular matrix are reviewed.

Some of the physiologic hallmarks of HF include decreased exercise tolerance, decreased contractile function, and pathologic remodeling of the left and right ventricles. These physiologic and anatomic changes lead to a devastating mortality from lethal arrhythmias and pump failure. This progression is, in part, mediated by five distinct modalities. These five basic mechanisms in progressive HF are:

(1) a decrease in contractile function and energetics;
(2) a decrease in total number of functional cells (myocytes and fibroblasts);
(3) perturbations in signal transduction mechanisms;
(4) alterations in genomic signaling and subsequent post-translational changes; and
(5) cytoplasmic regulatory factors including phosphorylation, nitrosylation and the inter-action of regulatory proteins that mitigate localization and temporal cellular changes.

It is also important to recognize that progressive HF is primarily due to pathologic per-turbations in two distinct areas of the heart. These areas are the ECM, or cytoskeleton, and the myocytes. Although HF can be precipitated by a multitude of etiologies, many of the basic mechanisms are applicable irrespective of the etiology, with some unique nuances for specific disease processes. This chapter focuses on the physiology, biochemistry and future therapeutics of interventions that affect the ECM in generalized HF.

David S. Feldman, MD, PhD, FACC, Associate Professor of Medicine, Director of Heart Failure and Cardiac Transplant, Division of Cardiology, Departments of Medicine, Physiology and Cell Biology, The Ohio State University, Columbus, Ohio, USA.

Francis G. Spinale, MD, PhD, Professor of Surgery and Physiology, Department of Surgery, Medical University of South Carolina, Charleston, South Carolina, USA.

Myocardial interstitium or ECM is now recognized to undergo significant alterations in structure and composition as HF progresses [1]. These changes have a profound impact on the heart's overall function, as it provides the skeleton for the remaining impaired myocytes. In addition, the ECM alters myocardial function as an active participant in many aspects of cell-to-cell signaling [2, 3] and should be regarded as a complex network of dynamic inter- actions between matrix, signaling, and trans-membrane proteins. The two structural compon- ents of the ECM are the basement membrane and the collagen network. The basement membrane provides a discrete barrier between the stroma and the myocyte membrane. This covalently-bonded polygonal framework is predominately composed of collagen type IV, and to a lesser extent, fibronectin and proteoglycans [4, 5]. A second polymer network of laminin is bridged to the collagen (type IV) by the sulfated glycoprotein nidogen.

The collagen network is the largest portion of the ECM, which is largely produced by myocardial fibroblasts. The secretion of α-chain collagen polypeptides coalesces into three tightly wound chains to form a highly organized skeleton around the myocytes composed primarily of types I and II collagen. This skeleton has three discrete components which include endomysial, perimysial, and epimysial collagen [1, 2]. Endomysial collagen binds individual myocytes to one another, while perimysial collagen binds bundles of myocytes and blood vessels together. Epimysial collagen provides the outer layer to these perimysial bundles. Modifications in the composition of the collagen network alter ventricular func- tion and geometry. With increased collagen deposition, hypertrophy and increased wall stiffness develop [6], while an attenuation of collagen deposition leads to decreased sup- port for the surrounding myocytes and subsequent remodeling [7].

Ongoing investigation by several laboratories has demonstrated that there are several potential therapeutic interventions which can alter the progression of HF by redirecting or blocking pathologic signaling. Examples of these interventions include the ability to block collagen cross-linking [8], an attenuation of collagen formation/distribution, or disruptions in post-translational glycation [9]. In addition to interventions that may alter ECM synthe- sis, there are also mechanisms that may alter the balance of the ECM breakdown.

MATRIX METALLOPROTEINASES

There are more than 25 proteins that can degrade the ECM known as MMPs. These endogen- ous proteins are essential for maintaining the integrity of the heart by regulating the normal turnover of the ECM. An imbalance of these MMPs produces pathologic phenotypes with progressive hypertrophy, HF or ischemia [10, 11]. MMPs are initially secreted as inactive pro-enzymes (zymogens) into the ECM, and thereafter remain biologically quiescent until their specific pro-peptide domain is cleaved [11]. Specifically, the interruption of a zinc- cysteine site leads to activation of the biologically inactive MMPs [12]. There has been multiple nomenclature changes as our understanding of these enzymes has evolved. In this chapter, we classify the MMPs based on their *in vitro* specificity and structure (Table 11.1). In addition to MMP's ability to degrade discrete portions of the ECM, there is now evolv- ing evidence that non-matrix proteins involved in cell growth and apoptosis may also be affected. The cross-communication between the multiple MMPs and other proteolytic enzymes frequently initiates cascades of signaling proteins. With this degradative system, there are multiple redundancies to initiate and inhibit these ECM signaling pathways [1, 13]. For example, zymogens can be activated by MMPs, membrane bound MMPs (MT-MMPs) [14] and serine proteases, which are frequently involved in adrenergic and cal- cium signaling. An additional layer of control is superimposed upon the MMPs by a series of regulatory proteins called TIMPs. There are currently four known TIMPs that competi- tively bind to MMPs and attenuate the MMP–ECM interaction and degradation [15]. The relevance of this stochiometric inhibition [15] has been demonstrated in a knockout mouse model. Deletion of TIMP-1 mice developed rapid pathologic remodeling in the absence of

Table 11.1 Representative matrix metalloproteinases found in the myocardium

MMP Number	Name	Substrate/function
Collagenases		
MMP-1	Interstitial collagenase	Collagens I, II, III, IV and basement membrane
MMP-8	Neutrophil collagenase	Collagens I, II, III and basement membrane
MMP-13	Collagenase-3	Collagens I, II, III
Gelatinases		
MMP-2	Gelatinase A	Gelatins, collagens I, IV, V, VII and basement membrane
MMP-9	Gelatinase B	Gelatins, collagens IV, V, XIV and basement membrane
Stromelysins		
MMP-3	Stromelysin 1	Fibronectin, laminin, collagens III, IV, IX and MMP activation
Membrane-type MMP		
MMP-14	MT1-MMP	Collagens I, II, III, fibronectin, laminin, Pro-MMPs-2 and -13

Adapted with permission from [13].

any noxious stimulus [16]. Perhaps the most expressed TIMP in the human myocardium is TIMP-4 [17]. MMPs are, in part, responsible for the observed phenotype in cardiac hypertrophy, dilated cardiomyopathies (DCM), and decreased ventricular function subsequent to a myocardial infarct.

In numerous studies to determine the role of MMPs in hypertrophy, investigators found reduced MMP plasma levels in patients with systemic hypertension [18]. Specifically, MMP-1 was found to be attenuated with an excessive deposition of collagen type I in a series of hypertensive patients, while in another cohort of untreated hypertensive patients, blood serum analysis revealed abnormal plasma levels of MMP-9 and TIMP-1. Other studies have noted an increased stochiometric ratio of TIMP-1 to MMP-1 in patients with severe ventricular hypertrophy [19]. Additional longitudinal studies have demonstrated progressive changes in MMP signaling with advanced hypertrophy and subsequent HF [20] (see additional studies in the next section). Several studies in animals suggest that initial hypertrophic changes are commensurate with mild up-regulation or no change of the TIMPs (protective mechanism) and no change in MMP activity. With progressive hypertrophy, an up-regulation of the MMPs and a decrease in TIMPs was noted, thus favoring pathologic remodeling. Taken together, these studies would suggest that an attenuation of MMPs, and an increase in TIMPs in hypertensive patients leads to an increase in ECM accumulation [20, 21].

In end-stage DCM, several studies have examined the relative contribution of MMPs and TIMPs in HF patients [22]. Both the zymogens and active MMPs have been found to be elevated in ischemic (MMP-9) and non-ischemic (MMP-3, -9, and -13) DCMs. In addition, there is a concordant dysregulation of TIMP-1 observed in DCM, and a lower affinity between TIMPs and their respective MMPs. Hence, there is not only an increase in certain MMPs, but the up-regulation of a specific MMP decreases the sensitivity of its endogenous antagonist (TIMP) and thereafter amplifies the degradation of the ECM and perpetuates progressive HF. The expression levels of TIMPs in DCM patients vary, suggesting differences in the etiology of DCM in these patients. These studies may suggest that the interaction of the MMPs and the TIMPs is more important than the actual expression levels of a TIMP. This generalization regarding the altered ratios of MMP/TIMP, and their relative affinities, is applicable to most DCM and this has a significant impact on pathologic remodeling [23–25].

Post-myocardial infarction remodeling represents an area of intense investigation with MMPs. Several studies have demonstrated increased levels of MMPs (MMP-2, -9 and TIMP-1) with acute coronary syndrome and after an acute infarct [26]. However, the initiation of the maladaptive MMP signaling and the temporal sequence of events remains largely unknown. To address these specific questions, researchers followed the pattern of MMP up-regulation subsequent to alcohol septal ablation ('controlled infarct'). This study demonstrated that in small–medium, 'controlled' infarcts, MMP-9 was elevated for up to 50 h subsequent to anterior-septal infarcts. Although patients' MMP-serum levels may not reflect myocardial tissue activity, these data may potentially help to determine the correct temporal sequence for a future therapeutic intervention. In addition, the lack of regulatory control of the TIMP has also been implicated in the pathogenesis of remodeling after a myocardial infarct. In animal models, TIMP levels were decreased with ischemia/reperfusion events. This disinhibition may act as a segue for enhanced MMP signaling immediately subsequent to an infarct [27, 28].

TRANSMEMBRANE PROTEINS

A distinct group of MMPs are membrane-bound. These proteins are sub-divided into MT-MMPs, disintegrins, metalloproteinases, and the integrins [1]. MT-MMPs are expressed in myocytes, fibroblasts, and invasive inflammatory cells. Membrane Type-1 MMP (MT1-MMP) is the best described of these proteins, and is known to be activated intracellularly *via* a furin-dependent pathway. Unlike the other MMPs, MT1-MMP is fully activated once it is embedded in the membrane. MT1-MMP can activate other MMPs and degrade fibronectin, laminin-I, as well as multiple collagens. In addition to the MT1-MMP's role in up-regulating ECM degradation, it affects non-ECM protein activity (e.g. tumour necrosis factor-α [TNF-α] and *vice versa*) [29]. Usually, animal models show minimal change in their cardiac phenotype when an MMP is genetically deleted; but the importance of these metalloproteinases (MT-MMPs) is demonstrated in a genomic deletion of MT1-MMP [30]. These animals develop severe hypertrophy and HF and die a few weeks after birth. In humans, DCM and ischemic HF models show more than a threefold increase in expression of this metalloproteinase. More recent studies have shown an increase in activation in ischemia and reperfusion [31, 32].

The disintegrins and metalloproteinases (ADAMs) are a family of cell surface proteins that function as signaling molecules to regulate proteolysis, adhesion and cellular communication [33]. ADAMs regulate cell-to-cell and ECM signaling. These proteins have been proposed to be involved in the progressive pathology of atrial fibrillation [34], myocarditis and pathologic remodeling. Although causal data linking these proteins to HF are limited, studies with aortic constriction mice suggest that antagonism of ADAM-12 [35] may attenuate a hypertrophic response. Finally, the integrins are a family of heterodimeric membrane proteins that link the ECM and the actin cytoskeleton. Like the other transmembrane proteins, the integrins serve as 'anchoring proteins', but are also actively involved in cell signaling. Of note, integrins are actively involved in the initiation of signaling cascades subsequent to stress-activated responses. These signaling pathways include the mitogen-activated protein kinases (MAPKs) [36]. Activation of these MAPKs can subsequently induce hypertrophy *via* ERK or pathologic remodeling perhaps through P-38 or JNK.

CLINICAL TRIALS ASSESSING THE IMPACT OF MMPs IN CARDIAC REMODELING WITH AVAILABLE THERAPEUTIC METHODS

Certainly, it is not possible to cover all of the MMP studies that have been performed. We have not attempted to be inclusive, but only to provide a basis for future consideration for more extensive clinical trials. Only studies related to cardiac disease have been included in this limited survey.

PRE-CLINICAL

Aldosterone antagonism

In diastolic HF, there is an increase in collagens I and III. One of the essential MMPs responsible for maintaining collagen breakdown is MMP-1. Studies would suggest that with HF there is an up-regulation of the renin–angiotensin system. With pathologic signaling, there is an increase in angiotensin II and aldosterone. Brilla *et al.* [37] demonstrated that rat myocytes treated with spironolactone decrease fibrosis. This may, in part, provide a mechanism to the improved survival results appreciated in the aldosterone antagonist trials.

Brain natriuretic peptide

Results of clinical trials with recombinant human brain natriuretic peptide (BNP) improve hemodynamic parameters in acute HF. These results may suggest that BNP exerts a direct cardio-protective effect and might be useful as an adjunct therapy in the setting of acute infarct. Kawakami *et al.* [38] used mice with genetically enhanced BNP levels to determine if BNP will alter pathologic remodeling subsequent to a myocardial infarct. Their results in this study suggested that elevated plasma BNP levels facilitated neutrophil infiltration of the infarcted area, and increased the activity of the MMP-9. This may suggest that BNP may play a role in ECM remodeling and wound-healing immediately after an infarct. A previous study [28] had been performed in swine to assess the impact of broad spectrum MMP inhibition on remodeling after an infarct. This study also attempted to address some of the timing concerns in the implementation of an MMPI. Results of this second study suggested that MMP-1 and -7 were not required to favorably alter ventricular remodeling subsequent to an infarct. In summary, these studies suggest that the timing for blocking MMPs subsequent to an infarct and which are the most important remains somewhat controversial [39].

ACE inhibitors and angiotensin receptor blockers

Researchers investigated the role of the renin–angiotensin system in the collagen gene expression by administration of an angiotensin-converting enzyme (ACE) inhibitor (ramipril) and an angiotensin receptor type I antagonist (losartan) in a post-infarct animal model [40]. These investigators noted an increase in the mRNA expression of collagen types I and III, 3 days after an infarct; and a zenith in collagen mRNA levels between 7 and 14 days. These increased collagen levels persisted when re-assessed at 1 and 2 months after the animals' infarcts. MMP activity was increased throughout the study in the infarcted animals, as compared to their matched controls. Subsequent to the completion of the study, losartan treatment was not associated with any normalization of elevated collagen mRNA levels, but decrease in cardiac fibrosis was noted with both therapies. These data suggest that these therapies are not likely to be mediated by the AT1 receptor; and perhaps the mechanism of ACE inhibition and losartan may reside at the level of post-translational/protein modification.

CLINICAL

HMG-CoA reductase inhibitors

Nakaya *et al.* [41] examined post-infarct patients, and thereafter attempted to determine if a decrease in MMP levels could be observed with patients utilizing conventional medical therapy. They proposed that the statin, pravachol, would have a significant impact on systemic MMP and on left ventricular remodeling, subsequent to an acute myocardial infarction. In

34 consecutive patients, serum levels of MMP-2 and TIMP-2 were measured immediately after reperfusion, on days 2, 3, 7, 30, and at 6 months. Echocardiograms were performed after reperfusion and at 4 weeks and 6 months. These investigators concluded that MMP-2 levels changed in a time-dependent manner following an acute infarction and correlated with ventricular size. They also noted that MMP-2 levels were significantly lower in the patients treated with pravachol.

Thiazolidinediones

Diastolic function is exacerbated by poor glucose control. Hence, this study was developed to assess the impact of pioglitazone and the treatment of insulin resistance in 30 patients with hypertensive heart disease [42]. The results from this pilot trial demonstrated an improvement of several echocardiographic parameters, with the most exaggerated improvement in the patients that had the worst diastolic function. The results appeared to be independent of glycemic control or ventricular mass regression. The investigators concluded that pioglitazone treatment significantly increased plasma levels of MMP-2 and improved diastolic function.

Ca^{2+} channel blockers and β-blockers

In the Anglo-Scandinavian Cardiac Outcomes Trial (ASCOT), investigators assessed the ability of a calcium channel blocker (CCB) or β-blocker to decrease cardiac events in hypertensive patients [43]. It was hypothesized that these hypertensive patients developed cardiac hypertrophy from a dysregulation of MMP-9 and TIMP-1 [44]. Thereafter, they proposed that these MMP circulating levels could be correlated with coronary heart disease (CHD) and stroke (CVA). At the conclusion of the trial, these investigators found that prior to treatment for hypertension, MMP-9 and TIMP-1 levels were significantly higher in patients with hypertension than in the normotensive patients. After therapy, plasma MMP-9 levels decreased, and TIMP-1 levels increased. In addition, MMP-9 levels correlated with CHD events, but not CVA events. They also noted no statistically significant difference between TIMP-1 and CVA or CHD events.

In a second trial of 72 hypertensive patients, researchers [45] attempted to assess the ability of felodipine or dilitiazem to attenuate vascular changes related to an MMP-mediated pathway. These investigators were unable to show any change in serum MMP-9 levels or an increase in MMP-2 levels with felodopine. The results of these collective data may suggest a greater degree of efficacy with dihydropyridines in pathologic states of proliferative ECM remodeling.

The impact of cardiopulmonary bypass on MMPs

Cardiopulmonary bypass (CPB) is known to induce the activation of neutrophils. Previous observational studies had observed an increase in MMP-9 in patients who have undergone CPB. Lin et al. [46] sought to determine whether CPB would increase neutrophil activation of MMP-9 or later TIMP-1 levels in 21 patients undergoing elective bypass surgery. In this study, the investigators found a significant increase in the plasma levels of MMP-9 2–6 h after CPB, and no significant change in patients with off-pump bypass surgery. Although the plasma levels of TIMP-1 gradually increased over this same period of time, the MMP-9/TIMP-1 ratio was increased suggesting increased cardiac tissue breakdown.

The impact of MMPs in aortic stenosis

Cardiac biopsies were procured from 36 patients with aortic stenosis (AS). These investigators hypothesized that TIMP and MMP levels were associated with increased ventricular hypertrophy in AS [47]. Microarray analysis revealed significantly increased mRNA expression of collagen types I, III, and IV in AS patients compared with controls, and was most pronounced in AS patients with severe diastolic dysfunction. Cardiac mRNA expression of TIMP-1 and -2 was significantly increased in AS compared with control patients, whereas MMP-1, -2, or -9 were not significantly changed. Cardiac TIMP-1 and -2 transcripts were also noted to be related to the degree of interstitial fibrosis and proportional to diastolic dysfunction in the AS patients.

FUTURE CONSIDERATIONS

With the conclusion of the Prevention of MI Early Remodeling (PREMIER) trial presented at the American College of Cardiology in 2005, the utilization of a broad-spectrum MMPI (PG-116800) fell short of investigators' expectations in a post-myocardial infarct population. PG-116800 was designed to target MMP-2, -3, -8, -9, -13 and -14. In this trial, ventricular remodeling was not significantly changed in the presence of the MMPI. There are several reasons why this study may have been confounded, including the late initiation of therapy (up to 2 days after the infarct), poly-pharmacy, or a lack of selective inhibition of targeted MMPs. This trial emphasizes the need to further delineate the timing of drug therapy, and a desire to sharpen our therapeutic interventions [13]. A recent study by Wagner *et al.* [48], suggest that MMP-9 levels are elevated subsequent to an infarct, and are predictive of future HF events. With continued efforts directed toward increasing our understanding of MMP signaling, clinicians should expect additional clinical trials with MMP-type inhibitors. The MMP signaling pathways represent several of the more promising therapeutic possibilities in the near future that target pathologic remodeling of the heart and may add to the treatment of progressive HF.

SUMMARY

- Do MMPs decrease pathologic remodeling? HMG-CoA reductase inhibitors may decrease ventricular remodeling subsequent to an infarct *via* the attenuation of MMP-2.
- Thiazolidinediones, dihydropyridines, and β-blockers may decrease diastolic dysfunction in select HF patients by altering MMP-2, -9 and TIMP-1 signaling.
- Aldosterone antagonists, natriuretic peptide, and several investigative compounds are among the possibilities that may be effective in altering progressive remodeling. Additional trials and investigation will be required to determine the specific type of MMP, and temporal sequence for therapeutic interventions in selective patients.
- Specific cardiothoracic surgical interventions may have a differential effect on MMP levels and subsequent remodeling.

REFERENCES

1. Deschamps AM, Spinale FG. Disruptions and detours in the myocardial matrix highway and heart failure. *Curr Heart Fail Rep* 2005; 2:10–17.
2. Weber KT, Sun Y, Tyagi SC, Cleutjens JP. Collagen network of the myocardium: function, structural remodeling and regulatory mechanisms. *J Mol Cell Cardiol* 1994; 26:279–292.
3. Geiger B, Bershadsky A, Pankov R, Yamada KM. Transmembrane crosstalk between the extracellular matrix–cytoskeleton crosstalk. *Nat Rev Mol Cell Biol* 2001; 2:793–805.
4. Yurchenco PD, Schittny JC. Molecular architecture of basement membranes. *FASEB J* 1990; 4:1577–1590.
5. Kalluri R. Basement membranes: structure, assembly and role in tumour angiogenesis. *Nat Rev Cancer* 2003; 3:422–433.
6. Jalil JE, Doering CW, Janicki JS, Pick R, Shroff SG, Weber KT. Fibrillar collagen and myocardial stiffness in the intact hypertrophied rat left ventricle. *Circ Res* 1989; 64:1041–1050.

7. Sutton MG, Sharpe N. Left ventricular remodeling after myocardial infarction: pathophysiology and therapy. *Circulation* 2000; 101:2981–2988.
8. Kato S, Spinale FG, Tanaka R, Johnson W, Cooper G, Zile MR. Inhibition of collagen cross-linking: effects on fibrillar collagen and ventricular diastolic function. *Am J Physiol* 1995; 269:H863–H868.
9. Asif M, Egan J, Vasan S et al. An advanced glycation endproduct cross-link breaker can reverse age-related increases in myocardial stiffness. *Proc Natl Acad Sci USA* 2000; 97:2809–2813.
10. Visse R, Nagase H. Matrix metalloproteinases and tissue inhibitors of metalloproteinases: structure, function, and biochemistry. *Circ Res* 2003; 92:827–839.
11. Creemers EE, Cleutjens JP, Smits JF, Daemen MJ. Matrix metalloproteinase inhibition after myocardial infarction: a new approach to prevent heart failure? *Circ Res* 2001; 89:201–210.
12. Van Wart HE, Birkedal-Hansen H. The cysteine switch: a principle of regulation of metalloproteinase activity with potential applicability to the entire matrix metalloproteinase gene family. *Proc Natl Acad Sci USA* 1990; 87:5578–5582.
13. Spinale FG. Matrix metalloproteinases: regulation and dysregulation in the failing heart. *Circ Res* 2002; 90:520–530.
14. Toth M, Hernandez-Barrantes S, Osenkowski P et al. Complex pattern of membrane type 1 matrix metalloproteinase shedding. Regulation by autocatalytic cells surface inactivation of active enzyme. *J Biol Chem* 2002; 277:26340–26350.
15. Brew K, Dinakarpandian D, Nagase H. Tissue inhibitors of metalloproteinases: evolution, structure and function. *Biochim Biophys Acta* 2000; 1477:267–283.
16. Roten L, Nemoto S, Simsic J et al. Effects of gene deletion of the tissue inhibitor of the matrix metalloproteinase-type 1 (TIMP-1) on left ventricular geometry and function in mice. *J Mol Cell Cardiol* 2000; 32:109–120.
17. Greene J, Wang M, Liu YE, Raymond LA, Rosen C, Shi YE. Molecular cloning and characterization of human tissue inhibitor of metalloproteinase 4. *J Biol Chem* 1996; 271:30375–30380.
18. Laviades C, Varo N, Fernandez J et al. Abnormalities of the extracellular degradation of collagen type I in essential hypertension. *Circulation* 1998; 98:535–540.
19. Hirono O, Fatema K, Nitobe J et al. Long-term effects of benidipine hydrochloride on severe left ventricular hypertrophy and collagen metabolism in patients with essential hypertension. *J Cardiol* 2002; 39:195–204.
20. Li H, Simon H, Bocan TM, Peterson JT. MMP/TIMP expression in spontaneously hypertensive heart failure rats: the effect of ACE- and MMP-inhibition. *Cardiovasc Res* 2000; 46:298–306.
21. Iwanaga Y, Aoyama T, Kihara Y, Onozawa Y, Yoneda T, Sasayama S. Excessive activation of matrix metalloproteinases coincides with left ventricular remodeling during transition from hypertrophy to heart failure in hypertensive rats. *J Am Coll Cardiol* 2002; 39:1384–1391.
22. Tyagi SC, Campbell SE, Reddy HK, Tjahja E, Voelker DJ. Matrix metalloproteinase activity expression in infarcted, noninfarcted and dilated cardiomyopathic human hearts. *Mol Cell Biochem* 1996; 155:13–21.
23. Thomas CV, Coker ML, Zellner JL, Handy JR, Crumbley AJ III, Spinale FG. Increased matrix metalloproteinase activity and selective upregulation in LV myocardium from patients with end-stage dilated cardiomyopathy. *Circulation* 1998; 97:1708–1715.
24. Spinale FG, Coker ML, Heung LJ et al. A matrix metalloproteinase induction/activation system exists in the human left ventricular myocardium and is upregulated in heart failure. *Circulation* 2000; 102:1944–1949.
25. Knauper V, Lopez-Otin C, Smith B, Knight G, Murphy G. Biochemical characterization of human collagenase-3. *J Biol Chem* 1996; 271:1544–1550.
26. Kai H, Ikeda H, Yasukawa H et al. Peripheral blood levels of matrix metalloproteases-2 and -9 are elevated in patients with acute coronary syndromes. *J Am Coll Cardiol* 1998; 32:368–372.
27. Mukherjee R, Brinsa TA, Dowdy KB et al. Myocardial infarct expansion and matrix metalloproteinase inhibition. *Circulation* 2003; 107:618–625.
28. Yarbrough WM, Mukherjee R, Escobar GP et al. Selective targeting and timing of matrix metalloproteinase inhibition in post-myocardial infarction remodeling. *Circulation* 2003; 108:1753–1759.
29. d'Ortho MP, Will H, Atkinson S et al. Membrane-type matrix metalloproteinases 1 and 2 exhibit broad-spectrum proteolytic capacities comparable to many matrix metalloproteinases. *Eur J Biochem* 1997; 250:751–757.
30. Spinale FG, Coker ML, Heung LJ et al. A matrix metalloproteinase induction/activation system exists in the human left ventricular myocardium and is upregulated in heart failure. *Circulation* 2000; 102:1944–1949.

31. Holmbeck K, Bianco P, Yamada S, Birkedal-Hansen H. MT1-MMP: a tethered collagenase. *J Cell Physiol* 2004; 200:11–19.

32. Deschamps AM, Yarbrough WM, Squires CE *et al*. Trafficking of the membrane type-1 matrix metalloproteinase in ischemia and reperfusion: relation to interstitial membrane type-1 matrix metalloproteinase activity. *Circulation* 2005; 111:1166–1174.

33. Seals DF, Courtneidge SA. The ADAMs family of metalloproteases: multidomain proteins with multiple functions. *Genes Dev* 2003; 17:7–30.

34. Arndt M, Lendeckel U, Rocken C *et al*. Altered expression of ADAMs (A Disintegrin And Metalloproteinase) in fibrillating human atria. *Circulation* 2002; 105:720–725.

35. Asakura M, Kitakaze M, Takashima S *et al*. Cardiac hypertrophy is inhibited by antagonism of ADAM12 processing of HB-EGF: metalloproteinase inhibitors as a new therapy. *Nat Med* 2002; 8:35–40.

36. Deschamps AM, Yarbrough WM, Squires CE *et al*. Trafficking of the membrane type-1 matrix metalloproteinase in ischemia and reperfusion: relation to interstitial membrane type-1 matrix metalloproteinase activity. *Circulation* 2005; 111:1166–1174.

37. Brilla CG, Schencking M, Scheer C, Rupp H. Spironolactone: renaissance of anti-aldosterone therapy in heart failure? *Schweiz Rundsch Med Prax* 1997; 86:566–574.

38. Kawakami R, Saito Y, Kishimoto I *et al*. Overexpression of brain natriuretic peptide facilitates neutrophil infiltration and cardiac matrix metalloproteinase-9 expression after acute myocardial infarction. *Circulation* 2004; 110:3306–3312.

39. Vanhoutte D, Schellings M, Pinto Y, Heymans S. Relevance of matrix metalloproteinases and their inhibitors after myocardial infarction: a temporal and spatial window. *Cardiovasc Res* 2006; 69:604–613.

40. Dixon IM, Ju H, Jassal DS, Peterson DJ. Effect of ramipril and losartan on collagen expression in right and left heart after myocardial infarction. *Mol Cell Biochem* 1996; 165:31–45.

41. Nakaya R, Uzui H, Shimizu H *et al*. Pravastatin suppresses the increase in matrix metalloproteinase-2 levels after acute myocardial infarction. *Int J Cardiol* 2005; 105:67–73.

42. Horio T, Suzuki M, Suzuki K *et al*. Pioglitazone improves left ventricular diastolic function in patients with essential hypertension. *Am J Hypertens* 2005; 18:949–957.

43. Oparil S. Long-term morbidity and mortality trials with amlodipine. *J Cardiovasc Pharmacol* 1999; 33(suppl 2):S1–S6.

44. Tayebjee MH, Nadar S, Blann AD, Gareth BD, MacFadyen RJ, Lip GY. Matrix metalloproteinase-9 and tissue inhibitor of metalloproteinase-1 in hypertension and their relationship to cardiovascular risk and treatment: a substudy of the Anglo-Scandinavian Cardiac Outcomes Trial (ASCOT). *Am J Hypertens* 2004; 17:764–769.

45. Zervoudaki A, Economou E, Pitsavos C *et al*. The effect of Ca2+ channel antagonists on plasma concentrations of matrix metalloproteinase-2 and -9 in essential hypertension. *Am J Hypertens* 2004; 17:273–276.

46. Lin TC, Li CY, Tsai CS *et al*. Neutrophil-mediated secretion and activation of matrix metalloproteinase-9 during cardiac surgery with cardiopulmonary bypass. *Anesth Analg* 2005; 100:1554–1560.

47. Heymans S, Schroen B, Vermeersch P *et al*. Increased cardiac expression of tissue inhibitor of metalloproteinase-1 and tissue inhibitor of metalloproteinase-2 is related to cardiac fibrosis and dysfunction in the chronic pressure-overloaded human heart. *Circulation* 2005; 112:1136–1144.

48. Wagner DR, Delagardelle C, Ernens I, Rouy D, Vaillant M, Beissel J. Matrix metalloproteinase-9 is a marker of heart failure after acute myocardial infarction. *J Card Fail* 2006; 12:66–72.

12

Erythropoietin analogs in the treatment of anemia in heart failure

Y.-D. Tang, S. D. Katz

INTRODUCTION

Anemia is common in chronic heart failure (CHF) patients and is independently associated with impaired ventricular function, reduced functional capacity and increased mortality. The underlying causes of anemia and the mechanisms that link anemia with increased mortality risk in CHF are not yet well-characterized. Small clinical trials with erythopoietic agents in anemic patients with CHF have demonstrated improved ventricular function, increased exercise capacity, and improved quality of life. The threshold hemoglobin (Hb) value for initiation of therapy, optimal Hb target during therapy, optimal dosing regimen for erythropoietic agents, and role of oral vs intravenous iron supplementation remains to be determined. Erythropoetic agents also have potential pro-thrombotic effects that have been associated with increased risk of adverse clinical outcomes in anemic patients with cancer and chronic kidney disease. Additional clinical trials in larger populations are ongoing to determine the safety and efficacy of erythropoietic therapy in anemic CHF patients. This chapter will summarize the potential therapeutic implications for treatment of anemia in CHF.

The pathogenesis of anemia in CHF has not been fully characterized, but observational studies indicate that several clinical factors are associated with greater risk of anemia. Advanced age, female gender, comorbid chronic kidney disease, inflammation, decreased body mass index and more advanced symptoms of CHF are associated with lower Hb values [1–7]. Other factors, such as use of angiotensin-converting enzyme inhibitors [8–10], hemodilution [11], and iron deficiency [12] also contribute to increased risk of anemia. Potential mechanistic pathways relevant to these clinical risk factors for anemia have been recently reviewed. Regardless of cause, anemia appears to be associated with adverse pathophysiologic consequences in CHF patients. Anemia is associated with greater impairment of functional capacity in CHF patients and may promote progression of pathologic left ventricular remodeling. Anemia has also been consistently linked to increased risk of adverse cardiovascular events in observational studies in patients with CHF. Whether or not the observed association between anemia and survival represents a true causal relationship is unknown. There are biologically plausible mechanisms by which anemia could directly or indirectly promote disease progression in CHF. Alternatively, anemia may be a marker of more severe underlying myocardial disease. Nonetheless, these observations provide sufficient reason to determine the impact of anemia treatment on functional capacity and clinical outcomes in CHF.

Yi-Da Tang, MD, PhD, Associate Research Scientist, Department of Internal Medicine, Section of Cardiovascular Medicine, Yale University School of Medicine, New Haven, Connecticut, USA.

Stuart D. Katz, MD, Associate Professor of Medicine, Yale University School of Medicine, New Haven, Connecticut, USA.

From a therapeutic standpoint, erythropoietin levels in anemic CHF patients, although in some cases above the normal range, are well below the physiologic levels expected in response to anemia [13–15]. Accordingly, exogenous supplementation of erythropoietic agents has been proposed as a therapeutic strategy to treat anemic CHF patients.

The physiologic and pharmacologic action of erythropoietin is mediated by specific receptors expressed on bone marrow erythroid precursors coupled to cytoplasmic and nuclear events *via* activation of the Janus Kinase-2 (JAK2) signal transducer and activator of transcription-5 (STAT5) signal transduction pathway [16, 17]. The primary mechanism by which erythropoietin promotes production of new red blood cells is by inhibition of apoptosis in bone marrow erythroid progenitor cells [16, 18].

There are three erythropoietic agents available for clinical use: epoetin α, epoetin β (both of which are forms of recombinant human erythropoietin [rHuEPO]) and darbepoetin α [19]. rHuEPO was first synthesized in 1985, only 2 years after the erythropoietin gene was cloned, and was approved for clinical use as a therapeutic agent for the treatment of anemia associated with end-stage chronic kidney disease in 1988 [20]. Initial results from studies in end-stage chronic kidney disease patients showed that intravenous or subcutaneous doses of 150–200 IU/kg/week (in 1–3 divided doses per week) increased Hb concentrations to 10–12 g/dl in the large majority of patients [21–24]. Plasma half-life of rHuEPO after intravenous dosing is 6–8 h. Approximately 25% of the administered dose is absorbed after subcutaneous dosing, but the plasma half-life is increased to >24 h [25, 26]. The amount of subcutaneous rHuEPO needed to achieve Hb targets in chronic kidney disease patients is approximately 25% less than that needed with intravenous dosing [26]. Darbepoetin α is a long-acting N-linked super-sialylated analog of human erythropoietin that was approved by Food and Drug Administration (FDA) for the treatment of anemia in patients with chronic kidney disease in 2001 [27, 28]. Compared to both native and recombinant erythropoietin, it has a stronger affinity for erythropoietin receptors and a longer plasma half-life of approximately 48 h, which in turn increases the time interval between doses to 1–2 weeks during maintenance therapy [28–30].

Several groups of investigators have published pilot studies on the effects of erythropoietic agents on clinical status in anemic CHF patients. The studies are summarized in Table 12.1 and are described in greater detail in the following paragraphs.

The clinical effects of rHuEPO treatment in anemic CHF patients were first reported by Silverberg *et al.* [31]. In this open-label study, 26 anemic CHF patients (New York Heart Association [NYHA] class III–IV and Hb <12 g/dl) were treated with subcutaneous rHuEPO (mean dose 5277 IU/week) and intravenous iron sucrose (mean dose 185 mg/month) with 4–15 months' follow-up duration (mean 7 months). The mean Hb increased from 10.2 to 12.1 g/dl. When compared with pre-treatment baseline values, rHuEPO therapy was associated with improved function class (3.66 ± 0.47 at baseline to 2.66 ± 0.7 post-treatment; $P < 0.05$), increased left ventricular ejection fraction (LVEF) (27.7 ± 4.8% at baseline to 35.4 ± 7.6% post-treatment; $P < 0.001$), and reduced the need for oral and intravenous furosemide [31]. The same group of investigators subsequently reported the findings of a randomized open-label trial to compare the effects of partial correction of anemia with subcutaneous rHuEPO and intravenous iron sucrose therapy vs usual care with a mean follow-up duration over 8 months in 32 patients with CHF and anemia (NYHA class III–IV and Hb <11.5 g/dl) [32]. When compared with usual care, rHuEPO therapy (4000 IU one to three times weekly subcutaneously plus iron sucrose 200 mg every 2 weeks intravenously) significantly increased Hb level (rHuEPO 10.3–12.9 g/dl vs usual care 10.9–10.8 g/dl; $P < 0.0001$), improved NYHA functional class (rHuEPO 3.8 ± 0.4 to 2.2 ± 0.7 vs usual care 3.5 ± 0.7 to 3.9 ± 0.3; $P < 0.0001$), and decreased hospitalization days during follow-up (rHuEPO 13.8 ± 7.2 to 2.9 ± 6.6 days vs usual care 9.9 ± 4.8 vs 15.5 ± 9.8 days; $P < 0.0001$) [32]. In a subsequent non-randomized clinical series of 179 patients with severe CHF, mild-to-moderate chronic kidney disease (pre-dialysis with mean serum Cr 2.1–2.4 mg/dl)

Table 12.1 Clinical trials of erythropoietic agents in anemic CHF patients

Trial	Clinicaltrial.gov identifier	n	Design	Inclusion criteria	Treatment	Endpoints	Results
Silverberg et al. [31]	–	26	Open-label, uncontrolled	NYHA III-IV CHF Hb <12 g/dl	EPO 2000 U/week SC titrated to Hb = 12 g/dl	Hb ≥12 g/dl; clinical status	NYHA class improved LVEF ↑, decreased hospitalization days
Silverberg et al. [32]	–	32	Open-label, randomized	NYHA III-IV CHF Hb <11.5 g/dl	EPO 4000 U/week SC titrated to Hb = 12.5 g/dl	Hb ≥12.5 g/dl; clinical status	NYHA class improved LVEF ↑, decreased hospitalization days
Silverberg et al. [33]	–	179	Open-label, uncontrolled	NYHA III-IV CHF Hb = 9.5-11.5	EPO 4000-5000 U/week SC titrated to Hb = 12.5 g/dl	Hb ≥12.5 g/dl; clinical status	NYHA class improved and LVEF ↑
Silverberg et al. [63]	–	40	Open-label, uncontrolled	NYHA III-IV CHF Hb <12 g/dl Age ≥80 years	EPO 4000-5000 U/week titrated to Hb = 12.5 g/dl	Hb ≥12.5 g/dl; clinical status	NYHA class improved and LVEF ↑
Silverberg et al. [64]	–	78	Open-label, uncontrolled	NYHA II-IV CHF Hb <12 g/dl	EPO SC titrated to Hb >13.5 g/dl	Hb ≥13.5 g/dl; clinical status	NYHA class improved LVEF ↑, decreased hospitalization days
Mancini et al. [35]	–	23	Single-blind, randomized, placebo-controlled	NYHA III-IV CHF Hct <35% Creatinine <2.5 mg/dl EPO level <100 IU/l	EPO 15 000-30 000 U/week SC; Hct >45%	Peak oxygen uptake	Peak oxygen uptake ↑, exercise duration ↑, quality of life ↑
Hampl et al. [34]	–	202	Open-label, uncontrolled	Optimized treatment of CHF ESRD on hemodialysis Hb <11 g/dl	EPO IV titrated to Hb 14.5 (M) and 13.5 g/dl (F).		LVH ↓ LVEF ↑ NYHA class improved

Table 12.1 (continued)

Trial	Clinicaltrial.gov identifier	n	Design	Inclusion criteria	Treatment	Endpoints	Results
A study of repeat dose SC darbepoetin α in subjects with congestive heart failure and anemia, and a single dose in healthy age- and sex-matched control subject	NCT00117247	33	Double-blind, randomized, placebo-controlled	CHF with Hb ≥12.5 g/dl and healthy controls	Darbepoetin 0.75 μg/kg IV and 2–5 μg/kg SC	Pharmaco-kinetics	No difference in pharmacokinetics between CHF and healthy controls
Impact of darbepoetin α on exercise tolerance and left ventricular structure in subjects with symptomatic congestive heart failure and anemia	NCT00117234	41	Double-blind, randomized, placebo-controlled	Symptomatic CHF ≥3 months Reduced LVEF Peak VO_2 ≤16 ml/kg/min Hb = 9–12 g/dl	Darbepoetin	Peak oxygen consumption	Enrollment completed; results presented in abstract form; exercise performance improved
A double-blind, randomized, placebo-controlled, multicenter study to evaluate the effects of treatment with two regimens of SC darbepoetin α (weight-based dosing and fixed dosing) or Hb concentration	NCT00086086	–	Double-blind, randomized, placebo-controlled	Symptomatic CHF ≥3 months Reduced LVEF Hb = 9–12.5 g/dl	Darbepoetin α	Rate of rise of Hb	Enrollment completed; results not published

response in subjects with symptomatic CHF and anaemia							
A double-blind, randomized, placebo-controlled, multicenter study to assess the impact of SC darbepoetin α treatment on exercise tolerance in subjects with symptomatic heart failure (CHF) and anemia (STAMINA-HeFT)	NCT00049985	300	Double-blind, randomized, placebo-controlled	Symptomatic CHF ≥3 months Limited exercise tolerance on a treadmill Reduced LVEF Hb = 9.0–12.5 g/dl	Darbepoetin α	Treadmill exercise duration	Enrollment completed; results not reported
Trial to assess the efficacy and safety of darbepoetin α treatment on mortality and morbidity in subjects with heart failure and anemia (HIPPOCRATES)	Not assigned		Double-blind, randomized, placebo-controlled		Darbepoetin α	Mortality	Announced on sponsor website

CHF = congestive heart failure; EPO = erythropoietin; Hb = hemoglobin; LVEF = left ventricular ejection fraction; LVH = left ventricular hypertrophy; NYHA = New York Heart Association; SC = subcutaneous

and coexisting anemia (Hb 9.5–11.5 g/dl), rHuEPO therapy for mean 11.8 ± 8.2 months was associated with clinical improvements in both diabetic and non-diabetic subjects as evidenced by increased functional capacity, improved LVEF, reduced hospitalizations, and evidence of slowing of progression of renal disease [33]. In an observational study of 183 anemic CHF patients (Hb <11.0 g/dl and NYHA class II–IV) and hemodialysis-dependent chronic kidney disease, treatment with rHuEPO to normal Hb target (14.5 g/dl in men, 13.5 g/dl in women) significantly decreased left ventricular hypertrophy, increased LVEF, and improved NYHA functional class when compared with pre-treatment values [34].

The lack of placebo control and non-blinded study design limit interpretation of these early studies. Mancini et al. [35] conducted a single-blind, randomized, placebo-controlled trial of rHuEPO therapy in 26 patients with advanced CHF and anemia (hematocrit [Hct] <35%). Patients received subcutaneous rHuEPO 5000–10 000 IU three times weekly adjusted to raise Hct to >45% for 3 months or a single subcutaneous injection of saline (2:1 random-ization ratio). Supplemental oral iron and folate were also given to the patients who received rHuEPO therapy. Compared with the placebo group, rHuEPO therapy was asso-ciated with significantly increased Hb (11.0 ± 0.5 vs 14.3 ± 1.0 g/dl; $P < 0.05$), peak oxygen uptake (11.0 ± 1.8 vs 12.7 ± 2.8 ml/min/kg; $P < 0.05$), and exercise duration (590 ± 107 vs 657 ± 119s; $P < 0.004$). The increases in Hb levels were significantly associated with the increases in peak oxygen uptake ($r = 0.53$; $P < 0.02$) [35]. Although the number of subjects in this study are small, these findings confirm the findings of previous uncontrolled obser-vational studies in a more rigorous study design.

Darbepoetin α, the long-acting erythropoietin analog, can be administered with less fre-quent dosing, a factor that may be important for clinical application in ambulatory non-dialysis populations. As discussed above for rHuEPO, the bulk of the clinical pharmacology data are derived from chronic kidney disease populations. In 122 anemic patients with end-stage chronic kidney disease not previously treated with erythropoietin, once weekly administration of darbepoetin α at a dose of 0.45–0.75 μg/kg (subcutaneous or intravenous) raised Hb 1 g/dl in 60–80% of patients within 4 weeks [30]. In an open-label study of 341 end-stage chronic kidney disease patients who were chronically treated with rHuEPO, darbepoetin α was substituted at a regimen based on the frequency and number of units of rHuEPO dosing (patients with 2–3 times weekly rHuEPO dosing received darbepoetin α once a week and patients with once-weekly rHuEPO dosing received darbepoetin α once every 2 weeks; for every 200 IU rHuEPO, patients received 1 μg darbepoetin α) without change in the route of administration [29]. The change to intravenous darbepoetin α was associated with a small but statistically significant increase in Hb of 0.58 g/dl [29].

The pharmacokinetic and pharmacodynamic profile of darbepoetin α was determined in 33 patients with symptomatic CHF and anemia (Hb ≤12.5 g/dl) and 30 healthy control sub-jects in two sequential studies [36]. In the first study, the pharmacokinetics of intravenous and subcutaneous darbepoetin α 0.75 μg/kg were found to be similar in anemic CHF patients when compared with healthy control subjects. This dose of darbepoetin did not change Hb levels [36]. In the second study, the effects of subcutaneous darbepoetin α administered once monthly at doses of 2, 3, and 5 μg/kg were compared with placebo. Two injections of darbe-poetin therapy over this dose range at a 1-month intervals produced a sustained increase in Hb concentration ranging 1.4–2.4 g/dl without evidence of a clear dose–response pattern and without severe, drug-related adverse events [36]. The effects of treatment with darbepoetin α on exercise tolerance in patients with CHF and anemia (Hb 9–12 g/dl) was reported in abstract form [37]. Forty-one eligible subjects were randomly assigned to active treatment (darbepoetin α administrated initially 0.7 μg/kg subcutaneously every 2 weeks for 26 weeks) or placebo groups. Darbepoetin therapy was associated with improved exercise tolerance and quality of life when compared with placebo [37]. There are two ongoing trials in larger populations that will provide additional information on the safety and efficacy of darbepo-etin α in cardiovascular disease populations. The Studies of Anemia in Heart Failure Trial

(STAMINA-HeFT) is a double-blind, placebo-controlled, randomized clinical trial designed to determine whether treatment of anemia with darbepoetin α can improve exercise capacity and quality of life in patients with CHF and anemia [38]. Approximately 300 anemic CHF patients (Hb <12 g/dl) were randomized to treatment (subcutaneous injections every 2 weeks for 1 year) with darbepoetin α or placebo. Exercise treadmill tests were performed at baseline and again after 13 and 27 weeks of study drug. Enrollment has been completed and it is anticipated that the findings of this study will be presented in late 2006 to early 2007 [38]. The Trial to Reduce Cardiovascular Events with Aranesp (darbepoetin α) Therapy (TREAT) is another ongoing randomized, double-blind, placebo-controlled trial designed to evaluate whether ameliorating anemia with darbepoetin α to a target Hb of 13 g/dl in patients with chronic kidney disease and type 2 diabetes mellitus will reduce the risk of death or major cardiovascular events [39]. Finally, plans to commence a study to determine the effects of darbepoetin α vs placebo on clinical outcomes in anemic CHF patients (HIPPOCRATES) have been announced on the sponsor's website, although further details of the study design are not yet listed in the clinical trials registry (see www.clinicaltrials.gov).

Although rHuEPO treatment has generally been well-tolerated in chronic kidney disease and other anemic populations, there are well-described side-effects of rHuEPO treatment that are of potential concern in CHF patients. Erythropoietin may increase risk of thrombosis through its effects on blood viscosity, platelets, or vascular endothelial cells [40–43]. In patients with end-stage renal disease and evidence or uremic platelet dysfunction, chronic rHuEPO therapy has been demonstrated to increase platelet count by 20%, normalize bleeding time, and increase *in vitro* platelet aggregation [44, 45]. Clinical studies on the incidence of thrombosis associated with chronic rHuEPO therapy in anemic patients with end-stage renal disease on dialysis have reported mixed findings [46–49]. Besarab and colleagues conducted a large randomized clinical trial in 1233 patients with hemodialysis-dependent end-stage chronic kidney disease and comorbid heart disease to compare the effects of treatment with rHuEPO to a low target Hct of 30% vs a normal range target Hb of 42%. Compared with patients treated to achieve a target Hct of 30%, the patients treated to achieve a target Hct of 42% had a non-significantly increased relative risk of death or non-fatal myocardial infarction (relative risk 1.3; 95% confidence interval [CI] 0.9–1.9). In a retrospective study of anemic patients with cervical cancer, chronic rHuEPO therapy was associated with increased risk of deep vein thrombosis that was independent of change in Hct [50]. rHuEPO therapy has also been associated with increased risk of all-cause mortality in two randomized, placebo-controlled trials of patients with breast cancer, and head and neck cancer. Although the findings in chronic kidney and cancer populations may not accurately predict risk in CHF patients, these findings emphasize the need for additional trials to determine the long-term safety and efficacy of erythropoietic agents in the CHF population. In the small clinical trials of anemic CHF patients summarized above, treatment with rHuEPO or darbepoetin α was not associated with increased risk of thromboembolic events or other adverse clinical outcomes [31–33, 35, 37]. Antiplatelet and anticoagulant medications are commonly used in CHF patients, and may protect against pro-thrombotic effects of erythropoietic agents.

rHuEPO therapy may also be associated with new onset or worsening of pre-existing hypertension [51]. In chronic kidney disease patients, risk factors for developing *de novo* hypertension or worsening of pre-existing hypertension include rapid increase in Hct during therapy, a low baseline Hct before rHuEPO administration, high doses and intravenous route of administration, the presence of native kidneys, and a genetic predisposition to hypertension [52]. In the study of anemic CHF subjects by Mancini *et al.* [35], treatment with rHuEPO did not change blood pressure at rest or during exercise and did not change forearm vascular resistance (measured with venous occlusion plethysmography) at rest or after 5 min of forearm ischemia. Rare serious side-effects reported with rHuEPO therapy include seizures and pure red cell aplasia due to antibody formation against erythropoietin.

Erythropoietin resistance, defined as poor responsiveness to the usual therapeutic doses of rHuEPO, is present in 10% of patients with chronic kidney disease and up to 40–50% of patients with cancer-associated anemia [27, 53]. Several factors have been recognized as contributors to erythropoietin resistance, such as absolute and functional iron deficiency, comorbid inflammatory conditions and infectious diseases, suboptimal dialysis, vitamin B12 and folate deficiency, and pro-inflammatory cytokine activation [27, 54, 55]. Three of 15 anemic patients with severe CHF in the study by Mancini *et al.* [35] who were randomized to the active treatment group did not respond to the initial dose of rHuEPO injection but did manifest a rise in Hb when the dose was doubled to 10 000 IU three times a week. Further work is needed to determine if resistance to erythropoietic agents will limit their clinical utility in anemic CHF patients.

Functional iron deficiency may contribute to erythropoietin resistance. Patients with functional iron deficiency do not manifest classic laboratory findings of iron deficiency, but administration of intravenous iron restores the hematopoietic response to erythropoietic agents. Although current clinical guidelines for chronic kidney disease patients recommend intravenous iron supplementation to augment the response to erythropoietic agents, possible side-effects of iron overload, including increased risk of infection and increased risk of cardiovascular events, raise concerns about the use of intravenous iron in CHF patients [56–60]. Much additional work is needed to determine whether intravenous or oral iron supplementation should be used alone or in conjunction with erythropoietic agents in anemic CHF patients with functional iron deficiency.

Current CHF treatment guidelines provide little practical information on anemia management [61, 62]. Based on available data, it is advisable to routinely measure Hb in CHF patients in order to identify anemic patients who may benefit from further assessment and treatment. In anemic patients, further laboratory studies to evaluate the cause of anemia including iron deficiency, folate or vitamin B12 deficiencies, and chronic kidney disease should be ordered. Whenever possible, the primary cause of anemia should be corrected. CHF patients with moderate–severe anemia (Hb <11 g/dl) and concomitant moderate-to-severe chronic kidney disease (estimated GFR ≤60 ml/min) meet the current guidelines and Medicare criteria for treatment with erythropoietic agents. Either rHuEPO or darbepoetin α can be administered at recommended doses with supplemental iron (oral or intravenous) to maintain a target Hb of 12 g/dl [57]. For CHF patients with less severe degrees of anemia and preserved renal function, treatment with erythropoietic agents is not recommended until more data on safety and efficacy are available.

SUMMARY

Anemia treatment in heart failure:

- Anemia represents an important comorbidity in heart failure and is associated with worse outcomes including mortality.
- The actual pathogenesis of anemia in heart failure has not been fully established.
- Preliminary data suggest that correction of anemia with erythropoietin analogs and possibly aggressive iron supplementation does improve surrogate measures of heart failure status including exercise capacity and quality of life but, to date, there are no data to suggest a survival advantage related to the treatment of anemia in heart failure.
- When anemia in heart failure is discovered, a search for the primary cause should be initiated and if a cause is identified it should be corrected. If current guidelines are met regarding renal insufficiency, erythropoietin analogs can be administered. However, the use of erythropoietin analogs as therapy for anemia in heart failure is not otherwise recommended.

REFERENCES

1. Komajda M. Prevalence of anemia in patients with chronic heart failure and their clinical characteristics. *J Card Fail* 2004; 10(suppl):S1–S4.
2. Okonko DO, Anker SD. Anemia in chronic heart failure: pathogenetic mechanisms. *J Card Fail* 2004; 10(suppl):S5–S9.
3. Horwich TB, Fonarow GC, Hamilton MA, MacLellan WR, Borenstein J. Anemia is associated with worse symptoms, greater impairment in functional capacity and a significant increase in mortality in patients with advanced heart failure. *J Am Coll Cardiol* 2002; 39:1780–1786.
4. Ezekowitz JA, McAlister FA, Armstrong PW. Anemia is common in heart failure and is associated with poor outcomes: insights from a cohort of 12 065 patients with new-onset heart failure. *Circulation* 2003; 107:223–225.
5. Means RT Jr. Advances in the anemia of chronic disease. *Int J Hematol* 1999; 70:7–12.
6. Bolger AP, Doehner W, Sharma R, Coats AJ, Anker SD. Anemia in chronic heart failure: the relationship to inflammatory cytokine production and prognostic importance. (Abstract). *Circulation* 2002; 106(suppl):S2819.
7. Herrera-Garza EH, Stetson SJ, Cubillos-Garzon A, Vooletich MT, Farmer JA, Torre-Amione G. Tumor necrosis factor-alpha: a mediator of disease progression in the failing human heart. *Chest* 1999; 115:1170–1174.
8. Albitar S, Genin R, Fen-Chong M, Serveaux MO, Bourgeon B. High dose enalapril impairs the response to erythropoietin treatment in haemodialysis patients. *Nephrol Dial Transplant* 1998; 13:1206–1210.
9. Katz SD. Mechanisms and treatment of anemia in chronic heart failure. *Congest Heart Fail* 2004; 10:243–247.
10. Macdougall IC. The role of ACE inhibitors and angiotensin II receptor blockers in the response to epoetin. *Nephrol Dial Transplant* 1999; 14:1836–1841.
11. Androne AS, Katz SD, Lund L et al. Hemodilution is common in patients with advanced heart failure. *Circulation* 2003; 107:226–229.
12. Anker SD, Chua TP, Ponikowski P et al. Hormonal changes and catabolic/anabolic imbalance in chronic heart failure and their importance for cardiac cachexia. *Circulation* 1997; 96:526–534.
13. Volpe M, Tritto C, Testa U et al. Blood levels of erythropoietin in congestive heart failure and correlation with clinical, hemodynamic, and hormonal profiles. *Am J Cardiol* 1994; 74:468–473.
14. Pham I, Andrivet P, Sediame S et al. Increased erythropoietin synthesis in patients with COLD or left heart failure is related to alterations in renal haemodynamics. *Eur J Clin Invest* 2001; 31:103–109.
15. George J, Patal S, Wexler D et al. Circulating erythropoietin levels and prognosis in patients with congestive heart failure: comparison with neurohormonal and inflammatory markers. *Arch Intern Med* 2005; 165:1304–1309.
16. Jelkmann W. Molecular biology of erythropoietin. *Intern Med* 2004; 43:649–659.
17. Farrell F, Lee A. The erythropoietin receptor and its expression in tumor cells and other tissues. *Oncologist* 2004; 9(suppl 5):18–30.
18. De Maria R, Zeuner A, Eramo A et al. Negative regulation of erythropoiesis by caspase-mediated cleavage of GATA-1. *Nature* 1999; 401:489–493.
19. Weiss G, Goodnough LT. Anemia of chronic disease. *N Engl J Med* 2005; 352:1011–1023.
20. Winearls CG. Recombinant human erythropoietin: 10 years of clinical experience. *Nephrol Dial Transplant* 1998; 13(suppl 2):3–8.
21. Bommer J, Kugel M, Schoeppe W et al. Dose-related effects of recombinant human erythropoietin on erythropoiesis. Results of a multicenter trial in patients with end-stage renal disease. *Contrib Nephrol* 1988; 66:85–93.
22. Eschbach JW, Abdulhadi MH, Browne JK et al. Recombinant human erythropoietin in anemic patients with end-stage renal disease. Results of a phase III multicenter clinical trial. *Ann Intern Med* 1989; 111:992–1000.
23. Sundal E, Kaeser U. Correction of anaemia of chronic renal failure with recombinant human erythropoietin: safety and efficacy of one year's treatment in a European multicentre study of 150 haemodialysis-dependent patients. *Nephrol Dial Transplant* 1989; 4:979–987.
24. Eschbach JW, Egrie JC, Downing MR, Browne JK, Adamson JW. Correction of the anemia of end-stage renal disease with recombinant human erythropoietin. Results of a combined phase I and II clinical trial. *N Engl J Med* 1987; 316:73–78.

25. McMahon FG, Vargas R, Ryan M et al. Pharmacokinetics and effects of recombinant human erythropoietin after intravenous and subcutaneous injections in healthy volunteers. Blood 1990; 76:1718–1722.
26. Fisher JW. Erythropoietin: physiology and pharmacology update. Exp Biol Med (Maywood) 2003; 228:1–14.
27. Macdougall IC, Cooper AC. Erythropoietin resistance: the role of inflammation and pro-inflammatory cytokines. Nephrol Dial Transplant 2002; 17(suppl 11):39–43.
28. Macdougall IC. Darbepoetin alfa: a new therapeutic agent for renal anemia. Kidney Int Suppl 2002; 61:55–61.
29. Locatelli F, Canaud B, Giacardy F, Martin-Malo A, Baker N, Wilson J. Treatment of anaemia in dialysis patients with unit dosing of darbepoetin alfa at a reduced dose frequency relative to recombinant human erythropoietin (rHuEPO). Nephrol Dial Transplant 2003; 18:362–369.
30. Macdougall IC, Matcham J, Gray SJ. Correction of anaemia with darbepoetin alfa in patients with chronic kidney disease receiving dialysis. Nephrol Dial Transplant 2003; 18:576–581.
31. Silverberg DS, Wexler D, Blum M et al. The use of subcutaneous erythropoietin and intravenous iron for the treatment of the anemia of severe, resistant congestive heart failure improves cardiac and renal function and functional cardiac class, and markedly reduces hospitalizations. J Am Coll Cardiol 2000; 35:1737–1744.
32. Silverberg DS, Wexler D, Sheps D et al. The effect of correction of mild anemia in severe, resistant congestive heart failure using subcutaneous erythropoietin and intravenous iron: a randomized controlled study. J Am Coll Cardiol 2001; 37:1775–1780.
33. Silverberg DS, Wexler D, Blum M et al. The effect of correction of anaemia in diabetics and non-diabetics with severe resistant congestive heart failure and chronic renal failure by subcutaneous erythropoietin and intravenous iron. Nephrol Dial Transplant 2003; 18:141–146.
34. Hampl H, Hennig L, Rosenberger C et al. Effects of optimized heart failure therapy and anemia correction with epoetin beta on left ventricular mass in hemodialysis patients. Am J Nephrol 2005; 25:211–220.
35. Mancini DM, Katz SD, Lang CC, LaManca J, Hudaihed A, Androne AS. Effect of erythropoietin on exercise capacity in patients with moderate to severe chronic heart failure. Circulation 2003; 107:294–299.
36. Cleland JG, Sullivan JT, Ball S et al. Once-monthly administration of darbepoetin alfa for the treatment of patients with chronic heart failure and anemia: a pharmacokinetic and pharmacodynamic investigation. J Cardiovasc Pharmacol 2005; 46:155–161.
37. Cleland JG, Coletta AP, Clark AL, Velavan P, Ingle L. Clinical trials update from the European Society of Cardiology Heart Failure meeting and the American College of Cardiology: darbepoetin alfa study, ECHOS, and ASCOT-BPLA. Eur J Heart Fail 2005; 7:937–939.
38. Mitka M. Researchers probe anemia-heart failure link. JAMA 2003; 290:1835–1838.
39. Mix TC, Brenner RM, Cooper ME et al. Rationale–Trial to Reduce Cardiovascular Events with Aranesp Therapy (TREAT): evolving the management of cardiovascular risk in patients with chronic kidney disease. Am Heart J 2005; 149:408–413.
40. Valles J, Santos MT, Aznar J et al. Platelet-erythrocyte interactions enhance alpha(IIb)beta(3) integrin receptor activation and P-selectin expression during platelet recruitment: down-regulation by aspirin ex vivo. Blood 2002; 99:3978–3984.
41. Diaz-Ricart M, Etebanell E, Cases A et al. Erythropoietin improves signaling through tyrosine phosphorylation in platelets from uremic patients. Thromb Haemost 1999; 82:1312–1317.
42. Fuste B, Serradell M, Escolar G et al. Erythropoietin triggers a signaling pathway in endothelial cells and increases the thrombogenicity of their extracellular matrices in vitro. Thromb Haemost 2002; 88:678–685.
43. Anagnostou A, Lee ES, Kessimian N, Levinson R, Steiner M. Erythropoietin has a mitogenic and positive chemotactic effect on endothelial cells. Proc Natl Acad Sci USA 1990; 87:5978–5982.
44. Cases A, Escolar G, Reverter JC et al. Recombinant human erythropoietin treatment improves platelet function in uremic patients. Kidney Int 1992; 42:668–672.
45. van Geet C, Hauglustaine D, Verresen L, Vanrusselt M, Vermylen J. Haemostatic effects of recombinant human erythropoietin in chronic haemodialysis patients. Thromb Haemost 1989; 61:117–121.
46. Besarab A, Bolton WK, Browne JK et al. The effects of normal as compared with low hematocrit values in patients with cardiac disease who are receiving hemodialysis and epoetin. N Engl J Med 1998; 339:584–590.

47. Foley RN, Parfrey PS, Morgan J et al. Effect of hemoglobin levels in hemodialysis patients with asymptomatic cardiomyopathy. Kidney Int 2000; 58:1325–1335.
48. Martino MA, Vogel KM, O'Brien SP, Kerstein MD. Erythropoietin therapy improves graft patency with no increased incidence of thrombosis or thrombophlebitis. J Am Coll Surg 1998; 187:616–619.
49. Churchill DN, Muirhead N, Goldstein M et al. Probability of thrombosis of vascular access among hemodialysis patients treated with recombinant human erythropoietin. J Am Soc Nephrol 1994; 4:1809–1813.
50. Wun T, Law L, Harvey D, Sieracki B, Scudder SA, Ryu JK. Increased incidence of symptomatic venous thrombosis in patients with cervical carcinoma treated with concurrent chemotherapy, radiation, and erythropoietin. Cancer 2003; 98:1514–1520.
51. Mann JF. Hypertension and cardiovascular effects – long-term safety and potential long-term benefits of r-HuEPO. Nephrol Dial Transplant 1995; 10(suppl 2):80–84.
52. Maschio G. Erythropoietin and systemic hypertension. Nephrol Dial Transplant 1995; 10(suppl 2):74–79.
53. Beguin Y. Prediction of response and other improvements on the limitations of recombinant human erythropoietin therapy in anemic cancer patients. Haematologica 2002; 87:1209–1221.
54. Rauchhaus M, Doehner W, Francis DP et al. Plasma cytokine parameters and mortality in patients with chronic heart failure. Circulation 2000; 102:3060–3067.
55. Gullestad L, Aukrust P. The cytokine network in heart failure: pathogenetic importance and potential therapeutic targets. Heart Fail Monit 2001; 2:8–13.
56. Day SM, Duquaine D, Mundada LV et al. Chronic iron administration increases vascular oxidative stress and accelerates arterial thrombosis. Circulation 2003; 107:2601–2606.
57. IV. NKF-K/DOQI Clinical Practice Guidelines for Anemia of Chronic Kidney Disease: update 2000. Am J Kidney Dis 2001; 37(suppl 1):S182–S238.
58. Kletzmayr J, Sunder-Plassmann G, Horl WH. High dose intravenous iron: a note of caution. Nephrol Dial Transplant 2002; 17:962–965.
59. Sullivan JL. Iron therapy and cardiovascular disease. Kidney Int Suppl 1999; 69:S135–S137.
60. Weinberg ED. Iron loading and disease surveillance. Emerg Infect Dis 1999; 5:346–352.
61. Hunt SA, Baker DW, Chin MH et al. ACC/AHA Guidelines for the Evaluation and Management of Chronic Heart Failure in the Adult: Executive Summary-A Report of the American College of Cardiology/American Heart Association Task Force on Practice Guidelines (Committee to Revise the 1995 Guidelines for the Evaluation and Management of Heart Failure): Developed in Collaboration With the International Society for Heart and Lung Transplantation; Endorsed by the Heart Failure Society of America. Circulation 2001; 104:2996–3007.
62. Swedberg K, Cleland J, Dargie H et al. Guidelines for the diagnosis and treatment of chronic heart failure: executive summary (update 2005): The Task Force for the Diagnosis and Treatment of Chronic Heart Failure of the European Society of Cardiology. Eur Heart J 2005; 26:1115–1140.
63. Silverberg DS, Wexler D, Blum M et al. Effect of correction of anemia with erythropoietin and intravenous iron in resistant heart failure in octogenarians. Isr Med Assoc J 2003; 5:337–339.
64. Silverberg DS, Wexler D, Blum M et al. Effects of treatment with epoetin Beta on outcomes in patients with anaemia and chronic heart failure. Kidney Blood Press Res 2005; 28:41–47.

Section V

Special topics in heart failure

13

Applying data from registries to improve outcomes in heart failure

G. C. Fonarow

INTRODUCTION

Heart failure (HF) remains a major public health problem, affecting 5 million patients in the US. HF is the leading cause of hospitalization in persons over 65 years of age with cost exceeding $29 billion annually. Despite the compelling scientific evidence that medications and HF device therapy reduce hospitalizations and mortality in patients with HF, these life-prolonging therapies continue to be underutilized. A number of registry studies in a variety of clinical settings have documented that a significant proportion of patients with HF are not receiving treatment with guideline-recommended, evidence-based therapies when guided by conventional care. Treatment gaps in providing other components of HF patient care including patient education have also been documented. Recent studies demonstrate that hospital-based performance improvement systems can improve medical care and education of hospitalized HF patients and accelerate use of evidence-based, guideline-recommended therapies by administering them before hospital discharge. Outpatient HF disease management programs have also been shown to improve HF treatment resulting in substantial reduction in hospitalizations and mortality. Application of validated and reproducible systems and disease management programs for patients with HF is an important step in maximizing interventions to improve outcomes in this patient population. Further efforts are clearly needed to ensure the implementation of effective strategies and disease management programs that increase the use of evidence-based therapies, to reduce the substantial HF morbidity and mortality risk.

HEART FAILURE BURDEN

HF affects 5 million Americans and 550000 new diagnoses are made each year [1]. HF is one of the few major cardiovascular conditions that is increasing in both its incidence and prevalence, which places a significant burden on the healthcare system [2–4]. The personal burden of HF includes debilitating symptoms, frequent hospitalizations, and high rates of mortality [2, 3]. Prognosis is very poor once a patient has been hospitalized with HF; the mortality risk after HF hospitalization is 11.3% at 30 days, 33.1% at 1 year, and well over 50% within 5 years [1, 2]. HF is the underlying or contributing cause of death in 286700 individuals annually in the US [1]. HF resulted in 1.1 million hospitalizations, which translates

Gregg C. Fonarow, MD, FACC, Eliot Corday Professor of Cardiovascular Medicine and Science, Director, Ahmanson-UCLA Cardiomyopathy Center, UCLA Division of Cardiology, David Geffen School of Medicine at UCLA, Los Angeles, California, USA.

into an annual estimated cost of $29 to $56 billion [1, 5, 6]. The almost 1.1 million hospital discharges due to HF in 2003 represent a 174% increase since 1979. In a study of almost 18 000 Medicare recipients, approximately 44% were rehospitalized at least once in 6 months following their index hospitalization [7]. A number of studies indicate that a significant proportion of rehospitalizations for HF appear to be preventable [2, 3, 6]. These statistics emphasize the need to develop and implement more effective strategies to manage HF.

THE GAP IN APPLYING GUIDELINE-RECOMMENDED THERAPY IN HEART FAILURE

There is compelling clinical trial evidence that all patients with HF due to left ventricular systolic dysfunction (LVSD), from asymptomatic to class IV symptoms, of any etiology, should be treated with angiotensin-converting enzyme (ACE) inhibitors and β-blocker therapy, in the absence of contraindications or intolerance [2–4, 8, 9]. HF patients with selected indications have also been shown to benefit from aldosterone antagonists, hydralazine long-acting nitrates, cardiac resynchronization and implantable cardioverter defibrillators [10–18]. Despite the wealth of scientific evidence and guideline recommendations regarding the benefits of HF therapies, there is an extensive body of evidence documenting that conventional management has left a substantial proportion of HF patients untreated with these prolonging therapies [19–23]. Longitudinal national data on outpatient use of ACE inhibitors for HF showed a modest increase in ACE inhibitor use from 24% to no more than 38% in the 12-year period between 1990 and 2002 [19]. This HF treatment gap is not just a problem in the US. The IMPROVEMENT international study of 1363 physician practices in 15 countries involving 11 602 chronic HF patients found that only 60% of these eligible patients were treated with ACE inhibitors [20]. In addition to the underuse of ACE inhibitors, sub-therapeutic dosages are commonly implemented [21].

The Acute Decompensated Heart Failure National Registry (ADHERE) was designed to bridge gaps in knowledge and care by prospectively studying the characteristics, management, and outcomes of a broad spectrum of patients hospitalized with acute decompensated HF. Participating community and university hospitals identified patients with a primary or secondary discharge diagnosis of HF and collected medical history, management, treatments, and health outcomes *via* secure web browser technology. ADHERE reported underuse of β-blockers in 2002–2003, with only 47% of chronic previously diagnosed systolic dysfunction HF patients receiving a β-blocker on an outpatient basis prior to admission to the hospital [23]. The international IMPROVEMENT survey showed that only 26% of chronic HF patients were being treated with β-blocker therapy [20]. A recent randomized trial conducted in the outpatient setting demonstrated that under conventional physician-directed care only 27% of eligible chronic HF patients were initiated on β-blocker therapy during the course of 1 year of follow-up [24]. Underuse of aldosterone antagonists in eligible patients has also been described [20].

Unfortunately, there is also a risk–treatment mismatch in HF: patients with severe HF or those with the highest risk of morbidity and mortality are less likely to receive therapy than those with lower risk. In a recent study of patients hospitalized with HF, drug administration rates at hospital discharge and 90 days after discharge, the highest-risk HF patients were much less likely to receive life-saving therapies [25]. Low-risk patients were more likely to receive ACE inhibitors or angiotensin receptor blockers (ARBs) (adjusted hazard ratio [HR] 1.61; 95% confidence interval [CI] 1.49–1.74) and β-receptor antagonists (HR 1.80; 95% CI 1.60–2.01) compared with high-risk patients (both $P < 0.001$) [25]. Because drug administration is inversely associated with risk, the potential benefit of HF pharmacotherapy will not be realized if current patterns continue. Greater quality improvement efforts aimed at increasing use of HF drugs in higher-risk patients are needed [25].

Gaps in the provision of other aspects of HF care have also been described. The Joint Commission on Accreditation of Healthcare Organizations (JCAHO) developed a disease-specific Heart Failure Core Measure Set [26]. The four HF performance measures in the set include use of ACE inhibitors in eligible patients, evaluation of left ventricular function (LVF), smoking cessation, and patient education (Table 13.1). Patient education comprises written instructions and educational material on diet, weight monitoring, activity levels, medications, and symptom management.

Data from more than 80 000 HF admissions to academic and non-academic hospitals in the US participating in the ADHERE registry were analyzed to determine the rates of conformity with the four core performance measures: discharge instructions (HF-1), assessment of LVF (HF-2), use of ACE inhibitors in patients with LVSD (HF-3), and smoking cessation counseling (HF-4) [23]. Across all hospitals, the median rates of conformity with HF-1, HF-2, HF-3, and HF-4 were 24.0%, 86.2%, 72.0%, and 43.2%, respectively. Rates of conformity at individual hospitals varied from 0% to 100%, with statistically significant differences between academic and non-academic hospitals. Figure 13.1 depicts the frequency distribution of conformity rates by lagging and leading hospitals in ADHERE [23]. For each measure, there were substantial clinically relevant differences in performance between hospitals at different percentile levels. For HF-1, there was a 100-fold difference in conformity between hospitals at the 10th and 90th percentiles. For HF-4, there was an 11.2-fold difference in conformity at these percentiles. In contrast, there was a 1.3- and a 1.5-fold difference in conformity between hospitals at the 10th and 90th percentiles for HF-2 and HF-3, respectively [23]. Academic and non-academic hospitals differed in their conformity with the four performance measures. Non-academic hospitals demonstrated significantly better median conformity with HF-1 than academic hospitals, whereas academic hospitals demonstrated slightly better median conformity than non-academic hospitals with HF-2 and HF-3 [23]. Thus, among the hospitals enrolled in ADHERE there was significant individual variability in conformity to quality-of-care indicators and a substantial gap in overall performance.

There was also marked variation in clinical outcomes observed between hospitals participating in ADHERE. Median hospital length of stay varied greatly ranging from 2.3 to 9.5 days. There was also substantial variation in the observed in-hospital mortality rates, varying from as low as 0% to as high as 11.1% [23]. Several studies have documented that processes of care provided in the hospital are strongly associated with rehospitalization rates and mortality [2, 3, 27]. Early HF re-admission and 30-day mortality are independently associated with the process of inpatient care. Explicit inpatient processes of care indicators shown to be associated with outcome include discharge on ACE inhibitors, measurement of left ventricular ejection fraction (LVEF), and discharge documentation. A case-controlled study at 12 Veterans Affairs hospitals demonstrated that the risk of early HF re-admission was increased nearly 2-fold when inpatient care was substandard (a readiness for discharge score below the 25th percentile) [27]. The gaps in care that exist in the outpatient and hospital setting suggest that new efforts targeting education and effective patient intervention are urgently needed in order to improve the overall quality of care for patients with HF.

ROLE OF HOSPITAL-BASED SYSTEMS TO IMPROVE QUALITY OF CARE AND OUTCOMES

A number of clinical studies have demonstrated an important role of hospital-based systems in improving the quality of cardiovascular care; moreover, such programs were substantially more effective than conventional guidelines and care [28, 29]. Based on this model, the Organized Program to Initiate Life-Saving Treatments in Patients Hospitalized with Heart Failure (OPTIMIZE-HF) was developed [30]. The key objective of OPTIMIZE-HF was to improve medical care and education of hospitalized HF patients. OPTIMIZE-HF consisted of a registry and performance improvement program. To provide optimal therapy, it was designed to promote the accelerated adoption of guideline-recommended therapies by starting these life-saving regimens before hospital discharge in suitable patients. In

Table 13.1 JCAHO core performance measures for heart failure (reprinted with permission from JCAHO [26])

Performance measure	Criterion met or acceptable alternative
HF-1. Discharged patients with HF with written instructions or educational materials given to the patient or caregiver at discharge or during the hospital stay that address all of the following: ■ Activity level ■ Diet ■ Discharge medications ■ Follow-up appointment ■ Weight monitoring ■ What to do if symptoms worsen	*Discharge instructions.* For discharge patients with or without home health services, documentation of written instructions or educational materials given to the patient or caregiver must address all of the following: ■ Activity level after discharge ■ Diet and fluid intake after discharge ■ Names of all discharge medications ■ Follow-up with a physician, nurse practitioner, or physician assistant after discharge ■ Weight monitoring after discharge ■ What to do if HF symptoms worsen after discharge
HF-2. Patients with HF with documentation in the hospital record that LVF was assessed before arrival or during hospitalization or that it is planned for after discharge	*LVF assessment.* In cases in which there is no reason documented by a physician, nurse practitioner, or physician assistant for not assessing LVF there must be: Documentation that an echocardiogram, appropriate nuclear medicine test, or cardiac catheterization with a left ventriculogram was performed during this hospital stay OR Documentation that one of the above diagnostic tests was performed any time before arrival OR Documentation of LVF, either as a ejection fraction or as a narrative qualitative description (e.g. 'Patient admitted with severe LV dysfunction') OR Documentation of a plan to assess LVF after discharge
HF-3. Patients with HF with LVSD and without ACE inhibitor contraindications who are prescribed an ACE inhibitor at hospital discharge	*ACE inhibitor.* Documentation that an ACE inhibitor was prescribed at discharge in patients with LVSD who are not participating in an ACE inhibitor alternative clinical trial at the time of discharge and where there is not documentation of a potential contraindication or reason for not prescribing an ACE inhibitor at discharge (e.g. ACE inhibitor allergy, moderate or severe aortic stenosis, or another reason documented by a physician, nurse practitioner, or physician assistant). LVSD is defined as documentation of an LVEF <40% or a narrative description of LVF consistent with moderate and severe systolic dysfunction. Where there are ≥2 documented LVF, the LVF closest to discharge is used

HF-4. Patients with HF with a history of smoking cigarettes who are given smoking cessation advice or counseling during the hospital stay

Adult smoking cessation advice or counseling. Documentation of smoking cessation advice or counseling in patients with a history of smoking cigarettes any time during the year before hospital arrival. Smoking cessation advice or counseling includes prescription of a cessation aid

ACE = angiotensin-converting enzyme; HF = heart failure; JCAHO = Joint Commission on Accreditation of Healthcare Organizations; LV = left ventricular; LVF = left ventricular function; LVSD = left ventricular systolic dysfunction

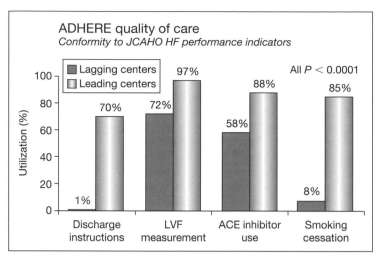

Figure 13.1 Conformity to Joint Commission on Accreditation of Healthcare Organizations (JCAHO) Heart Failure Performance Measure in ADHERE. Data from 81 142 admissions between 6/2002 and 12/2003 at 223 ADHERE hospitals grouped by leading (90th percentile) and lagging (10th percentile) performance (data from [23]).

addition, by studying variations in treatment use by patient and hospital characteristics, it aimed to increase understanding of the current barriers to initiation of evidence-based therapies in this patient population. The program encouraged hospital-based teams to implement the comprehensive OPTIMIZE-HF process-of-care improvement tools. The materials were based on the American College of Cardiology/American Heart Association (ACC/AHA) HF guidelines, recent clinical trials, and the collective expertise of the OPTIMIZE-HF Steering Committee members [30]. As part of an enhanced treatment and discharge plan, OPTIMIZE-HF provided evidence-based best practice algorithms, critical pathways, standardized orders, discharge checklists, pocket cards, chart stickers, and a variety of other elements to assist hospitals in improving HF management. The hospital teams collected data during hospitalization and at 60–90 days post-discharge to measure and improve the management and care of patients with HF as a primary or secondary diagnosis. The registry tracked the use of life-saving therapies before and after initiation, as well as hospital progress and discharge planning. Real-time reports and benchmark comparisons between institutions both regionally and nationally are provided, allowing participating institutions to share best practices. Preliminary data show substantial improvements in the use of evidence-based HF therapies both in the hospital and at 60–90 day follow-up. The percentage of patients that received the JCAHO HF performance measures, plotted over time, is shown in Fig. 13.2. Evidence-based medication use improved over time. The frequency of smoking cessation counseling and the use of discharge instructions improved greatly with the OPTIMIZE-HF program.

OPTIMIZE-HF provides further evidence that the use of in-hospital process-of-care improvement programs and critical pathways can increase the use of life-saving medications and adherence to quality measures. Hospital-based HF quality improvement is thus feasible on a national scale using largely pre-existing resources. The quality of HF care can thus be substantially improved if hospital teams implement processes such as those in OPTIMIZE-HF to insure the use of evidence-based therapies in their eligible HF patients prior to hospital discharge.

The AHA's Get With the Guidelines (GWTG) program is an acute-care hospital-based quality improvement program designed to help close the treatment gap in cardiovascular

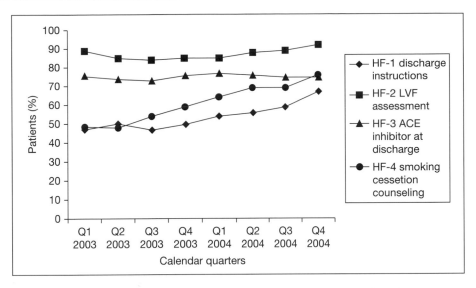

Figure 13.2 Joint Commission on Accreditation of Healthcare Organizations (JCAHO) performance measures in the Organized Program to Initiate Lifesaving Treatment in Hospitalized Patients with Heart Failure (OPTIMIZE-HF) over time. ACE-I = Angiotensin-converting enzyme inhibitors; LVF = left ventricular function.

disease, to significantly improve patient outcomes, and to move the AHA closer to its 2010 goal of reducing death, disability and risk by 25% [29]. The AHA initiated the GWTG program with a coronary artery disease module in July 2000, modeling the program in part after the UCLA Cardiac Hospitalization Atherosclerosis Management Program (CHAMP) system [28]. The GWTG program focuses on the use of treatment guidelines to ensure that patients are discharged on a regimen of appropriate medications and receive adequate counseling for risk factor modification. An integral part of the GTWG program is the use of the interactive AHA web-based data collection tool, the Patient Management Tool (PMT). The PMT, developed by Outcomes Inc. (Cambridge, Mass) is a customizable, web-based, interactive quality improvement reporting system used to prospectively collect data and measure program performance individually or against AHA's national benchmarks over time. Drop-down reminder screens provide immediate reference to the appropriate guideline and alert clinicians to omission of needed measurements and intervention before the patient leaves the hospital. Healthcare professionals can also generate patient education sheets and produce a letter to be sent to the patient's primary care physician, summarizing diagnosis, procedures, risk assessment, and interventions initiated during the hospitalization. The system may also be used to collect data for the JCAHO ORYX core measure sets for acute myocardial infarction, stroke, and HF. The AHA implemented a GWTG program module focused on HF in March 2005. Over 250 hospitals are currently participating. Preliminary data show improvement in HF performance measures in the first four quarters of participation.

Thus, implementation of hospital-based systems for HF has been shown to enhance adherence to established guidelines and core performance measures, reducing the treatment variability between hospitals. As a result, overall quality of care can be improved significantly, reducing the morbidity, mortality, and economic cost associated with this disorder.

Table 13.2 HF disease management components

- Multidisciplinary team: HF specialists, electrophysiologists, advance practice nurses, home nursing, pharmacists, medical social workers, nutritionists, administrative personnel
- Detailed assessment of HF etiology, potential reversible causes and related risks
- Optimization of HF medical therapy
- Evaluation of the need for and optimization of HF device therapy
- Assessment and management of patient comorbidities
- Close monitoring of volume status and application of non-invasive techniques to detect congestion
- Comprehensive HF education to patients and their family members in the hospital and outpatient settings
- Meticulous tracking of clinical status, laboratories, HF device data, and diagnostic testing
- Hospital discharge and continuity of care planning
- Increased outpatient access to healthcare professionals
- Long-term coordinated follow-up of patients

OUTPATIENT DISEASE MANAGEMENT PROGRAMS TO IMPROVE QUALITY OF CARE AND OUTCOMES

There has been much interest in identifying effective methods to improve the quality of outpatient care for HF patients, while reducing costs. The traditional model of outpatient care delivery is thought to contribute to frequent hospitalizations because in these brief, episodic encounters, little attention may be paid to the common, modifiable factors that precipitate many hospitalizations. We and others first studied the use of comprehensive HF management programs involving specialty care and a multidisciplinary team (Table 13.2); the goals of the HF disease management programs included optimization of drug therapy, intensive patient education, vigilant follow-up with early recognition of problems, and identification and management of patients' comorbidities [31–33]. HF patients who were cared for in these programs were shown to have significantly fewer rehospitalizations, lower healthcare costs, improved functional and symptom status, and better quality of life compared with either a pre-intervention time period or HF patients treated with conventional care [31–33].

However, as these initial studies of multidisciplinary disease management interventions were non-randomized, 'before and after' studies, concerns were raised about their interpretation. Rich *et al.* [34] were the first to provide randomized clinical trial evidence for the effectiveness of disease management in improving clinical outcomes in HF patients. They developed a nurse-directed, multidisciplinary disease management intervention to address risk factors for re-admission, including non-adherence to diet or medications, inappropriate medication prescribing, and failure to recognize HF exacerbations and seek appropriate care. In their single-center study of high-risk HF patients, they reported a reduction of HF re-admissions within 90 days by 56%, all re-admissions by 29%, and overall cost of care by $460 per patient [34].

Other studies of multidisciplinary disease management interventions confirmed these findings [35–39]. Stewart and Horowitz [35] reported on a randomized, controlled trial of a home-based HF specialty intervention in Australia in which they demonstrated that patients randomized to the intervention had a better survival rate and fewer rehospitalizations than those who received usual care. Krumholz *et al.* [36], in a single-center randomized study, tested a 1-year educational intervention without medical management in patients with HF. In intervention patients, there was a significant reduction in the primary endpoint of death or hospital re-admission. The Specialized Primary and Networked Care in HF (SPAN-CHF) study demonstrated a 52% reduction in HF hospitalizations with a 90-day nurse-driven HF disease management intervention delivered uniformly across a diverse provider system [37].

McAlister *et al.* [38] reviewed randomized trials of HF disease management programs published through 1999 and concluded that multidisciplinary teams providing direct specialized

Table 13.3 American College of Cardiology/American Heart Association performance measures for outpatients with chronic HF. Adapted with permission [42]

1. Initial laboratory tests
2. Left ventricular systolic function assessment
3. Weight measurement
4. Blood pressure measurement
5. Assessment of clinical symptoms of congestion
6. Assessment of clinical signs of congestion
7. Assessment of activity level
8. Patient education
9. β-blocker therapy in patients with HF and LVSD
10. ACE inhibitors or angiotensin receptor antagonists in patients with HF and LVSD
11. Warfarin therapy in patients with atrial fibrillation

follow-up care statistically significantly reduced hospitalization and healthcare costs, while studies that used telephone contact to coordinate primary care services seemed to have no effect. Since 1999, several more randomized trials have been published. In an updated analysis by McAlister *et al.* [39], HF disease management strategies that incorporated follow-up by a specialized multidisciplinary team (either in a clinic or a non-clinic setting) reduced mortality (risk ratio [RR] 0.75; 95% confidence interval [CI] 0.59–0.96), HF hospitalizations (RR 0.74; 95% CI 0.63–0.87) and all-cause hospitalizations (RR 0.81; 95% CI 0.71–0.92). In addition, 15 of the 18 trials reported that their disease management interventions were cost-saving with the other three trials reporting cost neutrality [39]. Strategies that employed telephone contact and advised patients to attend their primary care physician in the event of deterioration reduced HF hospitalizations, but not mortality or all-cause hospitalizations. Another recent meta-analysis including 18 trials published between 1993 and 2003 confirms that, overall, disease management interventions directed at recently hospitalized patients with HF significantly reduce rehospitalizations and healthcare costs with a trend toward lower all-cause mortality rates [40]. The authors concluded that, if applied on a national basis, multidisciplinary disease management strategies for HF have the potential to prevent 84 000 re-admissions with an estimated reduction in Medicare payments of $424 million per year [40].

Outpatient HF disease management programs reported to date have differed substantially in intervention focus (such as patient self-management, medication management, and care coordination), mode (telephone, home, or specialty clinic visit), timing in relation to index hospitalization, intensity (frequency and duration of contacts), disease manager training, cardiologist involvement, and nature and extent of interaction with the patient's primary care physician [38–40]. Furthermore, even with a similar focus, different disease management programs may substantially differ in their ability to implement change and improve health-related outcomes. Although some HF disease management programs have been proven to be effective, others have not. Significant additional attention is needed in developing, testing, and demonstrating best practices and sharing information on successful program components across a variety of care settings. Disease management programs should include ongoing and scientifically-based evaluation including consensus-driven performance measure and clinical outcomes (Table 13.3) [41, 42].

CONCLUSIONS

As reviewed in this chapter, HF poses a tremendous challenge and there are substantial opportunities to improve care. It has been clearly documented that not enough has been done to ensure the use of evidence-based, guideline-recommended therapies and optimize care in patients with HF. Despite compelling scientific evidence of the benefits of ACE inhibitor, β-blocker, and aldosterone antagonist therapy, a substantial proportion of HF patients are not on treatment. Similarly, there are currently large numbers of HF patients eligible for implantable cardioverter-defibrillator (ICD) and cardiac resynchronization therapy who have yet to receive these life-prolonging therapies. Substantial gaps in providing discharge instructions and HF patient education also exist. A review of the evidence from national registries and clinical studies provides a compelling argument for implementing evidence-based therapies and patient education as part of a systematic approach to address HF. Hospital-based systems have been effective in improving the quality of HF care and are associated with improved clinical outcomes. Outpatient HF disease management programs have accelerated the initiation of evidence-based medications, patient education, and other essential aspects of HF patient care, and thus patient adherence to recommended therapeutic regimens. The successful implementation of disease management for HF will enhance the quality of HF care and, as a result, substantially reduce the risk of hospitalizations and death in the very large number of HF patients.

SUMMARY

Does disease management matter in HF?

- Despite the compelling scientific evidence that HF medications and device therapy reduce hospitalizations and mortality in patients with HF, these life-prolonging therapies continue to be underutilized.
- Registry data from a variety of clinical settings have documented that a significant proportion of patients with HF are not receiving treatment with guideline-recommended therapies when guided by conventional care.
- Recent studies demonstrate that hospital-based performance improvement systems can improve medical care and education of hospitalized HF patients and accelerate use of evidence-based, guideline-recommended therapies.
- Outpatient HF disease management programs have also been shown to improve the quality of HF patient care resulting in substantial reduction in hospitalizations and mortality.
- Application of validated and reproducible systems and disease management programs for patients with HF is an important step in maximizing interventions to improve outcomes in this patient population.

Therapeutic strategies:

- Implement hospital-based systems for HF to enhance adherence to established guidelines and core performance measures, reduce the treatment variability between hospitals, and improve overall quality of care.
- As part of an enhanced treatment and discharge plan, apply evidence-based best practice algorithms, critical pathways, standardized orders, discharge checklists, pocket cards, chart stickers, and track treatment rates in a registry to improve HF management.
- Apply HF disease management programs which include a multidisciplinary team, optimization of HF drug and device therapy, intensive patient education, vigilant follow-up with early recognition of worsening symptoms, as well as identification and effective management of patients' comorbidities.
- Disease management programs should include ongoing and scientifically-based evaluation including consensus-driven performance measure and clinical outcomes.

REFERENCES

1. American Heart Association. *Heart Disease and Stroke Statistics – 2006 Update*. American Heart Association, Dallas, TX, 2006.

2. Hunt SA, Abraham WT, Chin MH *et al*. ACC/AHA 2005 Guideline Update for the Diagnosis and Management of Chronic Heart Failure in the Adult: a report of the American College of Cardiology/American Heart Association Task Force on Practice Guidelines (Writing Committee to Update the 2001 Guidelines for the Evaluation and Management of Heart Failure). *Circulation* 2005; 112:e154–e235.

3. Adams, KF, Lindenfeld J, Arnold JMO *et al*. Executive Summary: HFSA 2006 Comprehensive Heart Failure Practice Guideline. *J Card Fail* 2006; 12:10–38.

4. Swedberg K, Cleland J, Dargie H *et al*. Guidelines for the diagnosis and treatment of chronic heart failure: executive summary (update 2005): The Task Force for the Diagnosis and Treatment of Chronic Heart Failure of the European Society of Cardiology. *Eur Heart J* 2005; 26:1115–1140.

5. O'Connell JB. The economic burden of heart failure. *Clin Cardiol* 2000; 23:III6–III10.

6. Lee WC, Chavez YE, Baker T, Luce BR. Economic burden of heart failure: a summary of recent literature. *Heart Lung* 2004; 33:362–371.

7. Krumholz HM, Parent EM, Tu N *et al*. Readmission after hospitalization for congestive heart failure among Medicare beneficiaries. *Arch Intern Med* 1997; 157:99–104.

8. Garg R, Yusuf S. Overview of randomized trials of angiotensin-converting enzyme inhibitors on mortality and morbidity in patients with heart failure. Collaborative Group on ACE Inhibitor Trials. *JAMA* 1995; 273:1450–1456.

9. Packer M, Coats AJS, Fowler MB *et al*. Effect of carvedilol on survival in severe chronic heart failure. *N Engl J Med* 2001; 344:1651–1658.

10. Pitt B, Remme W, Zannad F *et al*. Eplerenone, a selective aldosterone blocker, in patients with left ventricular dysfunction after myocardial infarction. *N Engl J Med* 2003; 348:1309–1321.

11. Pitt B, Zannad F, Remme WJ *et al*. The effect of spironolactone on morbidity and mortality in patients with severe heart failure. Randomized Aldactone Evaluation Study Investigators. *N Engl J Med* 1999; 341:709–717.

12. Moss AJ, Zareba W, Hall WJ *et al*. Prophylactic implantation of a defibrillator in patients with myocardial infarction and reduced ejection fraction. *N Engl J Med* 2002; 346:877–883.

13. Bardy GH, Lee KL, Mark DB *et al*. Amiodarone or an implantable cardioverter-defibrillator for congestive heart failure. *New Eng J Med* 2005; 352:225–237.

14. Abraham WT, Fisher WG, Smith AL *et al*. Cardiac resynchronization in chronic heart failure. *N Engl J Med* 2002; 346:1845–1853.

15. McAlister FA, Ezekowitz JA, Wiebe N *et al*. Systematic review: cardiac resynchronization in patients with symptomatic heart failure. *Ann Intern Med* 2004; 141:381–390.

16. Young JB, Abraham WT, Smith AL *et al*. Combined cardiac resynchronization and implantable cardioversion defibrillation in advanced chronic heart failure: the MIRACLE ICD Trial. *JAMA* 2003; 289:2685–2694.

17. Bristow MR, Saxon LA, Boehmer J *et al*. Cardiac-resynchronization therapy with or without an implantable defibrillator in advanced chronic heart failure. *N Engl J Med* 2004; 350:2140–2150.

18. Cleland JG, Daubert JC, Erdmann E *et al*. The effect of cardiac resynchronization on morbidity and mortality in heart failure. *N Engl J Med* 2005; 352:1539–1549.

19. Stafford RS, Radley DC. The underutilization of cardiac medications of proven benefit, 1990 to 2002. *J Am Coll Cardiol* 2003; 41:56–61.

20. Cleland JG, Cohen-Solal A, Aguilar JC *et al*. Management of heart failure in primary care (the IMPROVEMENT of Heart Failure Programme): an international survey. *Lancet* 2002; 360:1631–1639.

21. Sueta CA, Chowdhury M, Boccuzzi SJ *et al*. Analysis of the degree of undertreatment of hyperlipidemia and congestive heart failure secondary to coronary artery disease. *Am J Cardiol* 1999; 83:1303–1307.

22. Havranek EP, Wolfe P, Masoudi FA *et al*. Provider and hospital characteristics associated with geographic variation in the evaluation and management of elderly patients with heart failure. *Arch Intern Med* 2004; 164:1186–1191.

23. Fonarow GC, Yancy CW, Heywood JT. Adherence to heart failure quality-of-care indicators in US hospitals: analysis of the ADHERE registry. *Arch Intern Med* 2005; 165:1469–1477.

24. Ansari M, Shilpak MG, Heindenreich PA *et al*. Improving guideline adherence. a randomized trial evaluating strategies to increase B-blocker use in heart failure. *Circulation* 2003; 107:2799–2804.

25. Lee DS, Tu JV, Juurlink DN *et al.* Risk-treatment mismatch in the pharmacotherapy of heart failure. *JAMA* 2005; 294:1240–1247.
26. Joint Commission on Accreditation of Healthcare Organizations. Overview of the Heart Failure (HF) Core Measure Set by Joint Commission on Accreditation of Healthcare Organizations. Available at: http://www.jcaho.org/pms/core+measures/hf_overview.htm; accessed 18 March, 2006.
27. Ashton CM, Kuykendall DH, Johnson ML, Wray NP, Wu L. The association between the quality of inpatient care and early readmission. *Ann Intern Med* 1995; 122:415–421.
28. Fonarow GC, Gawlinski A, Moughrabi S, Tillisch JH. Improved treatment of coronary heart disease by implementation of a Cardiac Hospitalization Atherosclerosis Management Program (CHAMP). *Am J Cardiol* 2001; 87:819–822.
29. LaBresh KA, Ellrodt AG, Gliklich R *et al.* Get with the guidelines for cardiovascular secondary prevention: pilot results. *Arch Intern Med* 2004; 64:203–209.
30. Fonarow GC, Abraham WT, Albert NM *et al.* Organized Program to Initiate Lifesaving Treatment in Hospitalized Patients with Heart Failure (OPTIMIZE-HF): rationale and design. *Am Heart J* 2004; 148:43–51.
31. Fonarow GC, Stevenson LW, Walden JA *et al.* Impact of a comprehensive heart failure management program on hospital readmission and functional status of patients with advanced heart failure. *J Am Coll Cardiol* 1997; 30:725–732.
32. Hanumanthu S, Butler J, Chomsky D, Davis S, Wilson JR. Effect of a heart failure program on hospitalization frequency and exercise tolerance. *Circulation* 1997; 96:2842–2848.
33. West JA, Miller NH, Parker KM *et al.* A comprehensive management system for heart failure improves clinical outcomes and reduces medical resource utilization. *Am J Cardiol* 1997; 79:58–63.
34. Rich MW, Becham V, Wittenberg C *et al.* A multidisciplinary intervention to prevent the readmission of elderly patients with congestive heart failure. *N Engl J Med* 1995; 333:1190–1195.
35. Stewart S, Horowitz JD. Home-based intervention in congestive heart failure. *Circulation* 2002; 105:2861–2866.
36. Krumholz HM, Amatruda J, Smith GL *et al.* Randomized trial of an education and support intervention to prevent readmission of patients with heart failure. *J Am Coll Cardiol* 2002; 39:83–89.
37. Kimmelstiel C, Levine D, Perry K *et al.* Randomized, controlled evaluation of short- and long-term benefits of heart failure disease management within a diverse provider network: the SPAN-CHF trial. *Circulation* 2004; 110:1450–1455.
38. McAlister FA, Lawson FME, Teo KK *et al.* A systemic review of randomized trials of disease management programs in heart failure. *Am J Med* 2001; 110:378–384.
39. McAlister FA, Stewart S, Ferrua S, McMurray JJ. Multidisciplinary strategies for the management of heart failure patients at high risk for admission: a systematic review of randomized trials. *J Am Coll Cardiol* 2004; 44:810–819.
40. Phillips CO, Wright SM, Kern DE *et al.* Comprehensive discharge planning with postdischarge support for older patients with congestive heart failure: a meta-analysis. *JAMA* 2004; 291:1358–1367.
41. Faxon DP, Schwamm LH, Pasternak RC *et al.* Improving quality of care through disease management: principles and recommendations from the American Heart Association's Expert Panel on Disease Management. *Circulation* 2004; 109:2651–2654.
42. Bonow RO, Bennett S, Casey DE Jr *et al.* ACC/AHA Clinical Performance Measures for Adults with Chronic Heart Failure: a report of the American College of Cardiology/American Heart Association Task Force on Performance Measures (Writing Committee to Develop Heart Failure Clinical Performance Measures): endorsed by the Heart Failure Society of America. *Circulation* 2005; 112:1853–1887.

14

Device therapy in heart failure

P. B. Adamson

INTRODUCTION

Clinical trial and basic science evidence demonstrate that ventricular electrophysiology, structure and function adversely remodel in response to neurohormonal activation in chronic cardiovascular disease, particularly in response to norepinephrine, aldosterone and angiotensin II. Electrophysiologic remodeling, a somewhat new concept in chronic heart failure pathophysiology, involves the production of both fixed and functional substrates conducive to lethal re-entrant arrhythmias. Arrhythmogenic substrates are many times coupled with interventricular conduction delay, which leads to abnormally dyssynchronous systolic and diastolic function and heightened risk for sudden cardiac death or progressive pump failure. Pharmacologic intervention instituted early after myocardial injury may prevent development of the anatomic components that comprise a fixed arrhythmogenic substrate, but there is no evidence that continued neurohormonal intervention in patients with heart failure can effectively reverse the fatty necrosis and fibrosis associated with mottled scars. Furthermore, neurohormonal intervention seldom results in a reversal of interventricular conduction delays.

It becomes apparent, then, that medical therapies in patients with heart failure may prevent adverse electrical remodeling, but once derangements in cardiac electrophysiology are established, the resultant risks for sudden death or pump failure mortality are optimally reduced by coupling medical therapy with implantation of appropriate devices designed specifically to address the electrical problem encountered in individual patients. This chapter will consider evidence and practical approaches to integration of device and drug therapies for patients with chronic heart failure.

Recommendations for therapeutic interventions in patients with chronic heart failure focus on achieving three main goals: (1) improve patients' well-being by reducing daily symptoms, which usually involves management of acute volume changes leading to classic left and right congestive heart failure symptoms; (2) improve ventricular function over time, which focuses on reversal of adverse ventricular remodeling associated with chronic neurohormonal activation; and (3) reduce the risk for early mortality, either by prevention of sudden cardiac death or progressive pump failure.

Major advances in the past 25 years have achieved dramatic success in meeting these three goals with multiple drug therapy classes targeting specific neurotransmitters or hormonal agents responsible for heart failure pathophysiology [1–3]. More recently, device therapies, such as implantable cardioverter-defibrillators (ICD) [4, 5], cardiac resynchronization

Philip B. Adamson, MD, FACC, Medical Director, Adjunct Associate Professor, The Heart Failure Institute at Oklahoma Heart Hospital, Oklahoma Foundation for Cardiovascular Research, Department of Physiology, University of Oklahoma Health Sciences Center, Oklahoma City, Oklahoma, USA.

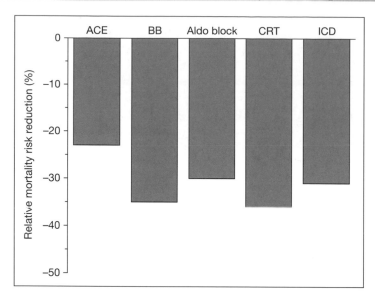

Figure 14.1 Synergy between neurohormonal blockade and device therapies in mortality risk reduction when applied to populations of patients with symptomatic chronic heart failure. ACE is compared to placebo while the other therapies are compared to the previous background therapies. Theoretically, mortality risk reduction is additive with the specific intervention's effect considered to be in addition to the background therapy effect. ACE = angiotensin-coverting enzyme; BB = β-blocker therapy; Aldo Block = aldosterone blockade with spironolactone; CRT = cardiac resynchronization therapy with biventricular pacing; ICD = implantable cardioverter-defibrillator. References: ACE [40], BB [26–30], Aldo Block [41, 47], CRT [9], ICD [4, 5].

devices [6–10] and implantable monitoring systems [11–16], have emerged to represent a new 'class' of heart failure therapy that is very effective in reducing heart failure mortality and morbidity (Figures 14.1 and 14.2). These advances have significantly increased the complexity of managing potential interactions between the polypharmacy of heart failure care with device implantation, function and informatics [17]. Complex interventions, however, are effective and worth the effort. In fact, the incredible advancement of heart failure therapies has called for new strategies for training heart failure providers [18] and, for the first time, a consideration of quantifying remission rates achieved in clinical trials involving heart failure patients. This is an impressive concept for a disease traditionally thought to be hopeless, with transplantation as the only intervention approximating a 'cure'.

The complexity of modern heart failure management requires special skill-sets that involve a rational integration of clinical trial data with an understanding of individual pathophysiology, comorbidities and estimates of longevity. The difficulty is usually not with which patient should be offered the hope of improvement with a medication or device, but identifying those individuals who are not likely to benefit from an invasive procedure or expensive medication. A rational approach requires a clear understanding of the pathophysiology being treated and an intimate knowledge of clinical trial evidence used to guide therapeutic recommendations.

MECHANISMS OF ELECTRICAL REMODELING IN CHRONIC HEART FAILURE

The two most common modes of cardiovascular mortality in patients with heart failure are sudden cardiac death, defined as death within minutes from the onset of symptoms in patients with otherwise stable symptoms, and progressive pump failure, which almost

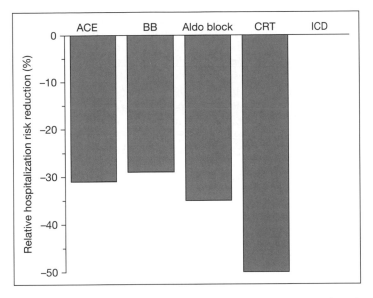

Figure 14.2 Reduction in relative risk for heart failure hospitalization with ACE compared to placebo, BB in combination with ACE, Aldo Block with background therapy of ACE and some BB, CRT in combination with ACE, BB, Aldo Block (when appropriate). ICD do not appear to reduce hospitalizations, but tend to result in increased hospitalizations. ACE = Angiotensin-coverting enzyme, BB = β-blocker therapy, Aldo Block = Aldosterone blockade with spironolactone, CRT = cardiac resynchronization therapy with biventricular pacing, ICD = implantable cardioverter-defibrillator. References: ACE [40], BB [29], Aldo Block [41, 47], CRT [7, 9], ICD [5].

always is associated with progressively worsening, refractory symptoms of left heart failure. Sudden death is thought to occur mostly from ventricular tachyarrhythmias, but brady-arrhythmias, great vessel rupture and pulmonary embolism also contribute to sudden cardiovascular collapse [19–24]. The clinical event of a ventricular tachyarrhythmia, however, is the culmination of multiple 'upstream' abnormalities that eventually serve to destabilize ventricular electrophysiology leading to ventricular fibrillation [25]. Exploring the 'upstream' mechanisms that are suppressed by chronic neurohormonal intervention in distinction to the 'event' therapies provided by ICD is essential to understand the synergy offered with pharmacologic and device therapies for preventing sudden cardiac death.

Lethal ventricular tachyarrhythmias require the presence of a substrate that can sustain re-entry coupled with a trigger that initiates the arrhythmia [21, 24, 25]. Neurohormonal interventions in chronic cardiovascular disease are thought to reduce the relative risk for sudden cardiac death both by preventing development of an arrhythmogenic substrate and, in the event the substrate is present, by suppressing the triggers responsible for initiating potentially lethal arrhythmias. β-blocker therapy effectively reduces the relative risk for sudden cardiac death [26–30] presumably by both preventing progressive fibrosis and decreasing the impact of adverse sympathetic activation on ventricular repolarization and activation. Sympathetic activation is well known to increase the risk of re-entrant arrhythmias, probably by enhancing the opportunity for late potential development and by production of heterogeneous regional repolarization, which constitutes the functional substrate for re-entry [25]. β-receptor antagonism using carvedilol, metoprolol succinate or bisoprolol probably blunts the end-organ response to sympathetic surges responsible for regional ventricular electrophysiologic abnormalities.

Cardiovascular neural and hormonal control systems' response to myocardial injury or dysfunction, however, tends to be determined on an individual basis [31], but usually includes some degree of generalized sympathetic neural activation with cardiac vagal withdrawal, coupled with increased renin–angiotensin–aldosterone activity. The neural and hormonal system responses are synergistic since increased sympathetic nerve discharge to the kidney increases renin elaboration [32] and increased levels of angiotensin II facilitate sympathetic activation by increasing the amount of norepinephrine release from sympathetic nerve terminals [33], decreasing the neurotransmitter reuptake [34] and increasing the firing rate of sympathetic nerve fibers [35]. This effect of angiotensin II is mediated through presynaptic angiotensin, AT2, receptors. Experimental and clinical data suggest unique inherent control system characteristics are present even before cardiovascular disease develops and, importantly, the immediate neural and hormonal response to injury may determine the type of electrophysiologic substrate an individual develops [31]. Therefore, prevention of a substrate conducive for lethal arrhythmogenesis must involve a strategy to provide neural and hormonal intervention early after myocardial injury to block deleterious long-term effects.

Myocardial fibrosis and fatty necrosis are stimulated by enhanced sympathetic nerve activity, angiotensin II and aldosterone activation. These effects influence both myocardial electrical activation and subsequent repolarization. For example, fractionated activation across mottled injury zones characterizes tissue from experimental and clinical subjects at high risk for sudden death [36–38]. Infiltration of non-conducting scar tissue in injury zones creates a surface area for delayed activation, unidirectional block and triggers with late excitation from the mottled area. This 'fixed' or permanent anatomic substrate can be further modified by the effects of continued sympathetic activation to increase the risk of triggered, late potential dependent arrhythmias arising from the injury zone. Angiotensin II, aldosterone and norepinephrine seem to play key roles in permanent substrate development and early use of angiotensin-converting enzyme (ACE) inhibitors, β-blockers and aldosterone antagonists can effectively reduce the relative risk for sudden cardiac death [39–41].

Repolarization changes are also important to consider in the chronic phase of cardiovascular disease. Down-regulation or dysfunction of inward rectifying potassium channels responsible for the rapid repolarization phase of cardiac cells in areas of hypertrophy, for example, produce dramatic repolarization heterogeneity and dispersion [38, 42]. This can be detected on the surface electrocardiogram by prolongation of the QT interval or abnormalities in the T wave (e.g. T wave alternans) [43, 44]. Experimental studies conclude that heterogeneous repolarization can exist either as a permanent or functional adverse electrical abnormality [38]. Furthermore, basic science data suggest that sympathetic activation plays a dominant role in developing functional abnormalities in repolarizing currents, which may lead to variable sudden death risk depending on the momentary state of sympathetic activation or consistency of β-blocker therapy. Finally, cell-to-cell electrical communication is deranged by alteration in gap-junction structure and function leading to increases in anisotropy with conduction defects developing over time [25]. Basic science evidence for neural or hormonal influences as key components in deleterious electrical remodeling is growing.

These concepts help explain the findings that early ACE inhibitor therapy after myocardial injury reduces sudden death risk by 20% [39], but an effect of ACE inhibition on sudden death risk in patients with long-standing heart failure is more difficult to demonstrate [40]. In contrast, β-blocker therapy reduces the relative risk for sudden death by 30% in patients with left ventricular dysfunction following myocardial infarction [45] and 41% in those with established heart failure [29]. β-blocker therapy prevents arrhythmogenic substrate development and effectively suppresses triggers that pose a continuous risk for initiating re-entrant arrhythmias [46]. Aldosterone antagonism, with either spironolactone [41] or eplerenone [47], in patients with left ventricular systolic dysfunction, effectively reduce the relative risk for sudden death, presumably by preventing functional arrhythmogenic substrates or triggers that initiate ventricular arrhythmias. Reversal of architectural and structural remodeling, characteristic of chronic heart disease, is also accomplished by neuro-hormonal interventions.

Risk for sudden death is reduced with appropriate medical therapy, but still remains high. In clinical trials examining potential benefits of β-blocker therapy in patients with heart failure, sudden death mortality risk was reduced, but was still the most common mode of cardiovascular mortality in those randomized to active drug therapy [48]. This gave rise to the hypothesis that the residual sudden death risk, which remains after maximal medical therapy, may be further altered with the use of ICD in patients with left ventricular dysfunction. The synergy between device and medical therapy to reduce sudden death risk is now demonstrated in multiple clinical trials [4, 5, 8]. Medical therapy suppresses adverse electrophysiologic substrate development and long-term risk for triggered activity, while ICD use terminates potentially lethal tachy- or bradyarrhythmias that occur despite neuro-hormonal intervention. Interestingly, the presence of interventricular conduction delay seems to increase the risk for sudden death mortality since cardiac resynchronization therapy (CRT) without ICD also reduces the relative risk for sudden death [9].

INTERVENTRICULAR CONDUCTION DELAYS

Progressive ventricular remodeling in heart failure patients may produce atrio-ventricular (AV) node or bundle branch dysfunction [49]. The result of interventricular conduction delays is to produce a spectrum of mechanical consequences that lead to increased symptoms, progressive heart failure, and increased risk for sudden death and pump failure mortality. CRT can be achieved using atrio-biventricular pacing systems that follow intrinsic sino-atrial node activity and deliver biventricular stimulation [6–9, 50–53]. Consideration of proposed mechanisms related to the benefit of CRT are the goal of other chapters, but improvements in mitral valve function, systolic efficiency, diastolic filling time and eventual improvement in cardiac autonomic control associated with reversal of adverse remodeling are associated with chronic CRT. Very importantly, mortality reduction, with an impact on both sudden and pump failure deaths, is achieved with long-term CRT.

The interaction between neurohormonal intervention and CRT is less clear. St. John Sutton et al. [53] have provided most of the systematic information comparing interaction between device and neurohormonal intervention in individuals randomized to CRT-on and CRT-off in the context of the Multicenter InSync Randomized Clincial Evaluation (MIRACLE) trial. CRT induced significant reversal of adverse remodeling, which was similar between those receiving β-blocker therapy and those unable to tolerate β-blockers.

Improvement in cardiac neural control, however, seemed more prominent in those receiving both β-blockers and CRT in the MIRACLE trial [11]. Heart rate variability measurements, markers of cardiac vagal control, suggested that improved parasympathetic control of the heart was more pronounced in those receiving β-blockers and CRT compared to CRT alone [11]. This may represent an insight into autonomic accentuated antagonism in patients with chronic heart failure. It is clear that both cardiac vagal withdrawal and sympathetic activation characterize patients with chronic heart failure. Pharmacologic therapies seem only to deal with the adverse effects of sympathetic activation, while device therapy using CRT is associated with improved vagal control. Therefore, a potential synergy between CRT and β-blocker therapy may relate to improved vagal control coupled with sympathetic antagonism, which undoubtedly improves overall ventricular function and decreases risk for sudden death.

An interesting reduction in sudden death mortality was observed in the Cardiac Resynchronization in Heart Failure (CARE-HF) study examining the long-term effects of CRT in patients with New York Heart Association (NYHA) class III and IV heart failure [9]. Patients randomized to the device limb of the study had a significant reduction in sudden death compared to medical therapy alone. This raises the possibility that electrophysiologic abnormalities created by interventricular conduction delays may increase the risk for ventricular arrhythmias leading to sudden death. An alternative hypothesis is that CRT may have prevented bradyarrhythmias that were possibly prevalent in patients randomized to medical therapy alone. Regardless of the mechanisms involved, CRT without an ICD reduces the incidence of sudden death compared to standard medical therapy with relative risk reductions that rival those of ICD trials.

In summary, interventricular conduction delay in the presence of left ventricular systolic dysfunction contributes to morbidity and mortality of the disease. CRT accomplished with biventricular pacing reduces mortality, heart failure symptoms, reverses adverse ventricular remodeling and improves cardiac autonomic control. No clear interactions with specific neurohormonal interventions can be proven based on clinical trial observations, suggesting that the electrical component of the disease may have an independent association with long-term morbidity and mortality. So far, CRT is the only effective therapy for this component of heart failure pathophysiology.

INTERACTIONS BETWEEN DEVICE AND MEDICAL THERAPIES

Improved output associated with correcting the impact of interventricular conduction delays using CRT results in improved renal blood flow and reduction in the primary stimulus for congestion. Therefore, diuretic therapy often has to be reduced to avoid volume depletion. In a recent algorithm for evaluating patients who do not appear to respond to CRT, an accurate volume assessment was suggested as a first consideration to ensure that the lack of improvement is not related to dehydration [53]. Accurate volume assessment should include orthostatic assessment of vital signs coupled with examination of jugular venous pressure, abdominal-jugular reflux and renal function. Diuretic dosing should then be closely monitored following CRT device implantation to avoid malaise associated with low-output volume depletion state (Tables 14.1 and 14.2).

Further improvements in cardiac output and rate support may allow increased doses of β-blocker therapy. It is clear that higher doses of evidence-based β-blocker therapy further improve overall ventricular function as measured by ejection fraction [54]. Only minimal synergism can be demonstrated between β-blocker therapy and CRT. Heart rate variability seems to improve more in patients receiving both CRT and β-blockers, but interactions between device and medical therapy are less apparent when considering long-term remodeling as patients with and without β-blocker therapy seem to have similar benefit. This may reflect the nature of clinical trial design, however, as almost all trials required randomized patients who tolerated β-blockers to have at least 3 months of stable β-blocker dose before enrollment in the trial. Little information is available about absolute dosing in most clinical trials so, theoretically, some patients may have tolerated up-titration after CRT hemodynamic and rate support, but these details are not yet available for consideration. Therefore, a beneficial interaction between devices and medications may be to support heart rate during up-titration of β-blocker therapy to doses that have proven effective in clinical trials. It is probable that improved cardiac output from CRT may also support those patients who have low blood pressure when neurohormonal intervention is applied. This may allow increased dosing of ACE inhibitor or angiotensin receptor blocker (ARB) therapies again to reach higher doses that may improve outcomes.

In summary, CRT improves cardiac performance in many ways that impact chronic medical management of heart failure. Important considerations should be given to volume, β-blocker therapy and dosing along with angiotensin–aldosterone interventions that may not have been possible prior to CRT.

MEDICATION INTERACTIONS WITH IMPLANTABLE CARDIOVERTER-DEFIBRILLATORS

ICD therapy has three general applications. First, patients who survive an out-of-hospital cardiac arrest without evidence for acute myocardial ischemia amenable to coronary

Table 14.1 Clinical interactions between devices and background medical therapies

- Cardiac resynchronization therapy
  - Enhanced pump performance with increased forward flow
    - Decreased mitral regurgitation
    - Improved diastolic filling time
    - Improved systolic contraction
  - Reversal of adverse remodeling
    - Decreased left ventricular end-systolic
    - Decreased left ventricular end-diastolic volume
    - Improved ejection fraction
  - Improved clinical outcomes
    - Enhanced quality of life
    - Improved exercise tolerance
    - Reduced need for hospitalization
    - Reduced mortality
- Implantable cardioverter-defibrillators
  - Improved clinical outcomes
    - Reduced total mortality
    - Presumed reduction in sudden death
    - Possible increase in hospitalizations
  - Reversal of adverse remodeling
    - None
  - Enhanced pump performance
    - None
    - Possibly reduced pump function with right ventricular apical pacing
- Monitoring devices (experimental)
  - Improved clinical outcomes
    - Possible decreased need for hospitalization
    - Mortality not investigated
  - Reversal of adverse remodeling
    - Not investigated
  - Enhanced pump performance
    - Not investigated

Table 14.2 Clinical considerations with medical and device therapy interactions

- Medication changes after cardiac resynchronization therapy
  - Volume management
    - With increased forward flow and improved renal perfusion consider reduction of diuretic dose
    - Assess for volume depletion within 30 days of implant
  - Neurohormonal intervention
    - Consider increased doses of β-blocker therapy after rate support and increased cardiac output from CRT
    - Consider increased ACE inhibitor dose following improved arterial blood pressure following CRT

revascularization have better long-term outcomes with ICD therapy compared to medical therapy alone [3]. Patients with structural heart disease and inducible ventricular arrhythmias during electrophysiologic (EP) study are also candidates for ICD implantation to further reduce sudden cardiac death risk [3]. Finally, in a broad application of implantable technology, patients with left ventricular systolic dysfunction (LVSD) (left ventricular ejection fraction [LVEF] ≤35%) of any etiology, have improved long-term outcomes when ICDs

Table 14.3 Interactions between device-based monitoring and clinical management

Parameter monitored	Clinical action
Incidence of atrial fibrillation and ventricular rate response	■ Assess need for anticoagulation ■ Adjust medication control of rate ■ Consider ablation procedures if rate is uncontrollable
Heart rate variability	■ Stratify risk for clinical events ■ Triage follow-up intervals
Activity	■ Implications concerning exercise activity ■ Review results with patient to encourage adherence to activity prescription
Day and night heart rate	■ Titrate β-blocker to control heart rate ■ Alter device-based rate support
Intrathoracic impedance	■ Stratify follow-up with remotely obtained data ■ Assess for volume overload and consider altering diuretics ■ Assess for pneumonia or other process that may change intrathoracic impedance

complement medications to prevent lethal arrhythmias [3–5]. The great interest in implantable devices to prevent sudden death should not obscure the benefits of medications to achieve the same goals. β-blocker therapy reduces sudden death risk by 41% [29], while coupling ICDs with maximal medical therapy theoretically reduces 1-year sudden death risk by up to 75% [16]. This incredible reduction in the relative risk for sudden death is demonstrable even after 5 years of therapy [4].

Overall, application of evidence-based medical therapies to individual clinical encounters would require institution of consensus-recommended neurohormonal intervention for the specific situation prior to a recommendation for device implantation. This is very important since neurohormonal interventions often increase ejection fraction and may take patients out of the range requiring device therapy.

MEDICAL MANAGEMENT INTERACTIONS WITH DEVICE INFORMATICS

Therapeutic devices now provide physiologic information that is helpful in the long-term management of patients with chronic heart failure [11–16] (Table 14.3). With the advent of internet-based information systems this information stream from therapeutic devices can be accessed remotely. The response to changes in physiologic information measured and accessed without examining the patient can be problematic. The difficult question of how medical therapies should be altered based on this new flow of information has led to a call for clinical trials to examine sensitivity and specificity of specific parameters that lead to remote medication changes. Remotely accessible information is in evolution and will eventually involve direct intracardiac or intrapulmonary hemodynamic monitoring to guide medical heart failure management [14–16]. A review of the parameters currently available will quickly become obsolete so a more useful review may involve understanding general concepts that guide use of remote data.

In general, it is important to understand whether a device-based information system is predictive of an event or represents a direct measurement of a parameter otherwise estimated by face-to-face encounters or physical examination. For example, implanted devices are capable of continuously measuring heart rate variability [12], which is a marker of cardiac autonomic control, and stratifies risk for clinical decompensation over time [12]. However, a decline in heart rate variability should not immediately trigger a change in medical management of the patient's heart failure. Instead, heart rate variability decline should serve as a trigger to identify patients who have started the progression to congestion [15]. Significant changes in heart rate variability herald clinical heart failure decompensation and precede hospitalization by an average of 17 days. Therefore, the recommended use of heart rate variability is to triage follow-up or serve as a trigger to interact with patients earlier than scheduled.

Continuous intrathoracic electrical impedance is an indirect marker of lung congestion and can be defined as the resistance to conduction of an electrical impulse from the ventricular lead to the pulse generator of an implanted system. Changes in intrathoracic impedance may identify the start of the progression to congestion [13]. Monitoring this parameter may be useful in alerting patients or providers to a meaningful change in clinical status [13]. Clinical studies suggest that significant changes in intrathoracic impedance occur up to 14 days prior to heart failure hospitalization, but the changes occur when patients are often totally asymptomatic [13]. Therefore, it is not clear if changing medical therapy based on remotely acquired or patient alert systems is safe or effective. Certainly, changing diuretic therapy in response to changes in intrathoracic impedance is not recommended without assessing the patient. Indirect markers such as heart rate variability or intrathoracic impedance should be viewed as 'triggers' that notify the provider or patient of an impending change in clinical status, but should be used to identify patients in need of assessment, rather than guides in medical therapy. Clinical trials are now in the planning stage to evaluate the possibility of guiding remote management of medical therapy in heart failure patients using device-based information. These trials promise to define true predictive value of intrathoracic impedance measurements to fully define their role in clinical practice. Until those trials are completed, the safest approach may be to use indirect markers to stratify risk of heart failure events.

Other parameters from implanted device-derived information streams include daytime and nighttime heart rate, ventricular rate response to atrial fibrillation, incidence of paroxysmal atrial or ventricular arrhythmias, and markers of patient activity. These parameters provide a reliable basis for changes in medical therapies. For example, a patient's ventricular rate response to atrial fibrillation may be well controlled during a clinical encounter, but examination of continuously acquired data may demonstrate poor control when the patient is active or engaged in activities of daily living. Medication adjustments may achieve better heart rate control and improve long-term outcomes. Other unexpected diagnoses are also possible with device-based information. Paroxysmal atrial fibrillation may be common in heart failure patients who are continuously monitored and may help elucidate the mechanisms involved in unexpected clinical decompensation or improve stroke risk assessment. Directly measured physiologic information can be clinically useful in guiding and tailoring heart failure therapies.

More direct measurements, such as intracardiac pressures, however, are capable of providing an exact measurement of a parameter that is merely estimated by daily weights or physical examination. Daily management of heart failure patients relies heavily on accurate assessment and estimation of ventricular filling pressures. Unfortunately, available tools intended to estimate filling pressure, physical examination and daily weights, are very insensitive when their ability to predict intracardiac pressures are critically examined [56, 57]. Therefore, currently the most important part of daily heart failure management is based on imperfect estimation of a parameter that is manipulated by potentially toxic medications, such as diuretic therapy. Newer experimental devices that continuously or intermittently measure intracardiac pressures to provide an exact measurement of the parameter being treated are in advanced stages of clinical development. These devices have the potential of directly guiding volume and neurohormonal management using very precise, remotely obtained information rather than gross estimations with weights or examination. They also have the advantage of remote acquisition, which may decrease the need for direct patient contact. Direct hemodynamic assessment may provide the basis for very specific tailoring of medical therapies in an unprecedented manner.

CLINICAL APPLICATION – PREDICTIVE VALUE

Understanding predictive value and the specific part of the clinical syndrome that is heralded by implanted device-based parameters is essential to safe clinical application. Parameters that herald potentially important clinical events, such as heart failure decompensation with accumulation of congestion may provide a rational means to remotely adjust diuretic dosing. Remote medication adjustment requires a clear understanding of how often the measured parameter changes without changes in congestion or what other disease processes result in similar changes. An example is intrathoracic impedance measured by an implanted device. Intrathoracic impedance decreases when fluid accumulates in the lung tissue between the intracardiac lead and the pacemaker pulse generator. This parameter changes predictably prior to hospitalization, but may also change with pneumonia or other lung diseases such as chronic obstructive pulmonary disease. Additionally, it is still unclear how many times intrathoracic impedance changes without attendant changes in congestion. Ongoing studies designed to elaborate these characteristics will clarify clinical use of intrathoracic impedance, but until data from these trials are available, the safest use of intrathoracic impedance is to notify the patient or provider of a potential change in clinical well-being.

As new device-based information systems are developed, practitioners will be challenged to integrate such information into their practice patterns and habits to both maximize patient outcomes and to make heart failure management more efficient. Cooperation between implanting physicians, device follow-up programs and heart failure practitioners is essential for seamless and efficient information exchange. Permission for heart failure practitioners to access internet-based information or to directly interrogate implanted devices to acquire heart failure diagnostics increases the likelihood that important information will be used by the appropriate clinical provider. This will require new strategies for infrastructural design and support, but has the promise of dramatically improving clinical outcomes.

FUTURE CONSIDERATIONS

Future devices to treat specific aspects of heart failure pathophysiology will undoubtedly include monitoring features that improve the value of the implanted device. For example, combining a hemodynamic monitoring device with an implantable cardioverter-defibrillator may reduce the need for hospitalizations by improving chronic volume management and avoiding congestion. This will be an important feature if device therapy is expected to become a mainstream component of heart failure care. Other combinations will likely include atrial, as well as ventricular rhythm control devices to treat the very common comorbidity of atrial fibrillation. Device therapies are an established component of chronic heart failure care and will continue to evolve to meet clinical challenges that arise as mortality continues to be positively impacted by both medical and device therapies.

REFERENCES

1. Packer M. The neurohormonal hypothesis: a theory to explain the mechanism of disease progression in heart failure. *J Am Coll Cardiol* 1992; 20:248–254.
2. Cohn JN. The management of chronic heart failure. *N Engl J Med* 1996; 335:490–498.
3. Hunt SA, Abraham WT, Chin MH *et al.* ACC/AHA 2005 guideline update for the diagnosis and management of chronic heart failure in the adult – Summary article. A report of the American College of Cardiology/American Heart Association task force on practice guidelines. *J Am Coll Cardiol* 2005; 46:1116–1143.
4. Bardy GH, Lee KL, Mark DB *et al.* Sudden Cardiac Death in Heart Failure Trial (SCD-HeFT) Investigators. Amiodarone or an implantable cardioverter-defibrillator for congestive heart failure. *New Engl J Med* 2005; 352:225–237.

5. Moss AJ, Zareba W, Hall WJ et al. Prophylactic implantation of a defibrillator in patients with myocardial infarction and reduced ejection fraction. N Engl J Med 2002; 346:877–883.

6. Cazeau S, Leclercq C, Lavergne T et al. for the Multisite Stimulation in Cardiomyopathies Study Investigators. Effects of multisite bi-ventricular pacing in patients with heart failure and intra-ventricular conduction delay. N Engl J Med 2001; 344:873–880.

7. Abraham WT, Fisher WG, Smith AL et al., for the MIRACLE Study Group. Cardiac resynchronization in chronic heart failure. N Engl J Med 2002; 346:1845–1853.

8. Bristow MR, Saxon LA, Boehmer J et al. Cardiac-resynchronization therapy with or without an implantable defibrillator in advanced chronic heart failure. N Engl J Med 2004; 350:2140–2150.

9. Cleland JG, Daubert JC, Erdmann E et al. The effect of cardiac resynchronization on morbidity and mortality in heart failure. N Engl J Med 2005; 352:1539–1549.

10. Freemantle N, Tharmanathan P, Calvert MJ et al. Cardiac resyncrhoronisation for patients with heart failure due to left ventricular systolic dysfunction – a systematic review and meta-analysis. Eur J Heart Fail 2006; 8:433–440.

11. Adamson PB, Kleckner KJ, VanHout WL. Cardiac resynchronization therapy improves heart rate variability in patients with symptomatic heart failure. Circulation 2003; 108:266–269.

12. Adamson PB, Smith AL, Abraham WT et al. Continuous autonomic assessment in patients with symptomatic heart failure: prognostic value of heart rate variability measured by an implanted cardiac resynchronization device. Circulation 2004; 110:2389–2394.

13. Yu CM, Wang L, Chau E et al. Intrathoracic impedance monitoring in patients with heart failure: correlation with fluid status and feasibility of early warning preceding hospitalization. Circulation 2005; 112:841–848.

14. Adamson PB, Magalski A, Braunschweig F et al. Ongoing right ventricular hemodynamics in heart failure: clinical value of measurements derived from an implantable monitoring system. J Am Coll Cardiol 2003; 41:565–571.

15. Adamson PB. Continuous heart rate variability from an implanted device: a practical guide for clinical use. Congest Heart Fail 2005; 11:327–330.

16. Adamson PB, Kjellström B, Braunschweig F et al. Ambulatory Hemodynamics from an implanted device: components of 24-hour pressures that correlate to supine resting conditions and acute right heart catheterization. Congest Heart Fail 2006; 12:14–19.

17. Adamson PB, Germany R. Therapy interactions in chronic heart failure: synergies and asynergies of device and medication therapies. Drug Discov Today: Ther Strateg 2004; 1:135–141.

18. Adamson PB, Abraham WT, Love C, Reynolds DW. The evolving challenge of heart failure management: a call for a new curriculum for training heart failure specialists. J Am Coll Cardiol 2004; 1354–1357.

19. Hinkle LE Jr, Thaler HT. Clinical classification of cardiac deaths. Circulation 1982; 65:457–464.

20. Zheng ZJ, Croft JB, Giles WH, Mensah GA. Sudden cardiac death in the United States, 1989 to 1998. Circulation 2001; 104:2158–2163.

21. Zipes DP, Wellens HJJ. Sudden cardiac death. Circulation 1998; 98:2334–2351.

22. Narang R, Cleland JG, Erhardt L et al. Mode of death in chronic heart failure. A request and proposition for more accurate classification. Eur Heart J 1996; 17:1390–1403.

23. Fox CS, Evans JC, Larson MG et al. A comparison of death certificate out-of-hospital coronary heart disease death with physician-adjudicated sudden cardiac death. Am J Cardiol 2005; 95:856–859.

24. Tomaselli GF, Zipes DP. What causes sudden death in heart failure? Circ Res 2004; 95:754–763.

25. Adamson PB, Barr RC, Callans DJ et al. The perplexing complexity of cardiac arrhythmias: beyond electrical remodeling. Heart Rhythm 2005; 2:650–659.

26. CIBIS-II Investigators. The Cardiac Insufficiency bisoprolol Study II (CIBIS-II). A randomized trial. Lancet 1999; 353:9–13.

27. Effect of metoprolol CR/XL in chronic heart failure: Metoprolol CR/XL Randomised Intervention Trial in Congestive Heart Failure (MERIT-HF). Lancet 1999; 353;2001–2007.

28. Willenheimer R, van Veldhuisen DJ, Silke B et al. Effect on survival and hospitalization of initiating treatment for chronic heart failure with bisoprolol followed by enalapril, as compared with the opposite sequence. Results of the Randomized Cardiac Insufficiency Bisoprolol Study (CIBIS) III. Circulation 2005; 112:2426–2435.

29. Hjalmarson A, Goldstein S, Fagerberg B et al. Effects of controlled-release metoprolol on total mortality, hospitalizations, and well-being in patients with heart failure: the Metoprolol CR/XL Randomized Intervention Trial in congestive heart failure (MERIT-HF). MERIT-HF Study Group. JAMA 2000; 283:1295–1302.

30. Nacarelli G, Lukas MA. Carvedilol's antiarrhythmic properties: therapeutic implications for patients with left ventricular dysfunction. *Clin Cardiol* 2005; 28:165–173.
31. Adamson PB, Vanoli E: Early autonomic and repolarization abnormalities contribute to lethal arrhythmias in chronic ischemic heart failure: characteristics of a novel heart failure model in dogs with postmyocardial infarction left ventricular dysfunction. *J Am Coll Cardiol* 2001; 37:1741–1748.
32. Schrier RW, Abraham WT. Hormones and hemodynamics in heart failure. *N Eng J Med* 1999; 341:577–585.
33. Boadle MC, Hughes J, Roth RH. Angiotensin accelerates catecholamine biosynthesis in sympathetically innervated tissues. *Nature* 1969; 222:987–988.
34. Khairallah PA. Action of angiotensin on adrenergic nerve endings: inhibition of norepinephrine uptake. *Fed Proc* 1972; 31:1351–1357.
35. Zimmerman BG, Gomer SK, Liao JC. Action of angiotensin on vascular adrenergic nerve endings: facilitation of norepinephrine release. *Fed Proc* 1972; 31:1344–1350.
36. de Bakker JM, van Capelle FJ, Janse MJ et al. Slow conduction in the infracted human heart. 'Zigzag' course of activation. *Circulation* 1993; 88:915–926.
37. Janse MJ. Infarct anatomy, baroreflex sensitivity and sudden death. *J Mol Cell Cardiol* 1993; 25:497–499.
38. Swann M, Nakagawa H, Vanoli E et al. Heterogeneity of endocardial repolarization and risk for lethal arrhythmias: components of a high risk myocardial substrate. *J Cardiovasc Electrophysiol* 2003; 14:1–7.
39. Domanski MJ, Exner DV, Borkowf CB et al. Effect of angiotensin converting enzyme inhibition on sudden cardiac death in patients following acute myocardial infarction. A meta-analysis of randomized clinical trials. *J Am Coll Cardiol* 1999; 33:598–604.
40. Garg R, Yusuf S. Overview of randomized trials of angiotensin converting enzyme inhibitors on mortality and morbidity in patients with heart failure. Collaborative Group on ACE inhibitor trials. *JAMA* 1995; 273:1450–1456.
41. Pitt B, Zannad F, Remme WJ et al. The effect of spironolactone on morbidity and mortality patients with severe heart failure. Randomized Aldactone Evaluation Study Investigators. *N Engl J Med* 1999; 341:709–717.
42. Volders PG, Sipidio KR, Vos MA et al. Down regulation of delayed rectifier K(+) currents in dogs with chronic complete atrioventricular block and acquirecd torsades de pointes. *Circulation* 1999; 100:2455–2461.
43. Chow T, Kereiakes DJ, Bartone C et al. Prognostic utility of microvolt T-wave alternans in risk stratification of patients with ischemic cardiomyopathy. *J Am Coll Cardiol* 2006; 47:1820–1827.
44. Bloomfield DM, Bigger JT, Steinman RC et al. Microvolt T-wave alternans and the risk of death or sustained ventricular arrhythmias in patients with left ventricular dysfunction. *J Am Coll Cardiol* 2006; 47:456–463.
45. Dargie HJ. Effect of carvedilol on outcome after myocardial infarction in patients with left-ventricular dysfunction: the CAPRICORN randomized trial. *Lancet* 2001; 357:1385–1390.
46. Brodine WN, Tung RT, Lee JK et al. Effects of beta-blockers on implantable cardioverter defibrillator therapy and survival in patients with ischemic dilated cardiomyopathy (from the Multicenter Automatic Defibrillator Implantation Trial II). *Am J Cardiol* 2005; 96:691–695.
47. Pitt B, Remme W, Zannad F et al. Eplerenone, a selective aldosterone blocker in patients with left ventricular dysfunction after myocardial infarction. *N Engl J Med* 2003; 348:1309–1321.
48. Kowey PR. A review of carvedilol arrhythmia data in clinical trials. *J Cardiovasc Pharmacol Ther* 2005; 10:S59–S68.
49. Hofmann M, Bauer R, Handrock R et al. Prognostic value of the QRS duration in patients with heart failure: a subgroup analysis from 24 centers of Val-HeFt. *J Card Fail* 2005; 11:523–528.
50. Saxon LA, De Marco T, Schafer J et al. Effects of long-term biventricular stimulation for resynchronization on echocardiographic measures of remodeling. *Circulation* 2002; 105:1304–1310.
51. Stellbrink C, Breighardt OA, Franke A. Impact of cardiac resynchronization therapy using hemodynamically optimized pacing on left ventricular remodeling in patients with congestive heart failure and ventricular conduction disturbances. *J Am Coll Cardiol* 2001; 38:1957–1965.
52. Yu CM, Chau E, Sanderson JE et al. Tissue Doppler echocardiographic evidence of reverse remodeling and improved synchronicity by simultaneously delaying regional contraction after biventricular pacing therapy in heart failure. *Circulation* 2002; 105:438–445.
53. St. John Sutton MG, Plappert T, Abraham WT et al. Effect of cardiac resynchronization therapy on left ventricular size and function in chronic heart failure. *Circulation* 2003; 107:1985–1990.

54. Aranda JM Jr, Woo GW, Schofield RS *et al*. Management of heart failure after cardiac resynchronization therapy: integrating advanced heart failure treatment with optimal device function. *J Am Coll Cardiol* 2005; 46:2193–2198.

55. Bristow MR, Gilbert EM, Abraham WT *et al*. Carvedilol produces dose-related improvements in left ventricular function and survival in subjects with chronic heart failure: MOCHA Investigators. *Circulation* 1996; 94:2807–2816.

56. Capomolla S, Ceresa M, Pinna G *et al*. Echo-Doppler and clinical evaluations to define hemodynamic profile in patients with heart failure: accuracy and influence on therapeutic management. *Eur J Heart Fail* 2005; 7:624–630.

57. Drazner MH, Rame JE, Stevenson LW, Dries DL. Prognostic importance of elevated jugular venous pressure and a third heart sound in patients with heart failure. *N Engl J Med* 2001; 345:574–581.

15

Ventricular replacement therapy for heart failure

R. Bogaev

INTRODUCTION

Cardiac transplantation remains the treatment of choice for ventricular replacement in patients who suffer from end-stage heart failure. Unfortunately, this type of therapy has been limited to merely 2200 recipients each year due to a dwindling donor pool and patient ineligibility from advanced age and comorbidities. Patients are more likely to die while awaiting heart transplantation than in the first 2 years following cardiac transplantation. Although xenotransplantation is technically feasible, societal, ethical, immunological, and infectious implications remain controversial barriers to this as an alternative biological replacement therapy. Steadily improving outcomes and efficacy with ventricular assist device (VAD) implantation in bridging patients to cardiac transplantation ushered in the application of mechanical circulatory support (MCS) as permanent ventricular replacement or destination therapy (DT) for the growing incidence of end-stage heart failure. In 2003, the Centers for Medicare and Medicaid Services and the Food and Drug Administration (FDA) approved left VADs (LVADs) for patients who meet certain inclusion criteria and are deemed ineligible for cardiac transplantation based on the results of the Randomized Evaluation of Mechanical Assistance for the Treatment of Congestive Heart Failure (REMATCH) trial. Only more recently, LVAD therapy been increasingly used as DT rather than as the traditional bridge to transplantation. Updated data from the DT registry highlights the importance of patient selection and risk stratification for DT. Low-risk patients who receive implants before the appearance of end-organ failure have significantly increased survival rates that rival those seen at 1-year post-cardiac transplantation. Strategies to augment DT success furthermore include optimizing patients' hemodynamics prior to VAD implantation, aggressive nutritional support, infection prevention, and right heart failure management. Multidisciplinary teams in the manufacturing industry are closely collaborating to develop improved designs, in particular smaller device size, increased durability, and improved biocompatibility. These improvements will soon afford more patients the option of ventricular replacement for end-stage heart failure.

In 1953, Dr John Gibbon [1], inventor of the cardiopulmonary bypass (CPB) machine launched the modern era of MCS when he utilized the CPB machine to correct an atrial septal defect (ASD) in an 18-year-old girl. After undergoing several modifications, the CPB machine revolutionized cardiac surgery [2].

The first cardiac allotransplant was performed by Dr Christiaan Barnard in December 1967. The initial worldwide enthusiasm for this landmark surgical success was soon tempered

Roberta C. Bogaev, MD, FACC, FACP, Medical Director, Advanced Heart Failure and Cardiac Transplantation, Texas Heart Institute at St Luke's Episcopal Hospital, Assistant Professor of Medicine, Section of Cardiology, Department of Medicine, Baylor College of Medicine, Houston, Texas, USA.

Table 15.1 Acute heart failure hemodynamics warranting consideration of MCS (with permission from [8])

- Cardiac index <2 l/min
- Systolic blood pressure <90 mmHg
- Left or right atrial pressure >20 mmHg
- Systemic vascular resistance >2100 dynes/s/cm

by early immunosuppressive complications and the limitations of long-term immunosuppressive agents. Infection and drug toxicity cascaded in a catastrophic 1-year survival rate of approximately 15%. By the 1970s, only two transplant centers, Stanford and the Medical College of Virginia, continued to pursue cardiac allotransplantation as a therapeutic strategy for cardiac replacement. Notwithstanding, the disappointment with cardiac transplant fueled a renewed quest for a long-term mechanical device as a replacement for the failing heart [3].

The Artificial Heart Program was established in 1964 by the National Heart Institute (now the National Heart, Lung, and Blood Institute, or NHLBI, reflecting expansion of functions) to promote the development of a total artificial heart (TAH) and other cardiac assist devices through the creation of research grants and contracts. In 1970, The Artificial Heart Program became the Medical Devices Application Branch of the National Heart and Lung Institute (NHLI). The objectives of the program were to develop cardiac assist systems to treat acute circulatory insufficiency, bridge patients to stabilization or recovery, or provide permanent support for the remainder of the patient's life, and to develop a totally implantable artificial heart to replace an irreversibly damaged heart [4]. John Watson, director of the Devices and Technology Branch of the NHLBI, issued two requests for proposals in 1977: one for the development of 'Left Heart Assist Pumps' [5] and the other for the 'Development of Electrical Energy Converters to Power and Control Left Heart Assist Devices' [6]. A third request for proposal was issued in 1980 for 'Development of an Implantable Integrated Electrically Powered Left Heart Assist System' to provide patient support in excess of 2 years [7]. The initial awardees of these requests, ABIOMED Inc., Baxter Healthcare, Thermo Cardiosystems Inc., and Thoratec, developed the first generation of left ventricular assist systems, which built the foundation for modern day devices in the field of MCS [4].

In the setting of acute heart failure, hemodynamic criteria warranting consideration of MCS include a cardiac index <2 l/min, a systolic blood pressure <90 mmHg, left or right atrial pressure >20 mmHg, and a systemic vascular resistance >2100 dynes/s/cm [8] (Table 15.1). However, these criteria do not accurately reflect the state of decompensation in those patients with chronic heart failure. The ability to achieve optimal outcomes is predicated by recognition of the patient's compromised hemodynamics and prompt referral to a center that offers MCS. In accordance with the objectives of the Artificial Heart Program, three major indications have emerged for MCS. The first indication is in patients whose ventricular function is anticipated to recover after a medium to short period of support. These patients, including those with acute viral myocarditis, acute myocardial infarction, or post-cardiotomy shock despite viable myocardium, are referred to as the *bridge to recovery* patients. Once hemodynamic stability has been restored, patients should be treated with optimal medical therapy, including ACE inhibitors, β-blockers, and aldosterone antagonists, to enhance the opportunity to reverse remodel their native hearts. Sir Magdi Yacoub demonstrated unparalleled success in bridging patients to recovery with his unique combination strategy of LVAD support to produce maximal unloading, standard medical therapy to produce maximal reverse remodeling, and pharmacologic therapy with clenbuterol, a selective β$_2$-adrenergic receptor agonist, to induce adaptive physiologic cardiac hypertrophy (the Harefield protocol) [9]. Following a period of myocardial unloading and optimization with standard medical therapy, the patient is weaned from the LVAD either at the

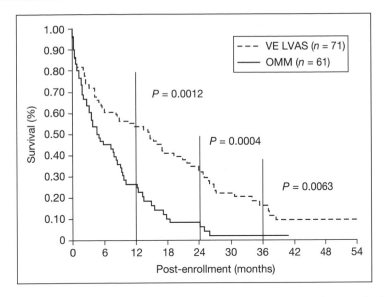

Figure 15.1 Mortality in patients who received the HeartMate® LVAS for DT vs patients randomized to optimal medical management (OMM). With permission from [12].

bedside or in the operating room under echocardiographic guidance. If the myocardial function remains preserved in the face of weaning support, the device may be explanted. If the patient develops hemodynamic instability or recurrent myocardial depression after device removal, a device for longer-term support should be implanted [10].

The second indication, known as *bridge to transplantation*, stabilizes those patients with progressive chronic heart failure who are actively awaiting cardiac transplantation. Patients are referred for LVAD support to prevent systemic effects of worsening heart failure such as progressive deterioration in renal function, development of pulmonary hypertension, or right heart failure with congestive cirrhosis, all of which can lead to ineligibility for cardiac transplantation. Patients with ventricular arrhythmias refractory to medical therapy and those with incessant defibrillator firings also benefit greatly from LVAD implantation. In light of the ACC/AHA guidelines which recommend avoiding continuous inotropic support with the exception of palliative care, transplant centers are initiating the use of MCS as a *bridge to transplantation* once patients are declared as inotrope-dependent [11].

The third indication is the use of an implantable LVAD as permanent therapy *or DT*. In a landmark study, the REMATCH trial demonstrated a 48% reduction in mortality in patients who received the HeartMate® LVAS for DT vs patients randomized to optimal medical therapy [12] (Figure 15.1). On 1 October 2003, the Center for Medicare and Medicaid Services approved DT for patients who meet criteria established by the REMATCH trial and who are deemed ineligible for cardiac transplantation [13]. The criteria require Stage C–D heart failure with NYHA class IV symptoms, LVEF <25%, a peak oxygen consumption <12 ml/kg/min, and a life expectancy <2 years. Additionally, patients must have significant functional limitations that are refractory to treatment with maximally tolerated doses of drugs, as outlined in the American College of Cardiology/American Heart Association (ACC/AHA) guidelines, for at least 60 of the 90 days before device implantation [12] (Table 15.2).

Appropriate patient selection has become paramount in achieving successful outcomes with VAD therapy. Multiple pre-operative risk scoring systems and criteria aid in identifying those patients for which VAD implantation would be contraindicated. Risk scoring can

Table 15.2 Eligibility criteria for destination therapy (with permission from [12])

- ■ Stage C–D heart failure
- ■ NYHA class IV symptoms
- ■ LVEF <25%
- ■ Peak oxygen consumption <12 ml/kg/min
- ■ Life expectancy from heart failure <2 years
- ■ Significant functional limitations, refractory to maximal medical therapy for at least 60 of the last 90 days

also guide the optimization of patients' conditions prior to surgery. In 1994, Swartz and colleagues [14] at St Louis University reported the use of 21 clinical variables, defining the patients' hemodynamic status, evidence of end-organ function, and hemostasis, to allocate patients into three different risk groups. The lowest-risk group had a survival rate of 100%, while 53% of the moderate-risk group and only 36% of the highest-risk group survived. Although this scoring system ignores factors such as previous open heart surgeries and the presence of diabetes, the stratification into high-, moderate-, and low-risk groups allows both the patient and the medical team a more realistic appreciation of the expected outcome with VAD therapy.

The first scoring system to predict more accurately which patients would have successful outcomes after LVAD implantation was developed in 1995 by investigators at the Cleveland Clinic Foundation and Columbia University. This LVAD screening score was revised in 2001 to reflect five clinically significant factors: ventilatory support, reoperative surgery, previous LVAD insertion, central venous pressure >16 mmHg, and prothrombin time >16 s. An LVAD score >5 correlates with a post-operative mortality of 47%; in contrast, a score ≤5 yields a post-operative mortality of 9% for those with a score <5 [15].

Lietz *et al.* [16] reviewed data on 195 LVAD patients enrolled in the Thoratec DT registry between November 2001 and March 2005. By univariate analysis, significant pre-operative risk factors for 30-day mortality included reflections of the severity of heart failure: serum Na <135 mmol/l, central venous pressure >10 mmHg, and systolic blood pressure <90 mmHg; evidence of end-organ dysfunction: aspartate aminotransferase >90 units/l, alanine transaminase >90 units/l, total bilirubin >1.3 mg/dl, and creatinine clearance <30 ml/min or serum creatinine >2.0 mg/dl; markers of malnutrition such as recipient body mass index <27 kg/m^2 or serum albumin <3.3 g/dl; hematologic abnormalities including white blood cell count >12 000/mm^3, platelet count <200 000/mm^3, and Hct <35%; recipient size: <80 kg, and advanced age >65 years. When DT candidates were stratified by the pre-operative risk score into extremely high-, very high-, high-, moderate- and low-risk categories, the 2-year survival ranged from 0%, 27.2%, 30.3%, and 54.2% to 72.4%, respectively [16] (Figure 15.2). To achieve optimal outcomes with VAD therapy, it is critical to adequately assess and optimize a patient's hemodynamic status, renal and hepatic function, nutrition, and coagulation as well as to mitigate inflammation and resolve any underlying infections. Although scoring systems assist in patient selection, each review is limited by the small number of patients included in the analysis. It is therefore difficult to firmly establish relative contraindications at this time. The ultimate decision to proceed with VAD implantation can only be made after a thorough assessment of the patient and all attempts to optimize the patient's hemodynamics and end-organ function.

Irreversible neurological injury, sepsis, irreversible renal failure, and uncorrectable hepatic dysfunction have emerged as absolute contraindications to VAD insertion. In the setting of cardiogenic shock, it may be initially impossible to determine all irreversible factors. Short-term support with either an intra-aortic balloon pump or percutaneous VAD will allow time to assess recovery of end-organ function. Those patients who develop acute

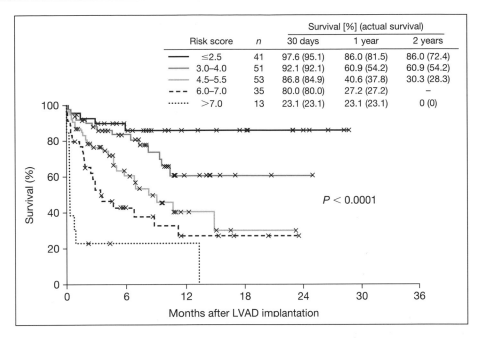

Figure 15.2 Two-year survival after LVAD implantation when DT candidates were stratified by the pre-operative risk score into extremely high, very high, high, moderate and low risk categories. With permission from [16].

renal failure and require hemodialysis post-operatively experience a higher incidence of LVAD infections due to the inherent need to maintain vascular access [9].

REMATCH identified infection, sepsis, bleeding, and mechanical device failure as the four major causes of death in the LVAD cohort. Pre-operative optimization of patients begins with a thorough analysis of the laboratory data to identify those with impending end-organ dysfunction [17]. Patients who remain volume overloaded should be diuresed aggressively in anticipation of reducing over distension of the right ventricle and decreasing hepatic congestion. Coagulation derangements are common and reflect the use of antiplatelet or anticoagulant therapy, nutritional deficits, and hepatic congestion. Screening for coagulopathy should include assessment of the prothrombin time, international normalized ratio, partial thromboplastin time, platelet count, platelet aggregation studies, and a bleeding time. Patients who have been exposed to heparin and most notably those who have undergone cardiac surgery should be screened for the development of heparin antibodies, which will predispose them to heparin-induced thrombosis and thrombocytopenia with re-exposure to heparin. Hyperbilirubinemia with elevated total bilirubin levels >3.6 mg/dl or direct bilirubin levels >1.2 mg/dl is an independent risk factor for death [18]. Great efforts must be made to correct the coagulation parameters and bilirubin levels before surgery.

Chronic renal insufficiency and anemia that is responsive to erythropoietin therapy are extremely common in patients with end-stage heart failure who may be candidates for VAD therapy. Inotropes, vasodilators, and a concomitant intra-aortic balloon pump should be used to augment the cardiac output to >2.0 l/min, reduce filling pressures to a CVP <12 mmHg and pulmonary capillary wedge pressure (PCWP) <24 mmHg, and increase renal blood flow to achieve a CrCl >30 ml/min.

Nutrition is one of the most under-valued aspects of a patient's pre-operative status, yet it is one of the most powerful predictors of post-operative mortality [19]. Poor nutrition portends poor wound healing and impaired T-lymphocyte function, predisposing the patient to a VAD infection. Screening for malnutrition entails testing of the serum albumin, pre-albumin, transferrin, and retinol binding protein levels. It is judicious to invest a few weeks into improving the patient's overall nutritional state through the use of multi-dose daily protein shakes or even continuous tube feeding [19]. On the other hand, those patients who are hemodynamically unstable or who develop systemic inflammatory response syndrome (SIRS) may not be able to tolerate tube feedings until they achieve hemodynamic restoration.

Infection was cited as the most common cause of mortality in the REMATCH trial, accounting for 41% of LVAD patient deaths. Infection prevention begins with proper patient selection and the good clinical practice of hand hygiene, and it continues with the prevention of surgical site infection, catheter-related bloodstream infection, and healthcare-associated pneumonia as outlined on the Centers for Disease Control and Prevention website [20]. Thoratec's Guidelines for Pre-operative Infection Prevention promote the administration of antibiotic prophylaxis customized per institutional flora and susceptibility patterns. The patient's nasal passages are cultured pre-operatively to identify colonization of methicillin-resistant *Staphylococcus aureus*. If the culture is positive, administration of mupirocin 2% nasal ointment is given twice daily (BID) for a 5-day course, starting the evening prior to surgery [21]. Adherence to these guidelines has lowered the sepsis-related death rate in DT patients at four high-volume institutions by 8.3 times [22].

Once the patient has been assessed for risk and all attempts have been made to optimize the patient's status, the team must select the most appropriate device to meet the patient's needs. Device selection is invariably influenced by the devices available at each institution, the physicians' and nurses' experience, and the clinical indication, as well as the patient's requirement for biventricular or univentricular support. The FDA has approved selected devices for all three clinical indications: bridge to recovery, bridge to transplantation and DT. Devices approved for *bridge to recovery* include ABIOMED's BVS® 5000 and AB 5000 Ventricle, and Thoratec's VAD and implantable VAD (IVAD™). For *bridge to transplantation*, the Thoratec® VAD, IVAD™, HeartMate® IP and XVE LVAD, Novacor® LVAS and CardioWest™ TAH are FDA-approved systems. The only device currently approved for *DT* is the HeartMate® XVE LVAD. A number of investigational devices, including the new-generation axial flow pumps – Jarvik 2000, HeartMate® II, and MicroMed DeBakey VAD® – are presently undergoing clinical trials and promise to expand and augment the clinical application of MCS.

Percutaneous MCS may be included as a component in the patient's pre-operative optimization to restore normal hemodynamics and improve end-organ function. The TandemHeart® Percutaneous Transseptal Ventricular Assist (PTVA®) system (CardiacAssist Inc., Pittsburg, PA) has a 510K approval by the FDA for temporary (≤6 h) left ventricular bypass. This continuous centrifugal pump can deliver up to 4 l/min of flow by diverting blood from the left atrium to the systemic circulation. A 21-F inflow cannula is inserted into the left atrium *via* a standard trans-septal puncture through a femoral venous sheath and a 15-F or 17-F outflow cannula placed in the femoral artery. Results from a trial that enrolled 18 patients with cardiogenic shock revealed a significantly reduced mortality rate of 41% compared to the 60% seen in the SHOCK trial registry [23]. The TandemHeart PTVA has also been used in selected cases at some institutions to support the right ventricle. For this application, a 21-F cannula is placed in the right atrium *via* the left femoral vein or subclavian vein, and a 21-F outflow cannula is placed over a guidewire into the main pulmonary artery from either a right internal jugular or a right femoral vein approach (Figure 15.3).

The BVS 5000 (ABIOMED Inc., Danvers, MA) is a short-term extracorporeal system composed of two polyurethane blood sacs separated by polyurethane valves. The device uses gravity to fill a pneumatic pump and eject blood. This straightforward engineering design eliminates the need for continuous monitoring by a perfusionist (Figure 15.4). The BVS 5000 was the first FDA-approved device for bridge to recovery for patients with reversible heart failure and has been widely used at over 600 institutions globally. The ease

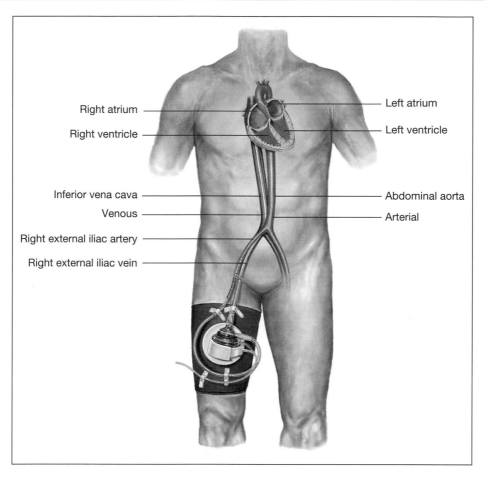

Figure 15.3 TandemHeart® Percutaneous Transseptal Ventricular Assist (PTVA®) System (CardiacAssist, Inc., Pittsburg, PA).

of insertion has generated the 'spoke and hub phenomenon', whereby the pump may be implanted at a non-transplant center and the patient subsequently transferred to an advanced cardiac center with the options of cardiac transplantation or DT. Most patients are supported for 5–7 days, after which point a decision to wean or convert to longer-term support is made. ICU monitoring, limited ability for patients to ambulate, and the need for continuous IV anticoagulation are placing this system at a disadvantage. However, a recently reported 10-year experience with the ABIOMED BVS at Columbia University revealed an overall 62% patient survival rate [24].

The AB 5000 Circulatory Support System (ABIOMED Inc., Danvers, MA) was approved by the FDA as an adjunct to the BVS system for short to intermediate support as a bridge to recovery (Figure 15.5). The AB 5000 ventricle is powered by a portable partial vacuum and partial pneumatic console, allowing patients to ambulate. This paracorporeal device uses the same cannulae as the BVS 5000 blood pump, thereby facilitating the transition from the BVS to the AB device when longer-term support is required. Hemolysis due to the presence of high-velocity flow at the inlet cannula was initially reported by the Texas Transplant Institute [25] but can be avoided with transesophageal guidance to prevent turbulence at the

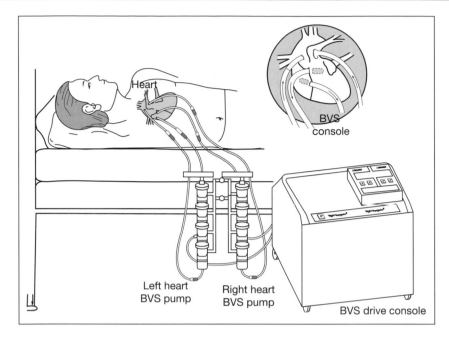

Figure 15.4 BVS® 5000 Blood Pumps (ABIOMED Inc., Danvers, MA).

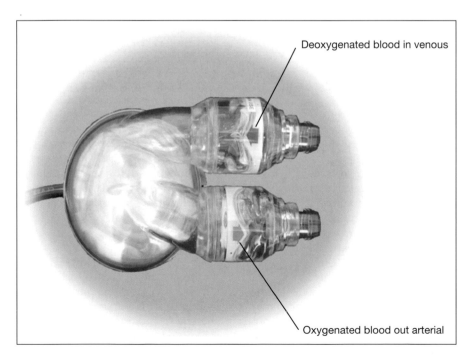

Figure 15.5 AB 5000 Ventricle (ABIOMED Inc., Danvers, MA).

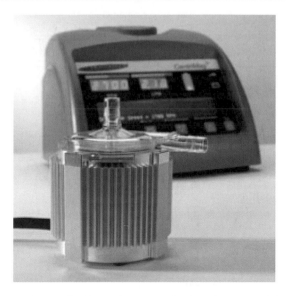

Figure 15.6 Levitronix® CentriMag® Blood Pumping System (Levitronix® Inc., Waltham, MA).

inflow cannula at the time of cannula placement. The AB 5000 console has subsequently been made to allow for adjustable vacuum if hemolysis develops following implantation.

The Levitronix® CentriMag® Blood Pumping System (Levitronix Inc., Waltham, MA) is designed to provide MCS for up to 14 days for patients suffering from severe, acute, but potentially reversible, cardiac failure. The magnetically levitated impeller in this pump eliminates the need for seals and bearings, which are known to cause hemolysis and promote thrombus formation (Figure 15.6). Because this design also avoids the use of flexing sacs, diaphragms, or valves, which are known to be prone to failure and thereby extends the longevity and reliability of the device. The CentriMag Short-Term Left Ventricular Assist System is FDA approved in the US for investigational use only but is CE-mark approved and commercially available throughout Europe [26].

The Thoratec VAD (Thoratec Corporation, Pleasanton, CA) is a commonly used pulsatile pump that consists of two mechanical valves and a polyurethane blood sac. The Thoratec VAD is FDA approved for bridging patients to recovery or transplantation. The paracorporeal position has facilitated left, right, or biventricular support of more than 2800 patients weighing from 17 kg to 144 kg (Figure 15.7) [27, 28]. An initially large and cumbersome console has been updated with a briefcase-sized TLC-II portable driver to allow patients to be discharged home while awaiting cardiac transplantation. Of note, the mechanical valves require patients to be on chronic anticoagulation therapy with warfarin. Longer waiting times have stimulated the design of an implantable iteration of the paracorporeal VAD. The Thoratec implantable VAD (IVAD), approved by the FDA in August 2004 for bridging to transplantation or treating post-cardiotomy shock, is about half the size of the paracorporeal version and has a smooth, polished, and contoured titanium alloy housing (Figure 15.8). A sensor on the TLC-II portable driver detects adequate filling and emptying of the blood sacs. The IVAD is versatile and can be used in either the paracorporeal or implantable position, as well as to support the left, right, or both ventricles [27]. El-Banayosy *et al*. [29] reviewed their experience with 104 patients supported by the Thoratec paracorporeal VAD. Although patients requiring biventricular support had worse outcomes than those who only needed univentricular support, powerful predictors of overall poor outcome included

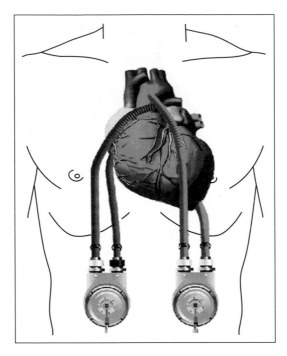

Figure 15.7 Thoratec® Ventricular Assist Devices (Thoratec Corporation, Pleasanton, CA).

pre-implant mechanical ventilation, hyperbilirubinemia, and age >60 years old. El-Banayosy's experience at Bad Oeynhausen highlights the importance of careful patient selection in achieving success with MCS.

The HeartMate® Left Ventricular Assist System (Thoratec Corporation, Pleasanton, CA) was initially FDA approved in 1994 as an implantable pneumatic (IP) device in bridging patients to transplantation. A more portable system with wearable batteries, the vented electric (VE), received FDA approval for commercial use in 1998. The most recent iteration, the XVE, which has a newly designed inflow valve, was FDA approved for bridge to transplantation in 2002 and subsequently approved for DT in 2003 [30]. Improvement in pump design, patient selection, and peri-operative management translated into improved survival, from 63.5% to 72.4%, when bridging patients to transplantation at Columbia University [31]. The HeartMate® is a simple pusher-plate pump with a diaphragm separating the blood compartment and air chamber. Titanium microspheres on the surface of the pump and textured polyurethane covering the flexible diaphragm promote the formation of a pseudo-intimal layer along the blood-contacting surfaces, obviating the need for chronic anticoagulation (Figure 15.9). Conversely, the textured surface has also been associated with the development of preformed reactive antibodies (PRAs) and T-cell dysfunction [32]. The Cardiac Transplant Research Database Research Group reviewed patients who received transplants from 1990 to 1997. Despite concerns about the elevated PRAs in VAD patients, Kaplan-Meier and multivariate Cox regression analyses showed no significant difference in post-transplant survival between the LVAD and medical therapy groups [33]. The HeartMate IP and XVE have been associated with very low thromboembolic rates of 3% and 6% respectively [34, 35]. Nonetheless, patients on the HeartMate LVAS may require chronic anticoagulation for other reasons such as atrial fibrillation, a hypercoaguable state, or the presence of a ventricular thrombus. The pump housing can be implanted in either a pre- or an intra-peritoneal position

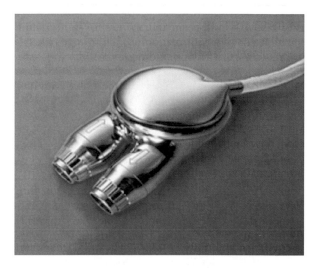

Figure 15.8 Thoratec® Implantable Ventricular Assist Device (IVAD™) (Thoratec Corporation, Pleasanton, CA).

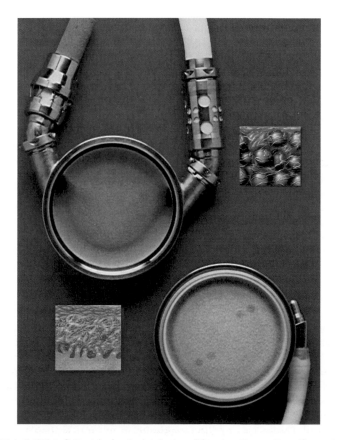

Figure 15.9 HeartMate® XVE Left Ventricular Assist System (Thoratec Corporation, Pleasanton, CA).

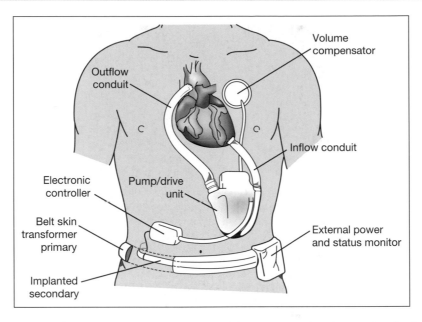

Figure 15.10 Novacor® Left Ventricular Assist System (World Heart Corporation, Ottawa, Ontario, Canada).

in the left upper quadrant with an external drive line, consisting of an air vent and electrical cable, traversing the abdomen to exit the skin in the right upper quadrant. This bulky pump is limited to patients with a body surface area (BSA) of >1.5 m². The HeartMate XVE remains the only device approved for DT. Growing experience with patient selection and management, as well as improvements in the HeartMate XVE LVAS, have allowed centers to improve outcomes to a level approaching those seen with cardiac transplantation [22].

The Novacor (World Heart Corporation, Ottawa, Ontario, Canada) LVAS is an implantable, wearable, pulsatile device that was first used at Stanford University in 1984 to bridge a patient to transplantation. Today, the Novacor® LVAS, implanted in more than 1600 patients, is the only MCS device to support a single patient for more than 6 years, thus earning its reputation as the most durable pump on the market (Figure 15.10) [36]. In this particular pump, dual pusher-plates compress a polyurethane sac, thereby ejecting blood into the aorta. Bioprosthetic valves are featured in the inflow and outflow grafts. The Novacor has been associated with thromboembolic events related to particulate matter in the inflow graft. Transitioning to an expanded polytetrafluoroethylene (PTFE) inflow conduit has decreased the embolic cardiovascular accident (CVA) risk to <10% by eliminating pannus formation along the inflow tract [36]. However, Novacor LVAS patients still require chronic anticoagulation with warfarin. Like the HeartMate, the pump is placed either in a pre-peritoneal pocket or the intra-peritoneal space, with a drive line tunneled across the lower abdomen and exiting in the right upper quadrant. For this reason, the device also requires a BSA of >1.5 m². Baran *et al.* [37], at Newark Beth Israel Medical Center, reviewed their cumulative experience with the Novacor LVAS as a bridge to transplantation. Twenty-six of 39 patients survived to transplantation with post-transplant survival rates of 80.4%, 75.7%, and 64% at 1, 3, and 10 years, respectively. In contrast to other VAD patients, those supported with the Novacor LVAS did not experience an increase in PRAs following VAD implantation, and they had rejection profiles after transplantation equivalent to those of non-VAD patients. The results of the Investigation of Non-Transplant Eligible Patients who are Inotrope Dependent (INTrEPID) feasibility study presented at the 2005 American

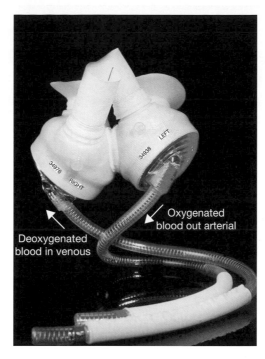

Figure 15.11 CardioWest™ Total Artificial Heart (SynCardia Systems, Tuscon, AZ).

Heart Association Scientific Sessions revealed an improved quality of life and improved survival among patients who received the Novacor LVAS vs those who were randomized to optimal medical therapy [38]. Following the INTrEPID study, World Heart began conducting the Randomized Evaluation of the Novacor LVAS In a Non-Transplant Population (RELIANT) trial to establish that the Novacor LVAS is superior to optimal medical therapy and equivalent to the HeartMate XVE for DT. The trial was later halted because of slow enrollment and clinicians' preferene for smaller, continuous-flow pumps.

The CardioWest™ TAH (SynCardia Systems, Tuscon, AZ) received FDA approval for temporary support to bridge patients to transplantation [39]. The CardioWest is a pneumatic pulsatile biventricular implantable system that replaces the native ventricles and all four valves in patients who are at risk of imminent death from biventricular failure (Figure 15.11). The device consists of two polyurethane chambers with a four-layer, pneumatically driven diaphragm, inflow and outflow conduits containing Medtronic Hall valves, and an externalized drive line. In the US, the CardioWest TAH is powered by a large console that tethers patients to the hospital, whereas facilities in Europe currently utilize portable drivers, which permit discharge from the hospital. A TAH may benefit patients with relative contraindications for an LVAD, including aortic regurgitation, intractable cardiac arrhythmias, and the presence of a left ventricular thrombus, a ventricular septal defect, or irreversible biventricular failure. A non-randomized prospective study conducted at five centers with the use of historical controls was performed to assess the safety and efficacy of the CardioWest TAH. Copeland *et al.* [40] reported a 1-year survival rate of 70% among patients who received the TAH as a bridge to transplantation compared to 31% among the control patients. After transplantation, the 1- and 5-year survival rates were 86% and 64% respectively.

The AbioCor Implantable Replacement Heart (ABIOMED Inc., Danvers, MA) (Figure 15.12) is the first totally implantable artificial heart. Because it fits inside the body without penetrating

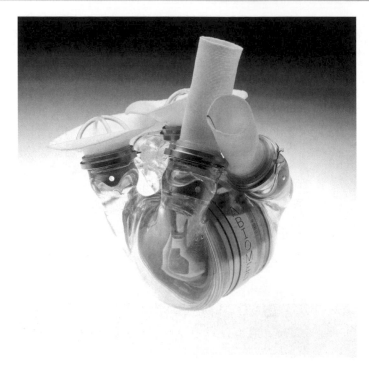

Figure 15.12 AbioCor Implantable Replacement Heart (ABIOMED Inc., Danvers, MA).

the skin, infection is avoided, and patients can maintain a relatively normal lifestyle. The AbioCor consists of an internal thoracic unit, which contains two artificial ventricles with their corresponding valves and a motor-driven hydraulic pumping system. The internal battery is recharged by a transcutaneous energy transmission (TET) system, or set of coils, one implanted internally and one placed externally overlying the internal coil, which transmits power across the skin without piercing it. This unique system gives the patient complete freedom from power base units and external battery packs, allowing them to move unrestrictedly. The initial clinical trial, which began in July 2001, enrolled 14 patients with end-stage biventricular failure who had exhausted all treatment options. Two patients died intra-operatively. Of the remaining 12 patients, 4 made excursions outside the hospital, and 2 were discharged to nearby facilities as a step toward discharge to home. These patients were able to go to restaurants, attend shows, sporting events, and religious services, and visit with family and friends at their homes. The longest-surviving patient was eventually discharged to home. The duration of support ranged from 56 to 512 days, with a cumulative duration exceeding 5.2 patient-years. On the basis of this experience, the AbioCor received a Humanitarian Device Exemption from the FDA in September 2006. The FDA now requires a Post Approval Study, which will consist of 25 patients in up to 10 US centers.

Axial flow pumps, a new generation of VADs, are currently in clinical trials for bridge to transplantation (BTT) and DT. This new generation of pumps is much smaller, approximately the size of a D-cell battery, and has few moving parts, so is much more silent (Figure 15.13). The continuous flow in axial flow pumps raises concern over the long-term effects of non-pulsatile flow. However, these effects are reduced when a patient's remaining heart function provides pulsatile flow and the axial pump only partially unloads the ventricle. In the event of device failure, the patient experiences hemodynamic perturbations similar to

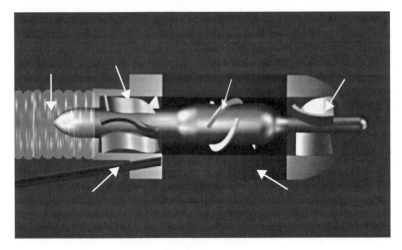

Figure 15.13 Axial flow pump (Courtesy of Texas Heart Institute, Houston, TX).

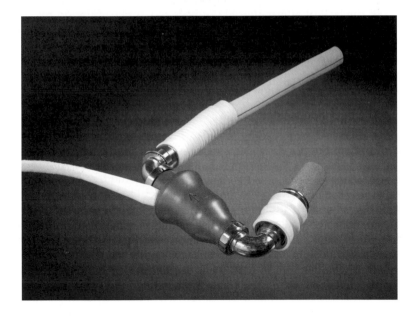

Figure 15.14 HeartMate® II LVAD (Thoratec Corporation, Pleasanton, CA).

those of acute aortic insufficiency, and emergent pump replacement is warranted. The Jarvik 2000 (Jarvik Heart® Inc., New York, NY) is the only intraventricularly positioned pump, and is fitted within the apex of the native left ventricle. Jarvik is currently enrolling up to 160 patients at 25 medical centers throughout the US in a pivotal trial for bridging to transplantation. The HeartMate II LVAD (Thoratec Corporation, Pleasanton, CA) (Figure 15.14) utilizes the TLC-II driver that is available for Thoratec VADs. The HeartMate Phase II clinical trial is evaluating bridge-to-transplant and DT patients in two separate arms.

Enrollment in the main bridge-to-transplant cohort has been completed for 133 patients at 26 sites, including 6-month follow-up. Seventy-five percent of the patients survived to transplantation, cardiac recovery, or ongoing support at 180 days while remaining transplant-eligible. Actuarial survival was 89% at 1 month, 75% at 6 months, and 68% at 12 months. During the support period (median 126 days, maximum 600 days), there were no mechanical blood-pump failures. Compared to the HeartMate I/VE experience, there was a significant decrease in adverse events: a 40% decrease in bleeding requiring surgery (0.78 vs 1.47 events/patient-year [pt-yr]), a 90% decrease in percutaneous lead infections (0.37 vs 3.49 events/pt-yr), and a 50% decrease in stroke (0.19 vs 0.44 events/pt-yr). These results were presented at the ACC meeting in March 2007, and a premarket approval application has been submitted to the FDA for use of the device as a bridge to transplantation.

Once a patient has been carefully selected, his or her status has been optimized pre-operatively, and the most appropriate device has been selected, success rests in the hands of the multidisciplinary operating room team, including a cardiac surgeon, cardiac anesthesiologist with transesophageal echocardiography (TEE) skills and a perfusionist, as well as surgical nurses and an MCS team. Although thrombocytopenia is relatively common in end-stage heart failure patients, one must be particularly cognizant of heparin-induced thrombocytopenia (HIT) syndrome. Each VAD program should develop an institutional protocol for managing HIT patients with alternative anticoagulants, especially because of the lack of alternative FDA-approved anticoagulation regimens for use with CPB. Aprotinin dose testing should also be performed prior to making the incision for the VAD implant. If the patient is sensitized to aprotinin, ε-aminocaproic acid administration may be appropriate to assist with hemostasis. All blood products must be leukocyte depleted and filtered. Prophylactic antibiotics should be completed 30–60 minutes prior to incision.

On the patient's arrival in the operating room, an initial TEE should be closely inspected for a patent foramen ovale (PFO) or an atrial septal defect (ASD); valve dysfunction, namely aortic regurgitation, mitral stenosis, and tricuspid regurgitation; right ventricular (RV) function, and the presence of an intra-cardiac thrombus. A PFO or ASD requires closure at the time of VAD implantation to avoid paradoxical embolus if right-sided pressures increase post-operatively. Mitral stenosis or even-mild-to moderate aortic regurgitation necessitates correction to permit LVAD filling and prevent backflow into the left ventricle, respectively. A mechanical prosthetic aortic valve requires either removal and oversewing of the valve or replacement of the mechanical valve with a bioprosthesis. Hemodynamic management calls for avoidance of right ventricular (RV) distention, administration of pulmonary vasodilators, and initiation of inotropic support to improve RV function, as well as to avoid systemic hypotension. De-airing the pump and weaning from CPB are critical steps that require careful attention and collaboration among the VAD team members to achieve optimal outcomes. RV failure is common in patients who receive an LVAD only and, when refractory to pharmacologic support, mandates placement of a right VAD [41].

Post-operative management of the LVAD patient is in reality RV management (Figures 15.15 and 15.16) [42]. The LVAD may be set at a lower flow rate initially to avoid an intraventricular septal shift, over-distention of the RV, and subsequent RV failure. The goals of mechanical ventilation should be to minimize pulmonary vascular resistance by increasing pH, optimizing arterial oxygen tension (PaO_2), and decreasing arterial carbon dioxide tension ($PaCO_2$) in addition to limiting positive end-expiratory pressure (PEEP). Patients should be weaned from mechanical ventilation as quickly as possible, with an aggressive pulmonary toilet, to prevent development of pneumonia. Additional pulmonary vasodilators, including inhaled nitric oxide, intravenous (IV) milrinone, and IV prostaglandins may be required. Correction of any coagulation derangements and notification to the cardiac surgeon when LVAD pocket drainage or chest tube drainage

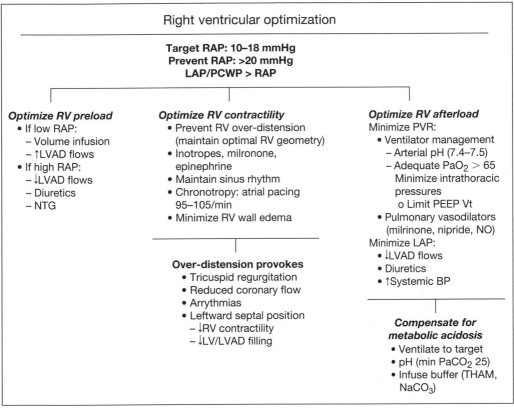

Figure 15.15 Right ventricular optimization. Adopted with permission from [42]. BP = blood pressure; LAP = left atrial pressure; LV = left ventricular; LVAD = left ventricular assist device; NaCO₃ = sodium carbonate; NO = nitrous oxide; NTG = nitroglycerin; PaO₂ = arterial oxygen tension; PaCO₂ = arterial carbon dioxide tension; PCWP = pulmonary capillary wedge pressure; PEEP = positive end-expiratory pressure; PVR = peripheral vascular resistance; RAP = right atrial pressure; RV = right ventricular; THAM = tromethamine; tris[hydroxymethyl]-aminomethane.

is >400 ml/h prevents excessive blood product administration. Arrhythmias may be treated pharmacologically or by cardioversion once the VAD is disconnected from the power source. Hypotension should alert the intensivist to possible RV failure, cardiac tamponade, SIRS, adrenal insufficiency, or LVAD dysfunction. Acidosis may cause pulmonary vasoconstriction and render inotropes ineffective and should therefore be corrected. Renal failure requires aggressive management with pharmacologic therapy or continuous veno–veno hemofiltration to avoid over-distention of the right ventricle and hypoxia. Agitation, delirium, and ICU psychosis, as well as adverse effects of sedatives and analgesics, can lead to neurologic dysfunction. These conditions are usually transient and will resolve once the patient's general condition has improved. The prophylactic antibiotic regimen should be completed and enteral nutritional support initiated as quickly as possible to promote wound healing and avoid infectious complications. Strict adherence to sterile technique with each dressing change and continual use of the immobilizer belt will dramatically reduce the risk of a drive-line infection. Either intensivists or cardiologists with expertise in MCS who can provide comprehensive detailed care in the ICU will greatly enhance the VAD patient's success post-operatively [42].

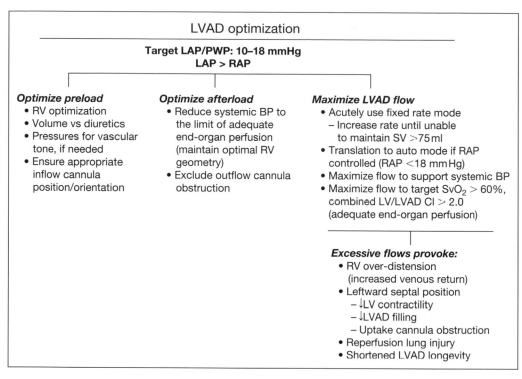

Figure 15.16 LAVD optimization. Adapted with permission from [42]. BP = blood pressure; CI = cardiac index; LAP = left atrial pressure; LV = left ventricular; LVAD = left ventricular assist device; RAP = right atrial pressure; RV = right ventricular; SV = stroke volume; SvO$_2$ = mixed venous oxygen saturation.

Optimal discharge planning begins at the initial evaluation of a patient for VAD support with a thorough assessment of the patient's psychosocial support system. The principal driver of success is a dedicated VAD coordinator who takes charge of the education of the patient and the patient's family support system. Facilitating discharge into the community of VAD patients involves the coordination of local physicians, emergency response teams, and community resources, and the management of ancillary equipment [43].

Since establishment of the Total Artificial Heart Program in 1964, MCS has had a tumultuous but progressive course. FDA-approved devices for bridging patients to recovery or transplantation, and for permanent therapy have become an integral part of the therapeutic armamentarium for end-stage heart failure. Devices are now available for support of the left or right ventricle, or for complete replacement of both ventricles. Systems can be implanted or inserted in a paracorporeal position to provide life-saving therapy to patients with diverse body sizes. The future holds much promise with improvements in patient selection, patient management, device durability, and miniaturization (Figure 15.17). Cellular-based therapy to augment reverse remodeling as an adjunct in restoring hemodynamic function with MCS, offers a new perspective in the advancing field of comprehensive treatment solutions for heart failure. With the melding of biology and technology, mechanical device therapy heralds the dawn of a new and exciting era in the treatment of end-stage heart failure.

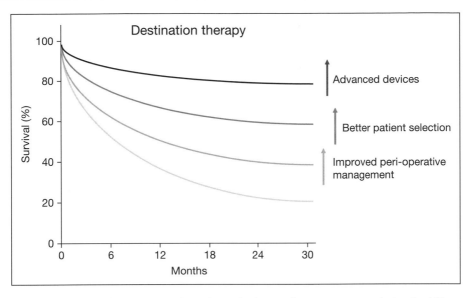

Figure 15.17 The effect of improvements in patient selection, patient management, device durability, and miniaturization on survival. Courtesy of James Long, MD, PhD. Latter Day Saints Hospital, Salt Lake City, UT.

SUMMARY

What is the role of ventricular replacement therapy for end-stage heart failure?

■ Mechanical devices are available to support heart failure patients for three major indications:
  ◆ Bridge to recovery.
  ◆ Bridge to transplantation.
  ◆ DT.
  ◆ Appropriate patient selection is paramount in achieving successful outcomes with VAD placement.
  ◆ Device selection is tailored by the expertise of the institution and the specific needs of the individual patient.
  ◆ A multidisciplinary approach to pre-operative optimization and peri-operative care by a dedicated VAD team has improved outcomes dramatically.
  ◆ Advances in device reliability, durability, and miniaturization will increase the number of patients who may benefit from MCS.

Therapeutic strategies for optimizing success with MCS include:

■ Recognizing hemodynamics in the acute heart failure patient that warrant MCS.
■ Identifying chronic heart failure patients who are candidates for DT.
■ Refering early to an implanting center before the development of end-organ dysfunction.
■ Maintaining open communication between referral centers and implanting centers to facilitate early transfer for MCS and early return of patients to their communities.

REFERENCES

1. Gibbon JH Jr. Application of a heart and lung apparatus to cardiac surgery. *Minn Med* 1954; 37:171–185; passim.
2. Frazier OH. Ventricular assist devices and total artificial hearts: a historical perspective. In: Samuels LE, Narula J, Crawford MH (eds). *Ventricular Assist Devices and the Artificial Heart. Cardiology Clinics.* W. B. Saunders Company, Philadelphia, PA, 2003, vol 21, pp 1–13.
3. Hunt SA, Kouretas PC, Balsam LB, Robbins RC. Heart transplantation. In: Zippes DR, Libby P, Bonow RO, Braunwald E (eds). *Heart Disease: A Textbook of Cardiovascular Medicine,* 7th edition. Elsevier Science, Philadelphia, PA, 2004, pp 641–651.
4. Frazier OH, Fuqua JM, Helman DN. Clinical left heart assist devices: a historical perspective. In: Goldstein DJ, Oz MC (eds). *Cardiac Assist Devices.* Futura Publishing Co, Inc, Armonk, NY, 2000, pp 3–13.
5. Department of Health and Human Services. National Institutes of Health. National Heart, Lung, and Blood Institute. Request for proposal. Left Heart Assist Blood Pumps. Bethesda, MD, 1977.
6. Department of Health and Human Services. National Institutes of Health. National Heart, Lung, and Blood Institute. Request for proposal. Development of Electrical Energy Converters to Power and Control Left Heart Assist Devices. Bethesda, MD, 1977.
7. Department of Health and Human Services. National Institutes of Health. National Heart, Lung, and Blood Institute. Request for proposal. Development of an Implantable Integrated Electrically Powered Heart Assist System. Bethesda, MD, 1980.
8. Norman JC, Cooley DA, Igo SR *et al.* Prognostic indices for survival during post-cardiotomy intra-aortic balloon pumping: methods of scoring and classification, with implications for left ventricular device LVAD utilization. *J Thorac Cardiovasc Surg* 1977; 74:709–720.
9. Hon JK, Yacoub MH. Bridge to recovery with the use of left ventricular assist device and clenbuterol. *Ann Thorac Surg* 2003; 75(suppl):S36–S41.
10. Naka Y, Chen JM, Rose EA. Assisted circulation in the treatment of heart failure. In: Zippes DR, Libby P, Bonow RO, Braunwald E (eds). *Heart Disease: A Textbook of Cardiovascular Medicine,* 7th edition. Elsevier Science, Philadelphia, PA, 2004, pp 625–639.
11. Hunt SA, Abraham WT, Chin MH *et al.* ACC/AHA 2005 Guideline Update for the Diagnosis and Management of Chronic Heart Failure in the Adult: A Report of the American College of Cardiology/American Heart Association Task Force on Practice Guidelines (Writing Committee to Update the 2001 Guidelines for the Evaluation and Management of Heart Failure) 2005. Available at http://www.acc.org/clinical/guidelines/failure/hf_index.htm.
12. Rose EA, Gelijns AC, Moskowitz AJ *et al.* Long term mechanical left ventricular assistance for end-stage heart failure. *N Engl J Med* 2001; 345:1435–1443.
13. Centers for Medicare & Medicaid Services. Available at: http://www.cms.hhs.gov/physicians.
14. Swartz MT, Votapka TV, McBride LR *et al.* Risk stratification in patients bridged to cardiac transplantation. *Ann Thorac Surg* 1994; 58:1142–1145.
15. Rao V, Oz MC, Flannery MA *et al.* Revised screening scale to predict survival after insertion of a left ventricular assist device. *J Thorac Cardiovasc Surg* 2003; 125:855–862.
16. Lietz K, Long J, Kfoury AG *et al.* Preoperative risk factors for early mortality following use of left-ventricular assist device as destination therapy for end-stage heart failure. *Surgical Treatment of Heart Failure I. American Heart Association Scientific Sessions.* 2005.
17. Park City Work Group. Candidate selection for destination therapy. In: *Advanced Practice Guidelines for HeartMate Destination Therapy.* 2004, pp 1–9.
18. Frazier OH, Rose EA, Oz MC *et al.* Heart LVAS Investigators Multicenter clinical evaluation of the HeartMate vented electric left ventricular assist system in patients awaiting heart transplantation. *J Thorac Cardiovasc Surg* 2001; 122:1186–1195.
19. Park City Work Group. Nutrition Management. In: *Advanced Practice Guidelines for HeartMate Destination Therapy.* 2004, pp 17–24.
20. Center for Disease Control in Atlanta. www.cdc.gov/handhygiene; www.cdc.gov/ncidod/hip/SSI/SSI_guideline.htm; www.cdc.gov/ncidod/hip/IV/IV.htm; www.cdc.gov/ncidod/hip/pneumonia/default.htm.
21. Park City Work Group. Guidelines for preoperative infection prevention. In: *Advanced Practice Guidelines for HeartMate Destination Therapy.* 2004, pp 29–37.
22. Long JW, Kfoury AG, Slaughter MS *et al.* Long-term destination therapy with the HeartMate XVE left ventricular assist device: improved outcomes since the REMATCH study. *Congest Heart Fail* 2005; 11:133–138.

23. Thiele H, Lauer B, Hambrecht R *et al*. Reversal of cardiogenic shock by percutaneous left atrial-to-femoral arterial bypass assistance. *Circulation* 2001; 104:2917–2922.

24. Morgan JA, Stewart AS, Lee BJ *et al*. Role of the Abiomed BVS 5000 device for short term support and bridge to transplantation. *ASAIO J* 2004; 50:360–363.

25. Bogaev RC, Schnitzler RN, Otero C. Hemolysis due to high shear rates at the inflow cannula site of the AB 5000 ventricle device. *ASAIO J* 2004; 50:134.

26. www.levitronix.com/Medical.php.

27. Riechenbach SH, Farrar SH, Hill JD. A versatile intracorporeal ventricular assist device based on the Thoratec VAD system. *Ann Thorac Surg* 2001; 71(suppl):S171–S175; discussion S183–S184.

28. www.thoratec.com/ventricular-assist-device/thoratec_imp.htm.

29. El-Banayosy A, Arusoglu L, Kizner L *et al*. Predictors of survival in patients bridged to transplantation with the Thoratec VAD device: a single center retrospective study on more than 100 patients. *J Heart Lung Transplant* 2000; 19:964–968.

30. www.thoratec.com/ventricular-assist-device/heartmate_lvas.htm#d.

31. Morgan JA, John R, Rao V *et al*. Bridging to transplant with the HeartMate left ventricle assist device: The Columbia Presbyterian 12-year experience. *J Thorac Cardiovasc Surg* 2004; 127:1309–1316.

32. Itesu S, Ankersmit JH, Kocher AA *et al*. Immunobiology of left ventricular assist devices. *Prog Cardiovasc Dis* 2000; 43:67–80.

33. Jaski BE, Kim JC, Naftel DC *et al*. Cardiac transplant outcome of patients supported on left ventricular assist device vs intravenous inotropic therapy. *J Heart Lung Transplant* 2001; 20:449–456.

34. Slater JP, Rose EA, Levin HR *et al*. Low thromboembolic risk without anticoagulation using advanced-design left ventricular assist devices. *Ann Thorac Surg* 1996; 62:1321–1327.

35. Frazier OH, Rose EA, Oz MC *et al*. Multicenter clinical evaluation of the HeartMate vented electric left ventricular assist system in patients awaiting heart transplantation. *J Thorac Cardiovasc Surg* 2001; 122:1186–1195.

36. www.worldheart.com/products/novacor_lvas/cfm.

37. Baran DA, Gass AL, Galin ID *et al*. Lack of sensitization and equivalent post-transplant outcomes with the Novacor left ventricular assist device. *J Heart Lung Transplant* 2005; 24:1886–1890.

38. Rogers, JR, Pierson RN, Butler J *et al*. Long term results of the Novacor Left Ventricular Assist Device in non-transplant candidates: results of the INTrEPID trial. *Surgical Treatment of Heart Failure: Assist Devices and Beyond. American Heart Association Scientific Sessions.* 2005.

39. www.fda.gov/cdrh/PDF3/P030011a.pdf.

40. Copeland JG, Smith RG, Arabia FA *et al*. Cardiac replacement with a total artificial heart as a bridge to transplantation. *N Engl J Med* 2004; 351:849–851.

41. Park City Work Group. Intra- and perioperative management. In: *Advanced Practice Guidelines for HeartMate® Destination Therapy*. Thoratec Corporation, Pleasanton, CA, 2004, vol 1, pp 38–47.

42. Rasmussen B, Holman WL, Buda T, Bogaev RC, Milano C. Postoperative management of the destination therapy patient. In: *Advanced Practice Guidelines for HeartMate® Destination Therapy*. Thoratec Corporation, Pleasanton, CA, 2004, vol 2, pp 4–19.

43. *HeartMate® LVAS Community Living Manual*. Thoratec Corporation, Pleasanton, CA. Available at: www.thoratec.com/medicalprofessionals/heartmate_lvas.htm.

16

Palliative and hospice care in heart failure

P. J. Hauptman, P. Mikolajczak

INTRODUCTION

The aging of the population, increasing prevalence of risk factors for congestive heart failure (HF), increasing prevalence of HF itself and a high mortality rate for patients who have advanced symptoms despite a multitude of available therapeutic strategies highlight the importance of evaluation and management of patients with progressive disease [1–3]. The implementation of a palliative care paradigm does not require the patient to be at end-of-life; rather, it is an approach that can be integrated with conventional HF care [4]. Hospice care, a specialized form of palliative care, can be employed when life-prolonging treatments are deemed to be inappropriate, meddlesome or in opposition to the goals of care established by the patient, the patient's family and providers.

EPIDEMIOLOGY

The epidemiology of HF demonstrates the potential for a major increase in the number of advanced cases. According to data from Medicare administrative files, the number of hospitalizations per 1000 Medicare beneficiaries has increased from 20.3 in 1990 to 22.1 in 2000 [5]. There is a clear age gradient with beneficiaries 85 years of age and older requiring 4.1-fold more hospitalizations than the 65–74-year-old cohort. In-hospital mortality has fallen [5, 6] but 30-day mortality may not have changed appreciably [6] and transfers from acute care hospitals to skilled nursing facilities rather than to home have increased. Numerical estimates from the American Heart Association heart disease and stroke statistics [7] include an annual number of discharges exceeding one million although this number is likely underestimated [8]. If a conservative estimate holds that 15% of these cases are advanced, the population of patients for whom palliative and ultimately hospice care should be considered may already exceed 750 000. However, the barriers to care and gaps in knowledge about best practices are significant.

PALLIATIVE CARE

The literature on palliative and hospice care is focused on oncologic diseases. This results in unique challenges for providers who care for HF patients with progressive symptoms. The lack of palliative care guidelines for HF is now recognized [9]. Unfortunately, clinical

Paul J. Hauptman, MD, Professor of Internal Medicine, Saint Louis University School of Medicine, Division of Cardiology, Saint Louis University Hospital, St. Louis, Missouri, USA.

Peter C. Mikolajczak, MD, Cardiology Fellow, Department of Medicine, Saint Louis University Hospital, Saint Louis, Missouri, USA.

trials in this area are unlikely to be supported. Industry-financed technologically advanced solutions are in vogue but often are not applicable to or appropriate for the vast majority of advanced HF patients. Uncertainties on the part of practitioners about the timing of referral remain significant. Nevertheless, the treatment goals are clear: relief of symptoms and maintenance of functional capacity. An algorithm has been constructed that demonstrates the integration of palliative care into the evaluation and management guidelines for patients with advanced HF (Figure 16.1). The key steps include continuous assessment of the clinical status of the patient. Progression of illness is defined by functional limitation or end-organ hypoperfusion and evidence for significant disease in the prior 6 months as demonstrated by recurrent hospitalizations and/or loss of ability to carry out many self-care and other daily activities.

A re-evaluation of the goals of care and the involvement of an expanded interdisciplinary team should be strongly considered when progression is identified. At the same time, the patient should be considered for advanced therapeutic options and even heart transplantation or destination therapy with a ventricular assist device if eligible and if the patient wishes to pursue these avenues of treatment.

Throughout all phases of care leading up to hospice, seamless transitions between sites of care are required in order to avoid unnecessary and costly hospitalizations. This is particularly true for patients with recurrent symptoms for whom non-compliance with standard medications, non-compliance with diet, inadequate discharge planning and lack of patient understanding about how to contact the care provider frequently lead to rehospitalization [10]. In that context, multidisciplinary management, whether or not part of a formal nurse-directed disease management team approach, can directly impact re-admission rates, resource utilization and quality-of-life. During the hospitalization, a statement of the goals of care may help facilitate earlier discharge. It is also conceivable that many patients who require a hospice can be identified at the time of admission or before admission, thereby preventing recurrent acute episodic care and interventions that are unlikely to prolong life.

FAILING THERAPY

The vast array of options for patients with progressive disease has complicated the decision-making that practitioners and patients face. Paramount in the process is the need to maximize proven medical therapies: angiotensin-converting enzyme inhibitors with or without the addition of an angiotensin receptor blocker approved for HF; β-adrenergic antagonists (carvedilol, metoprolol succinate and bisoprolol); the aldosterone antagonist spironolactone; and, in the African-American population, the use of oral nitrate and hydralazine therapy in combined formulation. Loop diuretic therapy, with or without adjuvant thiazide diuretic and digoxin may improve signs and symptoms of HF without definitive evidence for a survival benefit. These incontrovertible therapies have been developed for and applied in clinical practice; nevertheless, debates exist about the targeted dose, the best agent within any given class and the overall applicability of clinical trial data, specifically as it pertains to the elderly. While the mean age of patients with HF is over 75 years, clinical trials generally have not included elderly patients [11] who are at high risk for progressive HF and death.

The advent of device therapies has further complicated management. However, it is important to highlight the fact that implantable cardioverter-defibrillators are not indicated for patients with New York Heart Association (NYHA) functional class IV. Subgroup analysis from the Sudden Cardiac Death in Heart Failure (SCD-HeFT) trial suggested that patients with NYHA class III do not have a significant survival benefit, presumably because pump dysfunction, rather than sudden cardiac death, is the most likely outcome for these patients [12]. Further, patients who derived survival benefit in the Multicenter Automatic

Assess clinical status
(Particularly during or shortly after recovery from acute exacerbation)

- Assess LVF; document severe LV systolic dysfunction[1]
- Assess and treat exacerbating factors[2]
- Administer maximum tolerated medical therapy[3]
- Discuss prognosis and goals with patient and family
- Address all symptoms
- Coordinate care with interdisciplinary team

↓

Progression of illness

- Severe functional limitation[4] or end-organ hypoperfusion[5] present despite optimized medical therapy and
- Evidence for significant disease progression in the prior 6 months:
  - Multiple hospital admissions or emergency department visits or
  - Loss of abilities to perform activities of daily living

↓

- Reassess and treat exacerbating factors
- Reassess goals of care in light of diminished life expectancy
- Consider advanced therapeutic options[6]
- Readdress symptom control
- Consider expanded interdisciplinary team and expanded role for interdisciplinary team

↓

- Ineligible for or declines advanced therapeutic options[6]
- Ineligible for or declines destination therapy[7] or heart transplant
- Patient and family aware or prognosis and desire symptom relief but not further acute episodic care

↓

Hospice care

- Generally will include medical therapy, possibly including inotropic support, and will focus on symptom relief, directed by hospice/palliative care specialist
- Will not include an active ICD or acute care hospitalization for exacerbation

[1] Generally defined as left ventricular ejection fraction ≤20%.
[2] Common examples include hypothyroidism or hyperthyroidism, anemia, Ischemia, and depression.
[3] Generally consists of loop diuretic with dosing optimized, angiotensin-converting enzyme inhibitor or angiotensin receptor blocker if angiotensin-converting enzyme inhibitor is not tolerated, β-blocker, aldosterone antagonist, and digoxin.
[4] Generally defined as symptoms present at rest (NYHA class IV) and, whenever possible, documented cardiopulmonary exercise testing results should demonstrate maximal oxygen uptake ≤12 ml/kg/min.
[5] Includes clinically significant renal or hepatic dysfunction or abnormal mental status, each with no identifiable or reversible cause.
[6] Generally requires consultation with heart failure specialist or speciality clinic.
[7] Includes LV assist device or other mechanical circulatory aid.

Figure 16.1 Algorithm for integrating palliative care into the care of patients with advanced heart failure. ICD = Implantable cardiodefibrillator; LV = left ventricular; LVF = LV function. With permission [4].

Defibrillator Implantation (MADIT-II) trial were more likely to develop new or worsened HF requiring hospitalization than similar patients who did not receive a device for primary prevention [13]. Finally, the use of biventricular pacemakers is increasingly widespread but the magnitude of benefit in patients with very advanced symptoms has not been established.

Aggressive surgical approaches such as ventricular reconstruction and mitral valve repair or replacement have found advocates and may ultimately play a role in patient management. However, there are no well-designed randomized trials of these options. This has contributed to a lack of consensus about the appropriateness of these procedures in patients with very advanced HF. Further, cardiac transplantation is limited in number by the donor pool and by recipient age restrictions (generally 65 years of age); the number of these procedures performed in the US has remained stagnant for many years. The use of ventricular assist devices as destination therapy provides an opportunity to salvage those who are not heart transplant candidates (usually because of age). However, like transplant, the number of viable candidates is small as it is unlikely that many septuagenarians or octogenarians are candidates or select themselves for the surgery. Miniaturization of the devices and simplification of both the surgery itself and long-term management could potentially expand the population.

In summary, many aggressive approaches are not widely applicable to the HF population, despite the attention they engender in the medical literature and lay press [14]. However, even if selected, components of a palliative care model still apply given the significant morbidity associated with these procedures and the ongoing risk of mortality.

ASSESSING PATIENT PREFERENCES

It is important to recognize that for any given NYHA class or performance on a 6-minute walk test, older HF patients maintain a greater quality-of-life than younger patients [15], likely reflecting a more modest discrepancy between actual and desired health and functioning. The incorporation of quality-of-life measurement and a 'patient centered family focused' structure [9] are vital and can frame the approach to care for patients with advanced HF. Advance care planning can be facilitated by discussions of the patient's goals, the health states the patient finds undesirable and the outcomes that are likely in the event of an intervention. Cultural and individual differences among patients (and their families) do exist but involvement in decision-making and honest appraisal of the clinical course are usually sought. Unfortunately, a significant percentage of patients may not receive care that is consistent with their preferences [16]. Management of symptoms including pain and dyspnea and attention to quality-of-life are a major need [17] and should be the predominant focus of care when life-extending approaches are limited or no longer available.

GUIDELINES

The American College of Cardiology/American Heart Association (ACC/AHA) guidelines for the management of chronic HF emphasize the need to discuss end-of-life options with stage D patients [18]. The major class I indications (conditions for which there is evidence and/or general agreement that a given procedure or treatment is beneficial, useful, and effective) revolve around the need for patient and family education about prognosis, advance directives and palliative/hospice care. For hospice care, opiates, intravenous inotropes and diuretics are suggested options.

Perhaps equally important are the class III indications (conditions for which there is evidence and/or general agreement that a procedure/treatment is not useful/effective and in some cases may be harmful): partial left ventriculectomy (the 'Batista procedure') and empiric routine intermittent inotropic therapy for patients with refractory end-stage symptoms.

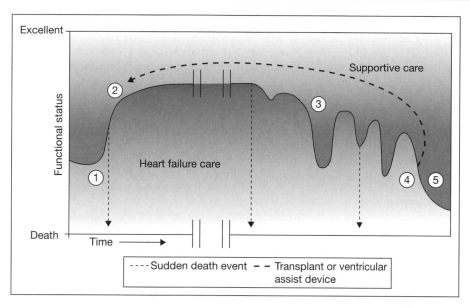

Figure 16.2 Schematic course of stages C and D HF. Sudden death may occur at any point along the course of illness. (1) Initial symptoms of HF can develop and HF treatment is initiated. (2) Plateaus of variable length may be reached with initial medical management or after mechanical support or heart transplant. (3) Functional status declines with variable slope, with intermittent exacerbations of HF that respond to rescue efforts. (4) Stage D HF, with refractory symptoms and limited function. (5) End of life. Adapted with permission from [9].

Further, intubation and implantation of a defibrillator are proscribed for NYHA class IV patients for whom clinical improvements are not anticipated. Dissemination of information about implantable cardioverter-defibrillator (ICD) deactivation is supported but the timing and best mode of communication has not been established. With thousands of devices implanted each year in patients with HF, clinical trial data suggesting an increase in progressive HF death in this population and impact of device discharge at the time of death [19], the magnitude of the problem of ICD deactivation is only now being recognized.

HOSPICE

Referral to hospice is a viable option for patients who have failed conventional therapy and are not candidates for or have refused advanced therapeutic and experimental approaches [9]. These patients may experience pain, fatigue and depression with a severity similar to end-stage cancer patients; in addition, the trajectory of the declines in functional status may be similar between the groups. Indeed, as many as 78% of advanced HF patients experience pain in the final weeks of life, a percentage comparable to those dying of lung or colon cancer [20]. Cardiac cachexia, defined as non-intentional, non-edema weight loss of 7.5% of previous normal weight over 6 months [21] is present in 16% of patients with advanced HF and is associated with a 50% mortality at 18 months [22]. Depression has been reported in over one-third and is correlated with risk of both hospitalization and mortality, although it is frequently unrecognized as a prominent symptom [23, 24]. Finally, 63% of advanced HF patients experience severe dyspnea in the last 3 days of life [25].

Despite these similarities with oncologic disease, advanced HF patients can experience a course of gradual decline that is interrupted by both recurrent exacerbation and partial recovery of function (Figure 16.2). In addition, a proportion of deaths will be sudden and unexpected, although when the patient has NYHA class IV symptoms, the categorization of 'sudden' should probably be seen as a misattribution.

The largest collection of patients referred to hospice has been evaluated from the Acute Decompensated Heart Failure National Registry (ADHERE) [26]. The data suggest that hospitals in the upper quartile of compliance with standard Joint Commission on Accreditation of Healthcare Organizations (JCAHO) indicators for HF also refer to hospice, alleviating concern that this subset of patients is undertreated. Further, preliminary analyses suggest that these patients can be identified early during the terminal hospitalization, allowing for timely risk stratification. However, no information can be derived from this or any other registry that addresses the therapeutic challenges implicit in the care of patients with advanced symptoms.

TREATMENT APPROACHES

Dyspnea is perhaps the most widely discussed and feared symptom at the end of life, although data suggest that significant percentages of patients experience metabolic death (e.g. renal or liver failure) rather than a 'drowning' with refractory pulmonary edema [27]. Multiple strategies are available: intravenous loop diuretics supplemented with oral thiazide diuretics, morphine sulfate, thoracentesis, and paracentesis. In general, HF specialists continue the use of angiotensin-converting enzyme inhibitors (with or without the addition of other vasodilators) and diuretics. To the extent feasible, adherence to a non-conventional and partly non-pharmacologic plan of care is also important. Options include continued sodium restriction, opiods for ongoing symptomatic dyspnea or pain, oxygen supplementation or continuous positive airway pressure (CPAP) for sleep disordered breathing, psychostimulants for palliation of fatigue and antidepressants. Most of these are not rated in the ACC/AHA guidelines nor have been subjected to rigorous study; this leaves providers to practice according to experience and local standards, which may not be enough to guarantee quality or uniformity of care.

The role of intravenous inotropic therapy remains controversial [28–30]. According to the ACC/AHA guidelines, continuous infusion of intravenous inotropes was accorded a class IIb rating (usefulness/efficacy is less well-established by evidence/opinion). This therapy may be appropriate for palliation, especially if a weaning trial has been attempted. Recurrence of the stigmata of a low-cardiac output state including hypoperfusion characterized by worsening renal function, inanition and deteriorating mental status may indicate the need for chronic infusions. Medicare coverage for inotropic therapy requires an increase in cardiac output or decrease in pulmonary capillary wedge pressure by 20% documented by pulmonary artery catheterization. Given the possibility of precipitating atrial and ventricular arrhythmias and ongoing controversy about increased mortality with use of these agents, a detailed discussion with the patient and family are necessary.

BARRIERS TO PALLIATIVE AND HOSPICE CARE

A prominent barrier to the adoption of a palliative care paradigm for HF is the belief among many providers that active care discontinues when palliative care starts. The concept of early-stage palliative care intervention, despite its potential to improve communication, address issues surrounding the possibility of sudden death, and identify patient and family goals and needs, may be particularly foreign to cardiologists, who have an acute care perspective. Further, there is legitimate concern that patients may not be offered the full spectrum of therapeutic options if palliative care is selected.

The employment of a palliative care paradigm has the additional problem of flagging reimbursement. Although there is increased interest in disease management approaches for chronic diseases on the part of the Centers for Medicare and Medicaid Services [31], there has been little to no progress in improving reimbursement for palliative care. These patients require focused care that can be facilitated by specially trained nurses. The multidisciplinary team approach has been most extensively studied; however, how such endeavors are funded remains unclear. In addition, the tasks associated with supportive care are time-consuming and cognitive. There are no procedure codes for participation in discussions with the patient and family about advance care planning or administration of serial quality-of-life assessments. One extreme example of the reimbursement problem is highlighted by the fact that while some patients obtain symptomatic relief from the initiation of intravenous inotropic therapy, hospice may not permit the therapy due to cost considerations [32].

There may also be misconceptions among providers about the way in which HF patients die. Preliminary data from a national survey suggest that physicians see parallels with chronic obstructive lung disease [33]; pain was infrequently perceived as a problem even though patient surveys suggest otherwise [20, 25]. It is highly likely that physician perception of the mode of death influences the selection of treatment options; this idea requires further investigation prior to implementation of an intervention designed to influence processes of care.

Data from research on hospice also suggest that there is a lack of coordinated approaches and significant knowledge gaps. In a recent survey, a minority of hospice medical directors described care plans that specifically apply to patients with terminal HF and few had formal training in HF management [34].

There is also implicit difficulty in assessing trajectory and predicting mortality within a 6-month period. The clinical variability of patients with advanced HF is significant in a brief time-frame such as 6 weeks [35]; this 'waxing and waning' of symptoms suggests that some patients may improve in a trajectory that has many dips and plateaus. The uncertainty about timing of referral can be best approached by the development of specific risk assessment tools that can provide both the patient and provider with a clearly delineated roadmap for the future.

FUTURE DIRECTIONS

Multiple areas of investigation are available to clinicians and researchers who have an interest in the palliative care paradigm. Many have been previously outlined [9]; they include explicit quantification of patient health status through the final stages of HF; analysis of the epidemiology of advanced HF symptoms and comorbid conditions; and evaluation of the costs of interventions and financial burdens associated with end-of-life care. Indeed, advocacy for a reimbursement system that recognizes the complexities of care of patients with chronic heart disease will become increasingly necessary. A solution to particularly vexing problems encountered by providers during the terminal management of HF will meaningfully impact care.

Greater insight into disease-specific therapies for the relief of dyspnea, pain and fatigue on both acute and chronic bases is clearly required. Further, the impact of various treatments and disease management strategies has not been evaluated for HF in its terminal phases. Educational models that will assist providers in ICD management need to be developed; specifically, the 'when' and 'how' of deactivation. The development and definition of quality indicators for care delivered during the terminal phases of HF would be helpful.

CONCLUSIONS

Despite the inclusion of end-of-life considerations in the ACC/AHA guidelines [18], the publication of a consensus statement on palliative and supportive care in HF [9] and the recognition that the epidemiology of the disease favors continued increases in prevalence, we are only now beginning to establish the foundations for well-designed studies that will assist providers in the care of advanced HF patients. Despite the advances in HF care, the disease is, for most patients, chronic and eventually progresses to death. Two seemingly opposing trends have come into play. There are a greater number of technically complicated options available; at the same time, we are increasingly recognizing our obligation to provide less proscriptive care that focuses on patient preferences and the impact of both the disease itself and those very options on quality-of-life. Attention to the palliative care paradigm can allow these trends to become better aligned, to the benefit of patients and patients' families.

REFERENCES

1. Gillum RF. Epidemiology of heart failure in the United States. *Am Heart J* 1993; 126:1042–1047.
2. Haldeman GA, Croft JB, Giles WH, Rashidee A. Hospitalization of patients with heart failure: National Hospital Discharge Survey, 1985 to 1995. *Am Heart J* 1999; 137:352–360.
3. Masoudi FA, Havranek EP, Krumholz HM. The burden of chronic congestive heart failure in older persons: magnitude and implications for policy and research. *Heart Fail Rev* 2002; 7:9–16.
4. Hauptman PJ, Havranek E. Integrating palliative care into heart failure care. *Arch Int Med* 2005; 165:374–378.
5. Brown DW, Haldeman GA, Croft JB, Giles WH, Mensah GA. Racial or ethnic differences in hospitalization for heart failure among elderly adults: Medicare, 1990 to 2000. *Am Heart J* 2005; 150:448–458.
6. Baker DW, Einstadter D, Thomas C, Cebul RD. Mortality trends for 23,505 Medicare patients hospitalized with heart failure in Northeast Ohio, 1991–1997. *Am Heart J* 2003; 146:258–264.
7. American Heart Association. Heart Disease and Stroke Statistics: 2007 Update. *Circulation* 2007; 115:e69–e171.
8. Goff DC Jr, Pandey DK, Chan FA, Ortiz C, Nichaman MZ. Congestive heart failure in the United States. Is there more than meets the I (CD Code)? The Corpus Christi Heart Project. *Arch Int Med* 2000; 160:197–202.
9. Goodlin SJ, Hauptman PJ, Arnold R et al. Consensus statement: palliative and supportive care in advanced heart failure. *J Card Fail* 2004; 10:200–209.
10. Vinson JM, Rich MW, Sperry JC, Shah AS, McNamara T. Early readmission of elderly patients with congestive heart failure. *J Am Soc Ger* 1990; 38:1290–1295.
11. Heiat A, Gross CP, Krumholz HM. Representation of the elderly, women and minorities in heart failure clinical trials. *Arch Int Med* 2002; 162:1682–1688.
12. Bardy GH. Amiodarone or implantable cardioverter defibrillator for congestive heart failure. *N Engl J Med* 2005; 352:225–237.
13. Moss AJ, Zareba W, Hall WJ et al. Prophylactic implantation of a defibrillator in patients with myocardial infarction and reduced ejection fraction. *N Engl J Med* 2002; 346:877–883.
14. Winslow R. The price of a broken heart. *Wall St J* 2005 (Nov 5/6), p A1.
15. Masoudi FA, Rumsfeld JS, Havranek EP et al. Age, functional capacity and health related quality of life in patients with heart failure. *J Card Fail* 2004; 10:368–373.
16. Teno JM, Fisher ES, Hamel MB, Coppola K, Dawson NV. Medical care inconsistent with patients' treatment goals: association with 1-year Medicare resource use and survival. *J Am Geriatr Soc* 2002; 50:496–500.
17. Walden JA, Dracup K, Westlake C, Erickson V, Hamilton MA, Fonarow GC. Educational needs of patients with advanced heart failure and their caregivers. *J Heart Lung Transplant* 2001; 20:766–769.
18. Hunt SA, Abraham WT, Chin MH et al. ACC/AHA 2005 guideline update for the diagnosis and management of chronic heart failure in the adult: a report of the American College of Cardiology/ American Heart Association Task Force on Practice Guidelines (Writing Committee to Update the 2001 Guidelines for the Evaluation and Management of HF). *Circulation* 2005; 112:e154–e235.
19. Goldstein NE, Lampert R, Bradley E, Lynn J, Krumholz HM. Management of implantable cardioverter defibrillators in end-of-life care. *Ann Int Med* 2004; 141:835–838.
20. McCarthy M, Lay M, Addington-Hall J. Dying from heart disease. *J R Coll Physicians Lond* 1996; 30:325–328.
21. Anker SD, Chua TP, Ponikowski P et al. Hormonal changes and catabolic/anabolic imbalance in chronic heart failure and their importance for cardiac cachexia. *Circulation* 1997; 96:526–534.
22. Pantilat SZ, Steimle AE. Palliative care for patients with heart failure. *JAMA* 2004; 291:2476–2482.

23. Gibbs JSR, McCoy ASM, Gibbs LME, Rogers AE, Addington-Hall JM. Living with and dying from heart failure: the role of palliative care. *Heart* 2002; 88:ii36–ii39.
24. Jiang W, Alexander J, Christopher E *et al*. Relationship of depression to increased risk of mortality and rehospitalization in patients with congestive heart failure. *Arch Intern Med* 2001; 161:1849–1856.
25. Levenson JW, McCarthy EP, Lynn J, Davis RB, Phillips RS. The last six months of life for patients with congestive heart failure. *J Am Geriatr Soc* 2000; 48:S101–S109.
26. Hauptman PJ, Goodlin SJ, Lopatin R, Costanzo MR, Fonarow GC, Yancy CW. Characteristics of patients hospitalized with acute decompensated heart failure who are referred for hospice care. *Arch Int Med* 2007 (in press).
27. Derfler MC, Jacob M, Wolf RE, Bleyer F, Hauptman PJ. Mode of death from congestive heart failure : implications for clinical management. *Am J Ger Cardiol* 2004; 13:299–306.
28. Ewy GA. Inotropic infusions for chronic congestive heart failure: medical miracles or misguided medicinals? *J Am Coll Cardiol* 1999; 33:572–575.
29. Bayram M, De Luca L, Massie BM, Gheorghiade M. Reassessment of dobutamine, dopamine and milrinone in the management of acute heart failure syndromes. *Am J Cardiol* 2005; 96(suppl):47G–58G.
30. Hershberger RE, Nauman D, Walker TL, Dutton D, Burgess D. Care processes and clinical outcomes of continuous outpatient support with inotropes (COSI) in patients with refractory end stage heart failure. *J Card Fail* 2003; 9:188–191.
31. Hauptman PJ, Bednarek H. The business concept of leader pricing as applied to heart failure disease management. *J Dis Manag* 2004; 7:226–234.
32. Rich MW, Shore BL. Dobutamine for patients with end-stage heart failure in a hospice program. *J Palliat Med* 2003; 6:93–97.
33. Hauptman PJ, Burroughs TE, Swindle J, Jans M, Biener L. Physician attitudes and beliefs regarding the care of patients with end-stage heart failure: insights from a national pilot study. *J Card Fail* 2005; 11:S169.
34. Kutner J, Goodlin SJ, Connor SR, Ryndes T, Houser J, Hauptman PJ. Hospice care for heart failure patients. *J Pain Symptom Manage* 2005; 29:525–528.
35. Hauptman PJ, Masoudi F, Weintraub W, Pina I, Jones P, Spertus J. Variability in the clinical status of patients with advanced heart failure. *J Card Fail* 2004; 10:397–402.

Postscript

As with any project that necessarily is longitudinal in nature, new discoveries and certain new perspectives emerge that merit comment and may either add or modify the information already presented.

Aliskiren is a first in class direct renin inhibitor. It appears to be an effective antihypertensive when use as monotherapy and may have its greatest utility when added to other agents, especially diuretics and other renin-angiotensin-aldosterone antagonists. Heart failure specific data using aliskiren are just beginning to emerge from the Aliskiren Observations of Heart Failure Treatment (ALOFT) trial. Important questions have recently emerged regarding the cardiovascular risk profile of thiazolidinedione (TZD) compounds, e.g. rosiglitazone and pioglitazone. No data are yet definitive but enhanced drug use warnings have been posted and more study is needed.

Regarding emerging and/or new therapies, several recent trials have been released: Follow-up Serial Infusions of Nesiritide (FUSION) II, Efficacy of Vasopressin Antagonism in Heart Failure Study with Tolvaptan (EVEREST) and the HeartMate® II, Pivotal Trial. FUSION II tested the potential benefit of nesiritide as adjunctive outpatient therapy for patients with advanced heart failure. There was no evidence of benefit in the setting of appropriate background therapy. The prevailing concerns regarding the use of nesiritide of nephrotoxicity and increased mortality were not however seen. The Acute Study of Clinical Effectiveness of Nesiritide in Decompensated Heart Failure (ASCEND-HF) trial has been initiated and will hopefully resolve many of the remaining questions regarding the use of nesiritide. EVEREST tested the benefit of tolvatpan, an oral arginine vasopressin receptor antagonist. The study demonstrated a modest benefit on dyspnea early in the course of hospitalization for decompensated heart failure and sustained weight loss but no long-term evidence of a reduction in the risk of death or recurrent hospitalization. There was no evidence of risk associated with tolvaptan. HeartMate® II is a smaller left ventricular assist device as described in chapter 15. The Pivotal Trial data now confirm its benefit as an effective bridge to heart transplantation with over 75% of candidates surviving long enough to undergo heart transplantation.

Two heart failure related registries have begun to generate important manuscripts and data outputs: Organized Program to Initiate Lifesaving Treatment in Hospitalized Patients with Heart Failure (OPTIMIZE-HF) and Registry to Improve the Use of Evidence-Based Heart Failure Therapies in the Outpatient Setting (IMPROVE-HF). The OPTIMIZE-HF data directly address quality of care issues in the inpatient setting with short-term follow-up at 60–90 days in 10% of the enrolled patient population. This registry has added important new perspectives to the importance of blood pressure, serum sodium assessments, the

Clyde W. Yancy, MD, FACC, FAHA, FACP, Medical Director and Chief, Cardiothoracic Transplantation, Baylor Heart and Vascular Institute, Baylor University Medical Center, Dallas, Texas, USA

James B. Young, MD, FACC, FAHA, FACP, Vice Chairman, Cardiovascular Medicine, The Cleveland Clinic, Cleveland, Ohio, USA

benefit of performance measures and the measurement of ejection fractions in patients admitted with decompensated heart failure. IMPROVE-HF addresses the quality of care in the outpatient setting – an area not previously investigated, and is just beginning to identify current practice in the outpatient care of patients with heart failure.

Clearly, heart failure is a dynamic disease process with new trials underway and new discoveries ongoing. Yet, we believe the information presented in this book represents a useable and clinically appropriate template that allows for the easy incorporation of new data and best application of appropriate therapy for patients with heart failure.

FURTHER READING

1. Oparil S, Yarows SA, Patel S, Fang H, Zhang J, Satlin A. Efficacy and safety of combined use of aliskiren and valsartan in patients with hypertension: a randomised, double-blind trial. *Lancet* 2007; 370:221–9

2. Nissen SE, Wolski K. Effect of rosiglitazone on the risk of myocardial infarction and death from cardiovascular causes. *N Engl J Med* 2007; 356:2457–2471. Epub 2007 May 21.

3. Yancy CW, Krum H, Massie BM *et al*. The Second Follow-up Serial Infusions of Nesiritide (FUSION II) trial for advanced heart failure: study rationale and design. *Am Heart J* 2007; 153:478–484.

4. Gheorghiade M, Konstam MA, Burnett JC Jr *et al*. Efficacy of Vasopressin Antagonism in Heart Failure Outcome Study With Tolvaptan (EVEREST) Investigators. Short-term clinical effects of tolvaptan, an oral vasopressin antagonist, in patients hospitalized for heart failure: the EVEREST Clinical Status Trials. *JAMA* 2007; 297:1332–1343. Epub 2007 Mar 25.

5. Konstam MA, Gheorghiade M, Burnett JC Jr *et al*. Efficacy of Vasopressin Antagonism in Heart Failure Outcome Study With Tolvaptan (EVEREST) Investigators. Effects of oral tolvaptan in patients hospitalized for worsening heart failure: the EVEREST Outcome Trial. *JAMA* 2007; 297:1319–1331. Epub 2007 Mar 25.

6. Fonarow GC, Stough WG, Abraham WT *et al*. OPTIMIZE-HF Investigators and Hospitals. Characteristics, treatments, and outcomes of patients with preserved systolic function hospitalized for heart failure: a report from the OPTIMIZE-HF Registry. *J Am Coll Cardiol* 2007; 50:768–777. Epub 2007 Aug 6.

7. Fonarow GC, Yancy CW, Albert NM *et al*. Improving the use of evidence-based heart failure therapies in the outpatient setting: the IMPROVE HF performance improvement registry. *Am Heart J* 2007; 154:12–38.

8. Miller LW, Pagani FD, Russell SD *et al*. HeartMate II Clinical Investigators. Use of a continuous-flow device in patients awaiting heart transplantation. *N Engl J Med* 2007; 357:885–896.

List of Abbreviations

AASK	African-American Study of Kidney Disease and Hypertension
ABCD	Appropriate Blood Pressure Control in Diabetes
ACC	American College of Cardiology
ACCOMPLISH	Avoiding Cardiovascular Events through Combination Therapy in Patients Living with Systolic Hypertension
ACE-I	angiotensin-converting enzyme inhibitor
ACTION	A Controlled Trial Investigating Outcomes of Exercise Training
ACTIV in CHF	Acute and Chronic Therapeutic Impact of a Vasopressin Antagonist in Congestive Heart Failure
ADH	antidiuretic hormone
ADAM	disintegrin and metalloproteinase
ADHERE	Acute Decompensated Heart Failure National Registry
AHA	American Heart Association
A-HeFT	African-American Heart Failure Trial
AIRE	Acute Infarction Ramipril Efficacy
ALLHAT	Anti-hypertensive and Lipid-Lowering Treatment to Prevent Heart Attack Trial
ALOFT	Aliskiren Observations of Heart Failure Treatment
AMP	adenosine monophosphate
ANBP	Australian National Blood Pressure
AQ-2	aquaporin 2
ARB	angiotensin receptor blocker
ASD	atrial septal defect
ASCEND-HF	Acute Study of Clinical Effectiveness of Nesiritide in Decompensated Heart Failure
ASCOT	Anglo-Scandinavian Cardiac Outcomes Trial
ATLAS	Assessment of Treatment with Lisinopril and Survival
ATP	adenosine triphosphate
ATP III	Adult Treatment Panel III
ATPase	adenosine triphosphatase
AV	atrioventricular
AVP	arginine vasopressin
BB	beta-blockade
BEST	Beta-blocker Evaluation of Survival Trial
BHAT	Beta-blocker Heart Attack Trial
BID	twice a day
BNP	brain natriuretic peptide/B-type natriuretic peptide *(check context)*
BP	blood pressure
BSA	body surface area
BTT	bridge to transplantation
BUN	blood urea nitrogen

CABG	coronary artery bypass graft
cAMP	cyclic adenosine monophosphate
CAPPP	Captopril Prevention Project
CARE-HF	Cardiac Resynchronization in Heart Failure study
CCB	calcium channel blocker
CHAMP	Cardiac Hospitalization Atherosclerosis Management Program
CHARM	Candesartan in Heart failure: Assessment of Reduction in Mortality and Morbidity
CHD	coronary heart disease
CHF	congestive/chronic heart failure *(check context)*
CI	confidence interval/cardiac index *(check context)*
CIBIS	Cardiac Insufficiency Bisopropol Study
CO	cardiac output
CoA	coenzyme A
COMET	Carvedilol versus Metoprolol European Trial
CONSENSUS	Cooperative North Scandinavian Enalapril Survival Study
CONVINCE	Controlled Onset Verapamil Investigation of Cardiovascular Endpoints
COPERNICUS	Carvedilol Prospective Randomized Cumulative Survival
CPAP	continuous positive airway pressure
CPB	cardiopulmonary bypass
CPT-1	carnitine palmitoyltransferase-1
Cr	creatinine
CRT	cardiac resynchronization therapy
CV	cardiovascular
CVA	cardiovascular accident
CVD	cardiovascular disease
CVP	central venous pressure
CXR	chest X-ray
DASH	Dietary Approaches to Stop Hypertension
DIG	Digitalis Investigation Group
DT	destination therapy
ECM	extracellular matrix
ED	Emergency Department
EDV	end-diastolic volume
EF	ejection fraction
eGFR	estimated glomerular filtration rate
ELITE	Evaluation of Losartan in the Elderly
EP	electrophysiologic
EPHESUS	Eplerenone Post-Acute Myocardial Infarction Heart Failure Efficacy and Survival Study
EPO	erythropoietin
ERK	extracellular signal-regulated kinase
ESV	end-systolic volume
EUROPA	European Trial on Reduction of Cardiac Events with Perindopril in Stable Coronary Artery Disease
EVEREST	Efficacy of Vasopressin Antagonism in Heart Failure Study with Tolvaptan
EWPHE	European Working Party on Hypertension in the Elderly
FACET	Flosequinan-ACE Inhibitor Trial
FDA	Food and Drug Administration
FUSION	Follow-up Serial Infusion of Nesiritide

GEMINI	Trial comparing the glycemic effects of carvedilol and metoprolol in hypertensive patients with diabetes
GFR	glomerular filtration rate
GLP-1	glucagon-like peptide-1
GLUT	glucose transporter
GWTG	Get With the Guidelines
HAAWG	Hypertension in African-Americans Working Guidelines
HAPPHY	Heart Attack Primary Prevention in Hypertension
Hb	hemoglobin
HCM	hypertrophic cardiomyopathy
Hct	hematocrit
HDFP	Hypertension Detection and Follow-up Program
HDL	high-density lipoprotein
HF	heart failure
HFSA	Heart Failure Society of America
Hippocrates	an ongoing study on cardiovascular risk and genetics in a general practice in Kerkrade, the Netherlands
HIT	heparin-induced thrombocytopenia
HOPE	Heart Outcomes Prevention Evaluation
HOT	Hypertension Optimal Treatment
IABP	intra-aortic balloon pump
ICD	implantable cardioverter-defibrillator
ICU	intensive care unit
IDNT	Irbesartan Diabetic Nephropathy Trial
IMGU	insulin-mediated glucose uptake
INSIGHT	International Nifedipine GITS Study: Intervention as a Goal in Hypertension Treatment
INTrEPID	Investigation of Non-Transplant Eligible patients who are Inotrope Dependent
INVEST	International Verapamil SR/Trandolapril Study
I-PRESERVE	Irbesartan in Heart Failure with Preserved Systolic Function
IRS-1	insulin receptor substrate-1
ISDN-HYD	isosorbide dinitrate and hydralazine
IV	intravenous
IVAD	implantable ventricular assist device
JCAHO	Joint Commission on Accreditation of Healthcare Organizations
JNC7	Seventh Report of the Joint National Committee on the Prevention, Detection, Evaluation and Treatment of High Blood Presure
LAP	left atrial pressure
LDL	low-density lipoprotein
LOS	length of stay
LV	left ventricle/ventricular
LVAD	left ventricular assist device
LVF	left ventricular function
LVEF	left ventricular ejection fraction
LVH	left ventricular hypertrophy
LVSD	left ventricular systolic dysfunction
MADIT-II	Multicenter Automatic Defibrillator Implantation Trial II
MAP	mean arterial pressure
MAPHY	Metoprolol Atherosclerosis Prevention in Hypotensives
MAPK	mitogen-activated protein kinase
MARVAL	Microalbuminuria Reduction with Valsartan

MCS	mechanical circulatory support
MERIT-HF	The Metropolol CR/XL Randomized Intervention Trial in Congestive Heart Failure
METEOR	Multicenter Evaluation of Tolvaptan Effect on Remodeling
MI	myocardial infarction
MIRACLE	Multicenter InSync Randomized Clinical Evaluation
MMP	matrix metalloproteinase
MMPI	matrix metalloproteinase inhibitor
mPAP	mean pulmonary artery pressure
MR	mitral regurgitation
MRNA	messenger ribonucleic acid
MT-MMPs	membrane-type matrix metalloproteinases
MWD	minute walking distance
NADPH	nicotinamide dinucleotide phosphate
Na^+-K^+	sodium-potassium
NAPA	Nesiritide Administered Peri-Anesthesia in Patients Undergoing Cardiac Surgery
NCEP	National Cholesterol Education Program
NEFA	non-esterified fatty acids
NHLBI	National Heart, Lung and Blood Institute
NICOLE	Nisoldipine in Coronary Artery Disease in Leuven
NICS-EH	National Intervention Cooperative Study in Elderly Hypertensives
NO	nitric oxide
NORDIL	Nordic Diltiazem
NOS	nitric oxide synthase
NSAID	non-steroidal anti-inflammatory drug
NSR	normal sinus rhythm
NTG	nitroglycerin
NYHA	New York Heart Association
OMM	optimal medical management
ONTARGET	Ongoing Telmisartan Alone and in Combination with Ramipril Global Endpoint Trial
OPTIMIZE-HF	Organized Program to Initiate Lifesaving Treatment in Hospitalized Patients with Heart Failure
PA	pulmonary artery
$PaCO_s$	partial pressure of carbon dioxide in the arterial blood
PAI-1	plasminogen activator inhibitor-1
PaO_s	partial pressure of carbon dioxide in the arterial blood
PCWP	pulmonary capillary wedge pressure
PDK	pyruvate dehydrogenase kinase
PEACE	Prevention of Events with Angiotensin Converting Enzyme Inhibition
PEEP	positive end-expiratory pressure (ventilation)
PFO	patent foramen ovale
PI-3	phosphatidylinositol 3-kinase
PMT	patient management tool
PPARγ	peroxisome proliferative activated receptor γ
PRA	preformed reactive antibody
PRAISE	Prospective Randomized Amlodipine Survival Evaluation
PREAMI	Perindopril and Remodeling in Elderly with Acute Myocardial Infarction
PRECEDENT	Prospective Randomized Evaluation of Cardiac Ectopy with Dobutamide or Natrecor Therapy

PREMIER	Prevention of MI Early Remodeling trial
PREVENT	Prevention of Recurrent Venous Thromboembolism
PROACTION	Prospective Randomized Outcomes study of Acutely Decompensated CHF treated Initially as Outpatients with Nesiritide
PROGRESS	Perindopril Protection against Recurrent Stroke Study
PROMISE	Prospective Randomized Milrinone Survival Evaluation
PROVED	Prospective Randomized Study of Ventricular Failure and the Efficacy of Digoxin
PTVA	Percuataneous Transseptal Ventricular Assist
PVR	peripheral vascular resistance
QD	every day
QOL	quality of life
QUIET	Quinapril Ischemic Event Trial
RAAS	renin–angiotensin–aldosterone system
RADIANCE	Randomized Assessment of Digoxin and Inhibitors of Angiotensin-Converting Enzyme
RALES	Randomized Aldactone Evaluation Study
RAP	right atrial pressure
RAS	renin–angiotensin system
RBF	renal blood flow
RCM	restrictive cardiomyopathy
RELIANT	Randomized Evaluation of the Novacor LVAS in a Non-Transplant Population
REMATCH	Randomized Evaluation of Mechanical Assistance for the Treatment of Congestive Heart Failure
RENAAL	Reduction of Endpoints in NIDDM with the Angiotensin II Antagonist Losartan
RESOLVD	Randomized Evaluation of Strategies for Left Ventricular Dysfunction
RHuEPO	recombinant human erythropoietin
RR	relative risk
RRR	relative risk reduction
RV	right ventricle/ventricular
SAP	systemic arterial pressure
SAVE	Survival and Ventricular Enlargement
SBP	systolic blood pressure
SC	subcutaneous
SCAT	Simvastatin/Enalapril Coronary Atherosclerosis Trial
SCD	sudden cardiac death
SCD-HeFT	Sudden Cardiac Death in Heart Failure Trial
SCOPE	Study on Cognition and Prognosis in the Elderly
SCr	serum creatinine
SENIORS	A Study of the Effects of Nebivolol Intervention on Outcomes and Rehospitalization in Seniors with heart failure
SHEP	Systolic Hypertension in the Elderly Program
SGC	soluble guanylate cyclase
SHOCK	SHould we emergently revascularize Occluded coronaries in Cardiogenic shocK?
SIADH	syndrome of inappropriate antidiuretic hormone
SNS	sympathetic nervous system
SOLVD	Study of Left Ventricular Dysfunction
SPAN-CHF	Specialized Primary and Networked Care in HF

STAMINA-HeFT	Studies of Anemia in Heart Failure Trial
STOP	Swedish Trial in Old Patients with Hypertension
SVR	systemic vascular resistance
TAH	total artificial heart
TCA	tricarboxylic acid
TEE	transesophageal echocardiography
TET	transcutaneous energy transmission
THAM	tromethamine; tris(hydroxymethyl)-aminomethane
TID	three times a day
TIMPs	tissue inhibitors of MMPs
TNF	tumor necrosis factor
TOHMS	Treatment of Mild Hypertension Study
TR	tricuspid regurgitation
TRACE	Trandolapril Cardiac Evaluation
TROPHY	Trial of Preventing Hypertension
TZDs	thiazolidinediones
UKPDS	UK Prospective Diabetes Study
VAD	ventricular assist device
V-HeFT	Vasodilator Heart Failure Trial
VAL-HeFT	Valsartan Heart Failure Trial
VALIANT	Valsartan in Acute Myocardial Infarction Trial
VALUE	Valsartan Antihypertensive Long-term Use Evaluation
VHAS	Verapamil Hypertension Atherosclerosis Study
VMAC	Vasoldilation in the Management of Acute CHF
VO_2	rate of oxygen uptake per minute

Index

A-HeFT (African-American Heart Failure
Trial) 53, 85, 100–2, 103
AB 5000 Circulatory Support System
197–9
abdominal obesity 26
AbioCor Implantable Replacement Heart
203–4
ACC/AHA
guidelines for palliative care 216–17
performance measures 173
ACE (angiotensin-converting enzyme)
inhibitors 10, 16, 30, 47, 54, 64, 67, 166,
178, 179
administration to HF patients 50–1
and anemia risk 151
clinical effects 48
clinical trials
combination therapy 11, 61
in heart failure 48–50
in hypertension 5
combination with beta-blockers 76–7
effect after MI 145
ethnic, age and gender considerations 53
in maximization of therapy 214
prevention of sudden cardiac death 180
recommended doses 50
response in African Americans 53, 96
side effects 52
underutilization 51–2
ACE escape 48, 58, 82
acebutolol, clinical trials 7
acidosis, after LVAD implantation 207
ACTIV in CHF trial 125, 126, 134–5
acute decompensated HF 69
digoxin therapy 43
nesiritide therapy (PROACTION) 112,
115–16
tolvaptan (ACTIV in CHF trial) 125
ADAMs (disintegrins and
metalloproteinases) 144

ADHERE (Acute Decompensated Heart
Failure National Registry) 166–7, 170, 218
adrenergic stimulation, role in insulin
resistance 29
adverse reactions see side effects
African-Americans 93, 103, 214
A-HeFT 53, 85, 100–2, 103
ACE inhibitor therapy 53
aldosterone levels 85
data from clinical trials 96–8
etiology of HF 94–5
HAAWG (Hypertension in African-
Americans Working Guidelines) 16
healthcare provision 103
NO bioavailability 100
prevalence of HF 94
relevance of clinical trials 93–4
AHA, GWTG (Get With the Guidelines)
program 170–1
AIRE (Acute Infarction Ramipril Efficacy)
trial 49–50
aldosterone 81
aldosterone antagonists 15, 81, 82, 166, 178,
179, 214
benefits 86
clinical trials 6, 82–3, 84
ethnic differences 85
gender differences 83, 85
guidelines for use 86–8
hyperkalemia 85–6
prevention of sudden cardiac death 180
see also spironolactone
aldosterone escape, ACE inhibitor therapy
48, 58, 82
aldosterone levels, effect of BNP
infusion 106
aliskiren 223
ALLHAT (Anti-hypertensive and Lipid-
Lowering Treatment to Prevent Heart
Attack Trial) 14, 16

ALOFT (Aliskiren Observations of Heart
    Failure Treatment) trial 223
alpha-blockers
    clinical trials 7
    in treatment of hypertension 14
ambulatory BP monitoring 9
amiloride, clinical trials 6, 12
amiodarone, use with digoxin 43
amlodipine, clinical trials 6
    combination therapy 11, 16
anemia 151–2
    management 158
angioedema
    in ACE inhibitor therapy 52, 54
    in angiotensin receptor blocker therapy 64
angiotensin, role in hypertension 4
angiotensin II 58, 180
    role in insulin resistance 29–30
angiotensin receptor blockers (ARBs) 10, 16,
    30, 47, 57, 66–7
    addition to ACE inhibitors 48
    clinical trials 5
        CHARM program 61–4
        combination therapy 11–12, 61
        ELITE II 59–60
        preliminary studies 58–9
        VAL-HEFT 60–1
    effect after MI 145
    in maximization of therapy 214
    pharmacology 57–8
    practical issues 64
    value in prehypertension 4
antidiuretic hormone see arginine vasopressin
aortic stenosis, impact of MMPs 146–7
aortic valve, mechanical prostheses 206
aprotinin dose testing 206
aquaporin 2 (AQP-2) water channels
    129, 131
    effect of lixivaptan 132
Aranesp see darbepoetin α
arginine vasopressin (AVP) 125, 129
    plasma levels 130–1
    role in heart failure 131–3
    vasopressin receptor antagonists 125–9
arrhythmias 177, 179–80
    effect of aldosterone antagonists 86
    management after LVAD implantation
    207
Artificial Heart Program 192, 208
ASCEND-HF (Acute Study of Clinical
    Effectiveness of Nesiritide in
    Decompensated Heart Failure) 120, 223

ASCOT (Anglo-Scandinavian Cardiac
    Outcomes Study) 16, 146
aspirin
    and aldosterone antagonist therapy 82
    combination with ACE inhibitors 51
atenolol
    clinical trials 7
    in combination therapy 12, 16
ATLAS (Assessment of Treatment with
    Lisinopril and Survival) trial 49, 50
atrial fibrillation
    digoxin therapy 43
    effect of RAS blockade 50
    value of device-based monitoring 185
atrial septal defect (ASD) 206
autonomic dysfunction 13
axial flow pumps 204–6

B-type natriuretic peptide (BNP) 105
    physiologic effects 105–6
    role in remodeling 145
    subcutaneous and oral administration 120
    see also nesiritide
baroreceptor dysfunction 13
baroreceptor mechanisms, action of digitalis
    glycosides 39–40, 42
basement membrane 142, 143
Batista procedure 216
benazepril
    clinical trials 5
    in combination therapy 11
bendroflumethazide, clinical trials,
    combination therapy 16
benzapril 48
BEST (Beta blocker Evaluation of Survival
    Trial) 72, 74–5, 94, 96, 97
beta-adrenergic stimulation, role in insulin
    resistance 29
beta-blockers 69, 78, 166, 178
    clinical trials 7, 72
        BEST 74–5
        CIBIS II 74, 75
        CIBIS III 77
        combination therapy 12, 61
        COMET 75–6
        COPERNICUS 73–4
        MERIT-HF 71
        SENIORS 76
        US Carvedilol Trials Program 71, 72
    combination with ACE inhibitors 51, 76–7
    early experience 70–1
    guidelines for use in HF 77, 78

interaction with CRT 181, 182, 183
in maximization of therapy 214
prevention of sudden cardiac death 179,
    180, 184
response in African-Americans 96
in treatment of hypertension 13–14
beta-cell function loss 24
beta-oxidation inhibition 32
betaxolol, clinical trials 7
bisoprolol 14, 75, 179, 214
    clinical trials 7
        CIBIS II 74, 75
        CIBIS III 51, 77
    in combination therapy 12
blood pressure
    effect of AVP 132, 133
    effect of rHuEPO treatment 157
    measurement 9
    relationship to cardiovascular disease
        risk 3
    see also hypertension
bradycardia, in calcium channel blocker
    therapy 13
bradykinin
    effect of ACE inhibitors 48, 58
    effect on insulin sensitivity 30
Braunwald panel recommendations,
    nesiritide 119
bridge to recovery, LVAD therapy 192–3,
    196–99
bridge to transplantation, LVAD therapy 193,
    196, 199–206, 223
bucindolol, BEST 72, 74–5, 96, 97
bumetanide, clinical trials 6
burden of heart failure 165–6
BVS 5000 device 196–7, 198

cachexia 217
calcium channel blockers 16
    clinical trials 6–7
        combination therapy 11
    effect on MMP-9 levels 146
    in treatment of hypertension 13
candesartan
    clinical trials 5
        CHARM 48, 61–4, 65
        RESOLVD 58–9, 65
    in combination therapy 11
    tolerability 64
    use in prehypertension 4, 16
captopril
    clinical trials 5

ELITE 58
    ELITE II 59–60, 65, 66
    in combination therapy 11
    effect on insulin sensitivity 30
    recommended dose 50
Captopril-Digoxin Multicenter Study 40
cardiac output, effect of AVP 132, 133
cardiac resynchronization 166, 174, 177–8,
    179, 181–2
    interactions with medical therapies 182, 183
cardiac steatosis 24
cardiac transplantation 191–2, 214, 216
cardiomyopathy
    insulin resistance as therapeutic target
        32–3
    relationship to insulin resistance 27
cardiopulmonary bypass, effect on MMPs 146
cardiopulmonary bypass machine 191
cardiovascular disease risk
    in metabolic syndrome 26
    relationship to blood pressure 3
CardioWest™ Total Artificial Heart 203
CARE-HF (Cardiac Resynchronization in
    Heart Failure) study 181
carteolol, clinical trials 7
carvedilol 14, 75, 179, 214
    benefits in insulin resistance 29
    clinical trials 7
        COMET 29, 72, 75–6
        COPERNICUS 72, 73–4, 96, 98
        US Carvedilol Trials Program 71, 72,
            96, 98
Centrimag® Blood Pumping System 199
CHAMP (Cardiac Hospitalization
    Atherosclerosis Management Program)
    171
CHARM (Candesartan Cilexitil in Heart
    Failure Assessment of Reduction in
    Mortality and Morbidity) trials 48, 65
    CHARM-Added trial 61–2, 64
    CHARM-Alternative trial 61, 62, 64
    CHARM-Overall program 64
    CHARM-Preserved trial 63–4, 66
chlorthalidone
    clinical trials 6
    in combination therapy 12
chlorthiazide, clinical trials 5
CIBIS (Cardiac Insufficiency Bisoprolol
    Study) II 72, 74, 75
CIBIS (Cardiac Insufficiency Bisoprolol
    Study) III 51, 77
clarithromycin, use with digoxin 43

clinical trials, extrapolation to African-
    Americans 93, 102
clonidine 14–15
    clinical trials 7
coagulopathy screening prior to LVAD
    therapy 195
collagen network, ECM 142, 143
collagenases 143
combination therapy 15–16, 66
    ACE inhibitors and beta-blockers 76–7
    with aldosterone antagonists 82–3
    clinical trials 11–12, 61
COMET (Carvedilol versus Metoprolol
    European Trial) 29, 72, 75–6
Comparative trial, nesiritide 107–8, 109
conivaptan 129
    clinical trials 127–8, 136–7
    properties 134
CONSENSUS (Cooperative North
    Scandinavian Enalapril Study) 47, 48–9, 76
COPERNICUS (Carvedilol Prospective
    Randomized Cumulative Survival) study
    72, 73–4, 96, 98
coronary artery bypass surgery, NAPA trial
    113, 117–18
coronary artery disease, role in etiology of
    HF 94
cough, ACE inhibitor-associated 10, 52
CPAP (continuous positive airway pressure)
    218
CPT-1 inhibitors 32
cyclosporine, use with digoxin 43

darbepoetin α 152
    clinical trials 154–5, 156–7
DASH (Dietary Approaches to Stop
    Hypertension) 16
demographic shift, US 93
depression 217
destination therapy 191, 193, 196
    choice of device 203–6
    eligibility criteria 194
    survival 209
diabetes, type 2 23
    development 24–5
    glycemic control 25
    treatment paradigm shift 31
DIG (Digitalis Investigation Group) trial 40,
    41, 42
digitalis glycosides 39–40
digoxin 39, 44, 214
    clinical trials 40–2

effect of aldosterone antagonists 82
gender differences 42
practical considerations 42–4
dihydropyridine calcium channel blockers 13
dilated cardiomyopathy
    relationship to insulin resistance 27
    role of MMPs 143–4
diltiazem 146
direct vasodilators
    clinical trials 8
    in treatment of hypertension 15
disease course 217, 219
disease management 174
    hospital-based care 167 170–1
    outpatient care 172–3
disintegrins 144
diuretics
    clinical trials 5–6, 11–12
    in combination therapy 11–12, 51
    interaction with cardiac resynchronization
        therapy 182, 183
    in treatment of hypertension 10, 13
dobutamine, comparison with nesiritide
    (PRECEDENT) 108, 110
dosage
    ACE inhibitors 50–1
    aldosterone antagonists 86–7
    digoxin therapy 43
doxazosin, clinical trials 7
dyspnea 217
    management 218

edema
    risk in TDZ therapy 31–2
    as side effect of calcium channel
        blockers 13
Efficacy trial, nesiritide 106–7, 109
elderly patients
    ACE inhibitor therapy 53
    SENIORS trial 76
electrophysiologic remodeling 177
    mechanisms 178–81
ELITE (Evaluation of Losartan in the Elderly)
    study 58
ELITE II 59–60, 65, 66
enalapril
    clinical trials
        CIBIS III 51, 77
        CONSENSUS 76
        in heart failure 48–9, 50
        in hypertension 5
        RESOLVD 58–9

in combination therapy 11
recommended dose 50
endomysial collagen 142
endothelial function, effect of aldosterone antagonists 86
enoximone 42
EPHESUS (Eplerenone Post-Acute Myocardial Infarction Heart Failure Efficacy and Survival Study) 82, 83, 84
epidemiology 165–6, 213
epimysial collagen 142
eplerenone 82, 180
clinical trials 6
EPHESUS 82, 83, 84, 85
eprosartan
clinical trials 5
in combination therapy 11
erythromycin, use with digoxin 43
erythropoetic agents 151, 152
clinical trials 152–7
side effects 157
erythropoetin levels 152
erythropoetin resistance 158
escape, ACE inhibitor therapy 48, 58, 82
esmolol, clinical trials 7
ethacrynic acid, clinical trials 6
ethnic differences
ACE inhibitors 53
aldosterone antagonists 85
see also African-Americans
etiology of HF, ethnic differences 94–5
etomoxir 32
EVEREST (Efficacy of Vasopressin Antagonism in Heart Failure Study with Tolvaptan) 125, 126, 135, 136, 223
exercise capacity, effect of darbepoetin α 157
extracellular matrix (ECM) changes 141, 142

felodipine 146
clinical trials 6
in combination therapy 11
fibronectin 142, 143
fibrosis, effect of spironolactone 145
filling pressure estimation 185
flosequinan 42
fosinopril
clinical trials 5
recommended dose 50
functional iron deficiency 158
furosemide
clinical trials 6

comparison with tolvaptan 134, 135
FUSION (Follow-Up Serial Infusion of Nesiritide) trial 111–12, 114–15
FUSION II 113, 116–17, 118, 120, 223

gelatinases 143
GEMINI trial 29, 30
gender differences
ACE inhibitor therapy 53
aldosterone antagonist therapy 83, 85
digoxin therapy 42
glitazones see thiazolidinediones (TZDs)
glomerular filtration rate, effect of BNP 106, 120
glucagon-like peptide-1 (GLP-1) 32–3
glucotoxicity 25, 33
glycemic control, type 2 diabetes 25
guanabenz, clinical trials 7
guanfacine, clinical trials 7
GWTG (Get With the Guidelines) program, AHA 170–1

HAAWG (Hypertension in African-Americans Working Guidelines) 16
heart failure
physiologic and anatomic changes 141
treatment paradigm shift 31
Heart Failure Core Measures, JCAHO 167, 168–9, 171
heart failure disease management components 172
heart rate, effect of AVP 132, 133
heart rate variability measurement 184–5
HeartMate® Left Ventricular Assist System 193, 200–2
HeartMate® II 205–6
HeartMate® II, Pivotal Trial 223
hemodynamic paradigm 69
hemodynamics, effect of AVP 132, 133
heparin-induced thrombocytopenia (HIT) syndrome 195, 206
hepatic steatosis 24
HIPPOCRATES trial 157
home BP measurement 9
HOPE (Heart Outcomes Prevention Evaluation) trial 47
hospice care, misconceptions 218–19
hospice referral 217–18
hospital stay, variation 167
hospital-based systems 167, 170–1, 174
HOT (Hypertension Optimal Treatment) study 16

hydralazine 15, 166
    benefit in African-Americans 96, 99,
        100–2, 103, 214
    clinical trials 8
hydrochlorothiazide
    clinical trials 6, 12
    in combination therapy 11, 12
hyperaldosteronism 15
hyperkalemia
    during ACE inhibitor therapy 52
    risk in aldosterone antagonist therapy 15,
        82, 82–3, 85–6
hypertension
    assessment of blood pressure 9
    classification 4
    diagnosis 3
    effect of rHuEPO treatment 157
    epidemiology 3–4
    mechanism leading to heart failure 4, 9
    role in etiology of HF 94, 95
    treatment 16
        aldosterone blockade 15
        alpha-blockers 14
        beta blockers 13 14
        centrally-acting drugs 14–15
        calcium channel blockers 13
        combination therapy 15–16
        direct vasodilators 15
        diuretics 10, 13
        RAS blockade 10
        sympathetic nervous system
            blockers 13
    treatment goals 16
    US treatment and control 9
    see also blood pressure
hypertensive urgency/emergency,
    treatment 14
hyponatremia
    effect of conivaptan 129, 137
    effect of lixivaptan 136
    effect of tolvaptan 134
hypotension
    after LVAD implantation 207
    during ACE inhibitor therapy 52

I-PRESERVE (Irbesartan in Heart Failure
    with Preserved Systolic Function)
    trial 63
implantable cardioverter defibrillators (ICDs)
    102, 166, 174, 177–8, 179, 181, 214
    deactivation 217
    medical interactions 182–4

implantable monitoring devices 178
    clinical application 186
    medical management interactions 184–5
IMPROVE-HF 223–4
IMPROVEMENT study 166
indapamide, clinical trials 6
infection prevention, LVAD therapy 196
initiation of therapy
    ACE inhibitors 50–1
    beta-blockers 77, 78
inotropic therapy 216
    intravenous 218
insulin resistance 23–5, 33
    metabolic syndrome 25–6
    role in heart failure 27–8
    role of RAS 29–30
    role of sympathetic nervous system 29
    therapeutic approaches 30–2
    as therapeutic target in cardiomyopathy
        32–3
insulin therapy 25
integrins 144
interactions, with digoxin 43
intracardiac pressure estimations 185
intrathoracic impedance 185, 186
intraventricular conduction delays
    181–2
intrinsic sympathomimetic properties,
    bucindolol 75
irbesartan
    clinical trials 5
        I-PRESERVE 64
    in combination therapy 11
iron deficiency, functional 158
ISDN/HYD (isosorbide dinitrate and
    hydralazine), benefit in African-Americans
    96, 99, 100–2, 103
isosorbide dinitrate benefit in African-
    Americans 96, 99, 100–2, 103
isradipine, clinical trials 6
itraconazole, use with digoxin 43

JCAHO (Joint Commission on Accreditation
    of Healthcare Organizations), Heart
    failure Core Measures 167, 168–9, 171
JNC 7 16

kidney function, effects of BNP 106

labetolol 14
    clinical trials 7
laminin 142, 143

left ventricular assist devices (LVADs) 191,
    209, 214, 216
    contraindications 194–5
    device selection 196–206
    indications for use 192–3
    optimization 208
    patient selection 193–4
    peri-operative management 206
    post-operative management 206–7
    pre-operative patient optimization 195–6
    two year survival 195
left ventricular hypertrophy (LVH) 9
    effect of ACE inhibitors 48
    role of MMPs 143
left ventricular systolic dysfunction 23
Levitronix® Centrimag® Blood Pumping
    System 199
lifestyle modification 16
lipid profile, effect of alpha-blockers 14
lipotoxicity 24, 25, 33
lisinopril
    clinical trials 5
        ATLAS 49, 50
    in combination therapy 11
    recommended dose 50
lixivaptan 125, 129
    clinical trials 126–7, 136
    effect on water balance 132
    properties 134
loop diuretics 214
    clinical trials 6
    in treatment of hypertension 10, 13
losartan 30, 145
    clinical trials 5
        ELITE 58
        ELITE II 59–60, 65, 66
    in combination therapy 11
    effect on bradykinin levels 58

macrovascular complications, type 2 diabetes
    25
MADIT (Multicenter Automatic Defibrillator
    Implantation) II trial 214, 216
malnutrition screening prior to LVAD
    therapy 95–6
matrix metalloproteinase (MMP) inhibitors
    141, 147
matrix metalloproteinases (MMPs) 142–4
    clinical studies 145–7
    pre-clinical studies 145
    transmembrane proteins 144
maximization of therapy 214, 216

mechanical circulatory support (MCS) 191,
    208, 209, 214, 216
    device selection 196–206
    indications 192–3
    percutaneous 196–7
    peri-operative management 206
    post-operative management 206–7
    see also left ventricular assist devices
        (LVADs)
membrane-bound MMPs 144
MERIT-HF (Metoprolol CR/XL Randomized
    Intervention Trial in Congestive Heart
    Failure) 71, 72, 94
metabolic syndrome 23, 24, 25–6, 33
METEOR (Multicenter Evaluation of Tolvaptan
    Effect On Remodeling) study 135
metformin 25, 31
methylclothiazide, clinical trials 6
methyldopa
    clinical trials 7
    in combination therapy 12
metolazone, clinical trials 6
metoprolol 14, 179, 214
    clinical trials 7
        COMET 29, 72, 75–6
        MERIT-HF 71
    in combination therapy 12
microvascular complications, type 2 diabetes
    25
milrinone 42
Milrinone-Digoxin Study 40
minoxidil 15
    clinical trials 8
MIRACLE (Multicenter InSync Randomized
    Clinical Evaluation) trial 181
mitochondrial dysfunction 28
mitral stenosis 206
mitral valve surgery 216
moexipril
    clinical trials 5
    in combination therapy 11
monitoring
    in ACE inhibitor therapy 53, 54
    in aldosterone antagonist therapy 87
monitoring devices, implantable 178
    clinical application 186
    medical management interactions 184–5
mortality
    African-Americans 94, 95, 96
        A-HeFT data 101
    effect of digoxin 42, 43
    effect of nesiritide 119

mortality rates, variation between hospitals
167
mortality reduction, synergy between device
therapies and neurohormonal blockade 178
mortality risk 93
MT1-MMP 143, 144
multidisciplinary management 172–3, 214,
219
ventricular assist device therapy
206, 209
myocardial energy deprivation 27
myocardial insulin resistance 23, 28
as therapeutic target 32–3
myocardium, effect of AVP 132–3

nadolol
clinical trials 7
in combination therapy 12
NAPA (Nesiritide Administered Peri-
Anesthesia in patients undergoing cardiac
surgery) trial 113, 117–18
nebivolol 14
SENIORS trial 76
NEFA (non-esterified fatty acids)
role in insulin resistance 24–5, 33
use by heart 27, 28
nesiritide 120–1, 223
Braunwald panel recommendations 119
Comparative trial 107–8, 109
comparison with dobutamine
(PRECEDENT) 108, 110
effect on mortality 119
Efficacy trial 106–7, 109
Emergency Department use
(PROACTION) 112, 115–16
NAPA trial 113, 117–18
outpatient use
FUSION I 111–12, 114–15
FUSION II 113, 116–17
renal effects 106, 118
VMAC trial 108, 110–11, 114
neurohormonal effects, digitalis glycosides
39–40, 42
neurohormonal paradigm 69–70
nicardipine, clinical trials 6
nifedipine, clinical trials 6
nisoldipine, clinical trials 7
nitric oxide (NO), synthesis and actions
99
nitric oxide (NO) deficiency 93
nitroglycerin, VMAC trial 108, 110–11, 114
nitroso-redox balance 99, 100

nocturia, in calcium channel blocker
therapy 13
non-dihydropyridine calcium channel
blockers 13
non-steroidal anti-inflammatory drugs
(NSAIDs), avoidance 51, 82
norepinephrine, role in remodeling 70
norepinephrine levels, effect of BNP infusion
106
Novacor® LVAS 202–3
nurse-driven multidisciplinary management
172
nutrition prior to LVAD therapy 95–6

obesity 23–4
in metabolic syndrome 26
olmesartan, clinical trials 5
OPC-41061 see tolvaptan
OPTIMIZE-HF (Organized Program to
Initiate Life-Saving Treatments in Patients
Hospitalized with Heart Failure) 167–71,
223
oral administration, BNP 120
osmolality, relationship to AVP levels 131
outpatient disease management programs
172–3, 174
oxfenicine 32
oxidative stress 93, 99–100

palliative care 213–14, 219–20
algorithm for integration into patient care
215
future directions 219
guidelines 216–17
hospice referral 217–18
management of progressive disease 214,
216
misconceptions 218–19
patient preferences 216
paraganglionic tumors 13
patent foramen ovale (PFO) 206
patient preferences 216
patient selection, LVAD therapy 193–4, 209
penbutolol, clinical trials 7
percutaneous mechanical circulatory support
196–7
performance measures, ACC/AHA 173
perhexiline 32
perindopril
clinical trials 5
combination therapy 16
recommended dose 50

perioperative use of nesiritide, NAPA trial
    113, 117–18
peroxynitrite production 99, 100
pheochromocytoma 13
pindolol, clinical trials 7
pioglitazone, effect on MMP-2 levels 146
platelet count, effect of rHuEPO treatment
    157
PMT (Patient Management Tool) 171
polythiazide, clinical trials 6
potassium-sparing diuretics
    clinical trials 6
    in treatment of hypertension 13
pravachol, effect on MMP-2 levels 146
prazosin, clinical trials 7
pre-operative patient optimization, left
    ventricular assist devices 195–6
PRECEDENT (Prospective Randomized
    Evaluation of Cardiac Ectopy with
    Dobutamine or Natreocor Therapy)
    108, 110
prehypertension 3, 4
    treatment 10, 16
PREMIER (Prevention of MI Early
    Remodeling) trial 147
preserved systolic function
    CHARM-Preserved trial 63–4, 66
    use of aldosterone antagonists 86
prevalence of HF, In African-Americans 94
PROACTION (Prospective Randomized
    Outcomes study of Acutely
    decompensated CHF Treated Initially as
    Outpatients with Nesiritide) 112,
    115–16
progressive disease
    disease course 217, 219
    maximization of therapy 214, 216
progressive pump failure 178–9
PROMISE (Prospective Randomized
    Milrinone Survival Evaluation) trial 42
propranolol
    clinical trials 7
    in combination therapy 12
proteinuria
    in calcium channel blocker monotherapy 13
    value of RAS blockade 16
proteoglycans, ECM 142
PROVED (Prospective Randomized study of
    Ventricular Failure and the Efficacy of
    Digoxin) study 40, 41, 43
pulmonary capillary wedge pressure, effect
    of AVP 132, 133

pulmonary vasodilators 206
pyruvate dehydrogenase kinase-4 inhibition
    32

quality of care, improvement 167, 170–1
quality-of-life 216
quinapril 48
    clinical trials 5
    in combination therapy 11
    recommended dose 50
quinidine, use with digoxin 43

RADIANCE (Randomized Assessment of
    Digoxin and Inhibitors of Angiotensin
    Converting Enzyme) study 40, 41, 43
RALES (Randomized Aldactone Evaluation
    Study) 82–3, 84
ramipril 48, 145
    clinical trials 5
        AIRE 49–50
    recommended dose 50
ranolazine 32
RAS (renin-angiotensin system)
    activation in heart failure 57–8, 70, 76
    role in insulin resistance 29–30
RAS (renin-angiotensin system) blockade
    10, 16
    see also ACE inhibitors; angiotensin
        receptor blockers (ARBs)
recombinant human erythropoetin (rHuEPO)
    152
    clinical trials 152, 153, 156
    side effects 157
registry studies 165
reimbursement problem, palliative care
    218–19
REMATCH (Randomized Evaluation of
    Mechanical Assistance for the Treatment
    of Congestive Heart Failure) trial 191, 193,
    195
remodeling
    effect of ACE inhibitors 48
    intraventricular conduction delays 181–2
    METEOR study 135
    PREMIER trial 147
    role of AVP 132–3
    role of MMPs 144, 145
    role of norepinephrine 70
    see also electrophysiologic remodeling
remote medication adjustment 185, 186
renal dysfunction, risk from nesiritide 118, 120
renal effects, BNP 106, 120

renal failure, management after LVAD
    implantation 207
renal insufficiency, during ACE inhibitor
    therapy 52
renal protection, RAS blockade 16
renin inhibitors 10
    aliskiren 223
repolarization changes 180
reserpine, in combination therapy 12
RESOLVD (Randomized Evaluation of
    Strategies for Left Ventricular
    Dysfunction) 58–9, 65
right ventricular function, in LVAD
    implantation 206
right ventricular optimization 206–7
risk-treatment mismatch 166

S-nitrosylation 99, 100
salt sensitivity 10
SAVE (Survival and ventricular Enlargement)
    study 131
SCD-HeFT (Sudden Cardiac Death in Heart
    Failure) trial 214
scoring systems, patient selection for LVAD
    therapy 193–4
SENIORS trial 72, 76
serum dioxin levels 43
SHOCK trial 196
side effects
    of ACE inhibitors 52, 61
    of aldosterone antagonists 82, 83
        hyperkalemia 85–6
    of alpha-blockers 14
    of angiotensin receptor blockers 57, 64
    of beta-blockers 14
    of calcium channel blockers 13
    of centrally-acting anti-hypertensives 15
    of digoxin 43
    of direct vasodilators 15
    of RAS blockade 10
    of recombinant human erythropoetin
        (rHuEPO) 157
    of thiazolidinediones 31–2
sodium excretion, effect of BNP 106
sodium intake 10
sodium-potassium ATPase inhibition,
    digitalis glycosides 39
SOLVD (Studies of Left Ventricular
    Dysfunction) trials 49, 76, 94, 96, 97
    AVP levels 130–1
SPAN-CHF (Specialized Primary and
    Networked Care in HF) study 172

spironolactone 82, 180, 214
    clinical trials 6, 12
    effect on fibrosis 145
    RALES trial 82–3, 84, 85
    see also aldosterone antagonists
STAMINA-HeFT (Studies of Anemia in Heart
    Failure Trial) 156–7
statins, pravachol, effect on MMP-2 levels
    146
stroke volume, effect of AVP 132, 133
stromelysins 143
subcutaneous administration, BNP 120
sudden cardiac death 178, 179–81
sulfonylureas 25, 31
superoxide, effect on S-nitrosylation 99
sympathetic nervous system
    action of digitalis glycosides 39
    effects of excessive activation 70
    role in insulin resistance 29
sympathetic nervous system blockers
    clinical trials 7
    in treatment of hypertension 13
symptom control 216, 218, 219
systemic vascular resistance, effect of AVP
    132, 133

TandemHeart® Percutaneous Transseptal
    Ventricular Assist (PTVA®) system 196,
    197
telephone contact, value in outpatient disease
    management 173
telmisartan
    clinical trials 5
    in combination therapy 11
terazosin, clinical trials 7
thiazides 214
    clinical trials 5–6
    in treatment of hypertension 10
thiazolidinediones (TZDs) 31–2
    pioglitazone, effect on MMP-2 levels 146
    cardiovascular risk profile 223
Thoratec® DT registry 194
Thoratec® VADs 199–200, 201
thrombosis, risk from rHuEPO treatment 157
timolol, clinical trials 7
TIMPs (tissue inhibitors of MMPs) 142–4
tissue-specific ACE inhibitors 48
tolvaptan 125
    clinical trials 126, 134–6, 223
    properties 133–4
torsemide, clinical trials 6
Total Artificial Heart 203

toxicity, digoxin 43
TRACE (Trandolapril Cardiac Evaluation)
    trial 49, 50
transcutaneous energy transmission (TET)
    system 204
trandolapril 48
    clinical trials 5, 11
        TRACE 49, 50
    recommended dose 50
transesophogeal echocardiography, prior to
    VAD implantation 206
transmembrane proteins 144
TREAT (Trial to Reduce Cardiovascular
    Events with Aranesp Therapy) 157
treatment gap 166–7, 174
triamterene, clinical trials 6, 12
trimetazidine 32
trimethiazide, clinical trials 6
TROPHY (TRial Of Preventing HYpertension)
    4, 10, 16

UKPDS (United Kingdom Prospective
    Diabetes Study) 25, 31
urine volume, effect of BNP 106
US Carvedilol Trials Program 71, 72, 94,
    96, 98

V-HeFT (Vasodilator Heart Failure Trials) 53,
    94, 96, 97
V_2 receptor antagonists 125, 129
VAL-HeFT (Valsartan Heart Failure Trial)
    60–1, 64, 65
valsartan
    clinical trials 5
    in combination therapy 12
vascular resistance in etiology of
    hypertension 4
vasodilator therapy, benefit in African-
    Americans 96, 99, 100–2, 103
vasodilatory effect, ACE inhibitors 48

vasopressin receptor antagonists 125, 129,
    133, 138
    clinical trials 126–8
        conivaptan 136–7
        lixivaptan 136
        tolvaptan 134–6
    future directions 137
    lixivaptan, effect on water balance 132
    properties 134
vasopressin receptors, pathophysiology
    129–30, 131
ventricular ectopy, effect of aldosterone
    antagonists 86
ventricular reconstruction 216
ventricular replacement therapy 191
    see also left ventricular assist devices
        (LVADs)
ventricular tachyarrhythmias 179–80
verapamil
    clinical trials 11
    use with digoxin 43
vesnarinone 42
VMAC (Vasodilatation in the Management
    of Acute CHF) trial 108, 110–11, 114,
    118, 120
VPA-985 see lixivaptan

waist circumference 26
water balance, effect of AVP 132
white coat hypertension 9
women
    ACE inhibitor therapy 53
    benefits of aldosterone antagonists 83, 85

xenotransplantation 191

YM-087 see conivaptan

zymogens 142